Unique Properties of Melanocytes

Pigment Cell

Vol. 3

Series Editor: V. RILEY, Seattle, Wash.

S. Karger · Basel · München · Paris · London · New York · Sydney

Proceedings of the 9th International Pigment Cell Conference
Houston, Tex., January 13–17, 1975 (Part II)

Unique Properties of Melanocytes

Editor: V. RILEY, Seattle, Wash.

224 figures, 1 color plate and 52 tables, 1976

S. Karger · Basel · München · Paris · London · New York · Sydney

Pigment Cell

Vol. 1: Mechanisms in Pigmentation. Proceedings of the 8th International Pigment Cell Conference, Sydney 1972. Editors: V. J. McGovern and P. Russell (Sydney) XIV + 414 p., 166 fig., 89 tab., 1973. ISBN 3-8055-1480-8

Vol. 2: Melanomas: Basic Properties and Clinical Behavior. Proceedings of the 9th International Pigment Cell Conference, Houston, Tex. 1975 (Part I). Editor: V. Riley (Seattle, Wash.)
XX + 456 p., 165 fig., 92 tab., 1976. ISBN 3-8055-2369-6

Cataloging in Publication
International Pigment Cell Conference, 9th, Houston, Tex., 1975
Proceedings of the 9th International Pigment Cell Conference, Houston, Tex., January 13–17, 1975
Editor, V. Riley. – Basel, New York: Karger, 1976
(Pigment cell; v. 2–3)
Contents: pt. 1. Melanomas: basic properties and clinical behavior. – pt. 2. Unique properties of melanocytes.
1. Melanoma – congresses 2. Melanocytes – congresses 3. Melanin – congresses
I. Riley, Vernon, 1914 – ed. II. Melanomas: basic properties and clinical behavior
III. Unique properties of melanocytes IV. Title V. Series
Wl PI24 v. 2–3/QZ 200 I6094 1975p
ISBN 3-8055-2371-8

Unique Properties of Melanocytes

Part II of the Proceedings of the 9th International Pigment Cell Conference, Houston, Tex., 1975.

For the contributions published in Part I of the Proceedings, appearing as Pigment Cell, Vol. 2, under the title 'Melanomas: Basic Properties and Clinical Behavior', see table of contents on page VIII of this volume.

Contents

Ultrastructure and Biochemical Organization of the Pigmentary System

Structure and Unique Properties of Melanoproteins

Enzymology of Melanin Formation and Transfer

Pigment Cell Genetics

Hormone and Prostaglandin Influences on Pigment Cells

Pigment Cell Photobiology and Control Mechanisms

Cell Culture of Melanocytes

Melanomas: Basic Properties and Clinical Behavior

Part I of the Proceedings of the 9th International Pigment Cell Conference,
Houston, Tex., 1975.
Published as Pigment Cell, Vol. 3.

Contents

Biochemical Properties of Melanoma

Genetics

Contents

Cell Culture of Malignant Melanocytes

Immunology of Experimental Melanoma

Immunology of Human Melanoma

Diagnosis and Physiological Influences of Melanoma

Experimental Therapy of Melanoma

Therapy of Melanoma

Epidemiology of Melanoma

Editorial

For the past thirty years the International Pigment Cell Conferences have convened periodically without the benefit of formal organization. The unstructured character of this interdisciplinary group was part of its special flavor and stimulating qualities. However, because of the increased interest in research on the pigment cell, and its application to the problems of biology including cancer, as represented by the malignant melanocyte, there is accumulating evidence that research in these areas might benefit by the establishment of an appropriate vehicle for the orderly perpetuation of the conferences, and by providing a stable literary means for publishing the proceedings of the conferences as well as interim papers of investigators working on the pigment cell.

As a consequence, the conference organizer undertook a mail survey to objectively assess the opinion of individuals who participated in previous conferences, or were otherwise identified with an interest in the field. Their views were specifically solicited concerning the formation of a pigment cell society, and whether a society journal would be desirable. The following responses were received from 143 scientists and physicians involved with pigment cell research or related clinical problems: approval was expressed by 86 percent for the formation of a Pigment Cell Society, while 11% felt that the present informal arrangements were satisfactory and should not be changed. Three percent were undecided. In respect to the question of a society journal, 65 percent were in favor of this additional means for publishing the diverse interdisciplinary papers bearing upon pigmentation chemistry and pigment cell problems. Twenty-eight percent were against adding another journal to the world's crowded literature.

Based on the personal experiences of the editor and conference organizer, the practical accomplishment of these expressed preferences depends largely upon the availability of a physician or investigator who is not only familiar with the pigment cell field but also has available the extensive time required, as well as the interest and skills necessary to produce a journal of high quality. Special circumstances are essential to carry out the time-consuming requirements of organizing conferences and managing the business needs of such a society. Further discussion would be welcome from individuals in the field concerning practical solutions to the transformation of an organization that has served a valuable purpose in the scientific community, and deserves to be perpetuated in an appropriate manner. It would be particularly relevant to receive information about individuals whose limited teaching load, or other circumstances such as forthcoming retirement, would provide a long-term candidate to carry out the organization of such a society, and to assume primary responsibility for the organization of future International Pigment Cell Conferences.

VERNON RILEY, Series Editor
Chairman, Department of Microbiology
Pacific Northwest Research Foundation
Member, Fred Hutchinson Cancer Research Center
1102 Columbia Street, *Seattle, WA 98014* (USA)

Preface

What qualities are there about pigment cells that can attract 200 scientists from all parts of the world to meet for a 5-day conference at periodic intervals? In respect to the historical importance of these cells, it has been suggested that in terms of evolutionary survival, a few pleasant sunny days might destroy mankind with his naked vulnerable skin were it not for the special protection of melanocytes, the pigment-producing cells in our skin.

The visually conspicuous product of these cells is melanin, the natural pigment synthesized by these highly specialized cells that are embryologically related to brain and other cells of the central nervous system.

This pigmented umbrella of melanin shades the cells that lie beneath the melanocytes and those special cells which gratuitiously acquire the newly synthesized and packaged melanin. Many of the subcellular elements are sensitive to ultraviolet radiation and thus require protection. The mitochondria in the cytoplasm with their UV-sensitive enzymes provide the essential energy that drives the multiple cellular activities. Perhaps the most vital subcellular entity requiring protection from ultraviolet radiation is DNA, composed of fragile linear molecules that carry the genetic code upon which all replication depends. Thus without pigment cells and their light-screening melanin, all cells in the surface of man's naked skin would be exposed to damaging solar radiation.

But in addition to their intrinsic importance to life processes, pigment cells are also independently useful as models for studying universal cellular activity. As an indication of the wide variety of interests and activities of pigment cell scientists, it will be noted that this monograph describes experiments on mammals, avians, and amphibians, Negroes and Caucasians, both *in vivo* and *in vitro*. Life forms that offer entrancing models include chickens, gerbils, guppys, various strains of mice, sea urchins, piebald-spotted dogs, teleosts, salamanders, and New Guinean aborigines, as well as albinos of various species. These are but a few of the biological models that have been employed in the endeavor to better understand all living processes. The acquision of this knowledge is sufficient unto itself for many of the dedicated investigators of this fraternity, however for others, it provides a valued means for obtaining clues to various pathological processes which still plague mankind.

VERNON RILEY

Acknowledgements

The following physicians and investigators reviewed the glossary terms for accuracy and relevance to pigment cell studies: PHILLIP BANDA, MARSDEN BLOIS, JAMES BOWMAN, JOHN BRUMBAUGH, GARY ELMER, M. A. FITZMAURICE, BERNARD GOFFE, JOYCE HAWKS, FUNAN HU, GEORGE ODLAND, GEORGE SANTISTEBAN, and CARL WITKOP. Editorial assistance was provided by M. A. FITZMAURICE, who also compiled the subject index and glossary. Administrative assistance by HEATHER MCCLANAHAN greatly lessened the burden for the Editor. Without the organizational skills of Professor ELEANOR J. MACDONALD, and her associates in Houston, the Ninth International Pigment Cell Conference could not have taken place, and thus this monograph is a product of their activities. Thanks go to these individuals and the other unnamed contributors who made this monograph possible.

Ultrastructure and Biochemical Organization of the Pigmentary System

Pigment Cell, vol. 3, pp. 1–12 (Karger, Basel 1976)

Ultrastructure of the Human Melanocyte System in the Newborn, with Special Reference to 'Racial' Differences

INGER ROSDAHL and GEORGE SZABO

Laboratory of Electron Microscopy, Harvard School of Dental Medicine, and Departments of Anatomy and Dermatology, Harvard Medical School, Boston, Mass.

Introduction

Melanocytes are derived from the neural crest and can be recognized ultrastructurally in the human epidermis by the 8th week of gestation [5]. The melanocyte population density remains stable after the 5th fetal month [11]. It is not known when melanocytes begin to produce pigment, but electron microscopic studies have shown [5] that in Caucasoids non-melanized melanosomes are present in the melanocytes by the 8th week of gestation, and by the 10th week early stages of melanization can be detected. At this stage, there is no indication of pigment donation to melanocytes. Light microscopic studies by ZIMMERMAN [12], have shown that keratinocytes contain melanosomes in the 5-month-old Negro fetus.

The purpose of our study has been to investigate, on the ultrastructural level, the epidermal pigmentary system at birth, with special reference to the formation, melanization and distribution of melanosomes. Previous analyses of the ultrastructure of the epidermal melanin unit have dealt with adult skin which may already have been exposed to sunlight [4]. Since sun exposure has a profound influence on pigmentation, it was hoped that an investigation of unexposed foreskins from newborns would help to differentiate the role of genetic and external factors in the development of the epidermal pigmentary system.

One aspect of this problem is the role of ultraviolet irradiation in the development of 'racial' color differences. It has been shown that there is no difference in the melanocyte population density in skin from newborns or adults of various races [1, 4]. The difference in skin color is rather due to differences in the number of melanosomes, their degree of melanization and their pattern of distribution [6]. Interestingly, a Caucasoid skin can assume the ultrastructural characteristics of Negroid skin following psoralen (TMP) administration and ultraviolet light stimulation [6, 7].

Therefore, our question is whether the susceptibility to ultraviolet stimulation is the primary agent in bringing about the ultrastructural differences in the epidermal melanin unit in different racial groups, or whether the differences are already present at birth before ultraviolet stimulation. In other words, does the genetic control of the ultrastructural features express itself through differences in light susceptibility, or does it *directly* influence the morphological pattern? To answer this question, we have compared the ultrastructure of foreskins from newborns of different racial groups with that of the adult skin.

Materials and Methods

This investigation is based on 14 foreskin specimens which were removed during circumcision of newborns at Beth Israel Hospital. The circumcisions were performed 1–4 days after birth. The donors were all healthy and normal babies without visible pigmentary disturbances. Some had a 'Mongolian spot' on the lower part of the back, and some had a slightly raised serum bilirubin. The skin samples removed had not been exposed to sunlight or even to visible light for any length of time. We obtained specimens from 5 American Negroid (with skin color of the parents ranging from heavily to moderately dark), 5 Caucasoid and 5 Mongoloid children. Since we could not obtain any exact geneological data, we do not claim to deal with 'pure' populations of the different racial groups.

The outer part of the foreskin was immediately dissected into small slices and put into Ito-Karnovsky fixative [2]. The tissue was then washed with phosphate or cacodylate buffer, postfixed in osmium tetroxide and blockstained with uranyl acetate. The specimens were dehydrated through a graded series of ethanols and embedded in Epon. The grids were stained with uranyl acetate and lead citrate and examined in an AEI 6B or an AEI Corinth 275 electron microscope.

Fig. 1. Survey electromicrograph of basal regions of the epidermis from Caucasoid skin. × 2,800. D = Dermis; M = nucleus of melanocyte; K = nucleus of keratinocyte; → = pigment granules in complexes.

Fig. 2, 3. Survey electromicrographs of basal regions of the epidermis. Figure 2, Negroid skin (moderately pigmented). × 2,800. Figure 3, Mongoloid skin. × 2,800. D = Dermis; M = melanocyte.

Fig. 4, 5. Melanocyte from Negroid skin (same specimen). Figure 4, parikaryon. × 11,000. Figure 5, dendrite. × 19,000. D = Dermis; M = nucleus of melanocyte; K = keratinocyte.

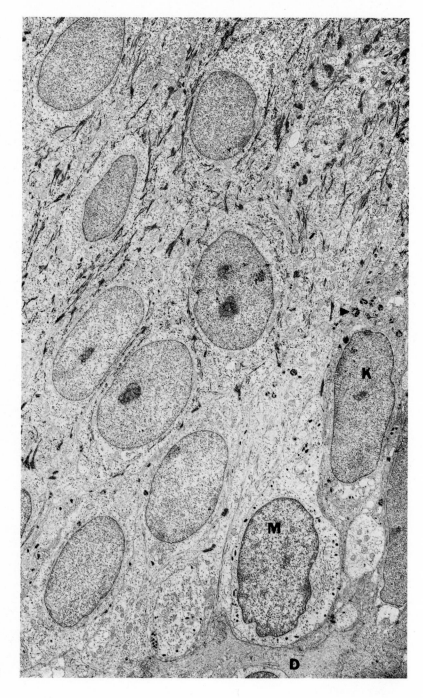

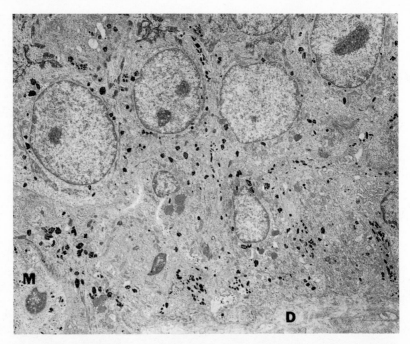

2

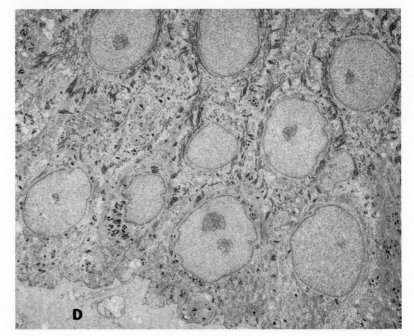

3

For legends, see p. 2.

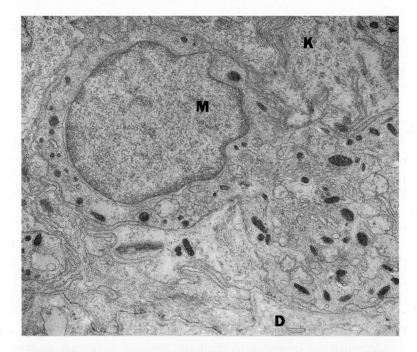

4

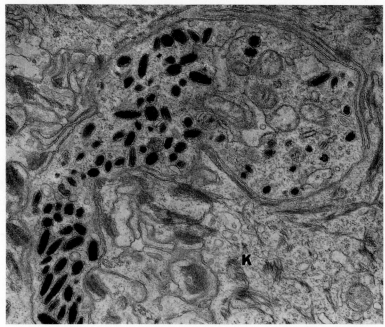

5

For legends, see p. 2.

Results and Discussion

In the foreskins of newborns of all racial groups, melanosomes are found in melanocytes as well as in keratinocytes (fig. 1–3). The melanocytes contain individually dispersed melanosomes in different stages of development, including fully melanized stage IV melanosomes (fig. 4–7) [8]. The melanosomes in the perikaryon of the melanocytes are, on the whole, less melanized than in the dendrites (fig. 4, 5). The keratinocytes contain mostly fully melanized melanosomes in the Negroid and Mongoloid skin. However, in the Caucasoid skin melanosomes in stage II and III are also transferred into keratinocytes (fig. 8–11). The melanosomes of newborns are not as numerous as in the adult skin. They are also somewhat smaller in size than those of the adult unirradiated skin from corresponding racial groups [6, 7]. The melanosomes appear to be randomly dispersed throughout the cytoplasm of the keratinocytes (figs. 1–3, 8, 9). This is in contrast to previous reports of clustering of melanosomes in the perinuclear area of the keratinocytes [3]. As in adult unirradiated skin, the melanosomes are present mainly in the basal regions of the epidermis (fig. 1–3) [3].

Although the overall activity of the newborn epidermal pigmentary system seems to be somewhat less than that of the adult, our findings demonstrate that the epidermal melanin unit is a mature and functioning system at birth. Thus, melanosomes are formed, melanized and transferred into keratinocytes. External influences, such as ultraviolet light, are consequently only stimulating factors in skin pigmentation, and not prerequisites for any step in the process.

Macroscopically there is a visible difference in the color of foreskins of different racial groups at birth. On the ultrastructural level, less melanosomes are found in the melanocytes and keratinocytes in the white skin than in the black skin (fig. 1–3). Table I illustrates the proportions of melanosomes in different stages of melanization in melanocytes of different racial groups. These estimates are based on a qualitative evaluation using the classification of Toda and Fitzpatrick [8]. As in the adult [4], melanosomes in Negroid melanocytes are predominantly in stage IV, whereas in Caucasoid melanocytes they are predominantly in stages II and III.

Fig. 6, 7. Melanocyte from Mongoloid (fig. 6; × 8,800) and Caucasoid (fig. 7; × 10,600) skin. D = Dermis; K = nucleus of keratinocyte.

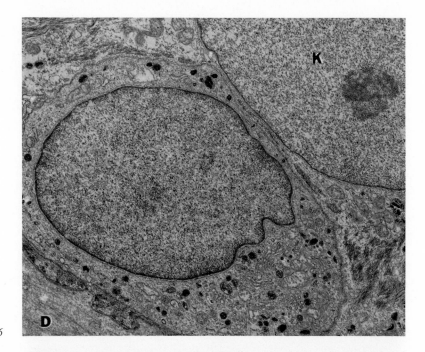

6

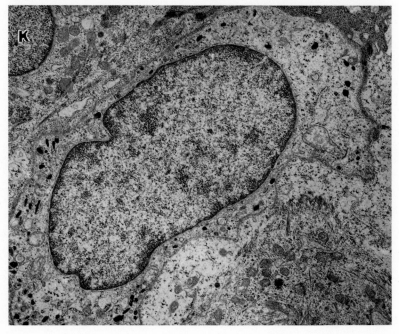

7

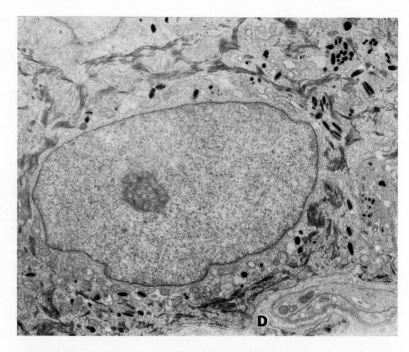

8

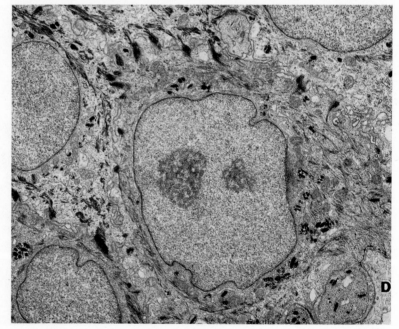

9

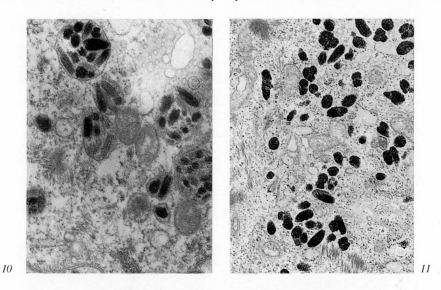

Fig. 10, 11. Melanosome distribution in keratinocytes. Figure 10, Caucasoid skin. × 15,000. Figure 11, Negroid skin (heavily pigmented). × 15,000.

Table I. Illustrating the percentage of melanosomes in different stages of melanization in representative melanocytes of different racial groups. These estimates are based on a qualitative evaluating using the classification of TODA and FITZPATRICK [8]

Negroid skin (5 individuals) melanosome stages		Caucasoid skin (5 individuals) melanosome stages		Mongoloid skin (4 individuals) melanosome stages	
II–III	IV	II–III	IV	II–III	IV
4	96	47	53	79	21
9	91	73	27	43	57
16	84	56	44	66	34
30	70	85	15	80	20
62	38	77	23		

Fig. 8, 9. Keratinocyte from heavily pigmented Negroid (fig. 8; × 7,500) and Mongoloid (fig. 9; × 6,400) skin. D = Dermis.

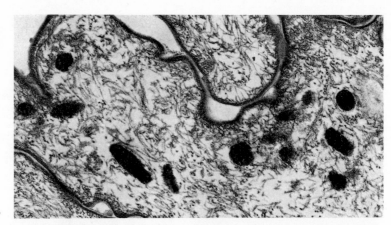

12

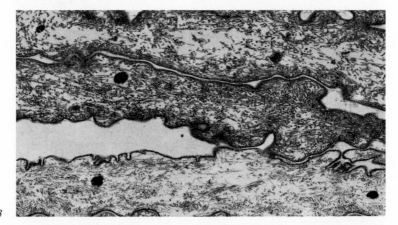

13

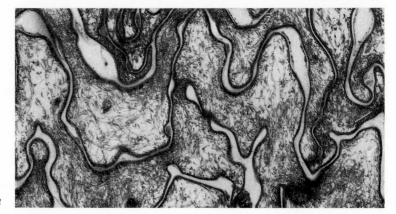

14

The melanosomes are differently distributed in the keratinocytes of various racial groups in the newborn, as in the adult [4, 10]. The keratinocytes of Negroid skin of newborns contain mostly single, large melanosomes, but occasional complexes of 2–3 melanosomes are also found. In lighter Negroid skin, more melanosomes are found in groups than in heavily pigmented Negroid skin (fig. 2, 8, 11). In the Caucasoid keratinocytes, the melanosomes exist in complexes surrounded by a membrane (fig. 1, 10). Mongoloid skin occupies an intermediate position between Negroid and Caucasoid skin in respect to the number of melanosomes present and their pattern of dispersion (fig. 3, 6, 9).

The melanosome-containing keratinocytes are mainly localized in the basal layer, and in the lower portion of the stratum spinosum. In the higher strata, the melanosomes rapidly diminish in number, and in white skin almost disappear. The Negro skin, however, contains some small melanosomes in the uppermost layers of the epidermis and, occasionally, also in the stratum corneum (fig. 12–14). The melanosomes higher in the epidermis are not as numerous as in adult skin. This difference may also be related to the postnatal darkening of Negroid skin [9].

All these observed differences in the structure of the epidermal melanin unit in the foreskin of newborns of different racial groups are similar to those of adult skin. Thus, the principal racial pattern of melanosome distribution is present at birth, and is not due to racial differences in the response to ultraviolet light stimulation.

Summary

The ultrastructure of the epidermal pigmentary system was investigated in newborn human foreskins of different racial groups (Caucasoid, Mongoloid, and Negroid). As in adults, the melanocytes contain melanosomes in all stages of development, and melanosomes have already been transferred to keratinocytes. In the keratinocytes of Mongoloid and Caucasoid skin, the melanosomes are mostly in complexes, whereas in Negroid skin they are mostly dispersed as single units. The melanosomes are more numerous and more melanized in the Negroid than in the Caucasoid skin. Thus, the main features of the epidermal melanin unit develop independently of ultraviolet light stimulation.

Fig. 12–14. Representative electromicrographs showing the number of melanosomes present in the keratin. Figure 12, Negroid skin (heavily pigmented). × 32,000. Figure 13, Mongoloid skin. × 17,000. Figure 14, Caucasoid skin. × 22,000.

Acknowledgements

We want to thank the residents of the Department of Obstetrics and Gynecology at Beth Israel Hospital for providing the specimens. We also thank Evelyn Flynn for technical assistance and Elsie Rosenfield for editing and typing the manuscript. This investigation was supported by USPHS Grant No. DEO 1766-13, National Institute of Dental Research and the John A. Hartford Foundation.

References

1 Glimcher, M. E.; Kostick, R. M., and Szabo, G.: The epidermal melanocyte system in newborn human skin. A quantitative histologic study. J. invest. Derm. 61: 344–347 (1973).

2 Ito, S. and Karnovsky, M. J.: Formaldehyde-glutaraldehyde fixatives containing trinitro compounds. J. Cell Biol. 39: 168a–169a (1968).

3 Pathak, M. A.; Hori, Y.; Szabo, G., and Fitzpatrick, T. B.: The photobiology of melanin pigmentation in human skin; in Kawamura, Fitzpatrick and Seiji Biology of normal and abnormal melanocytes, pp. 149–169 (University of Tokyo Press, Tokyo 1971).

4 Szabo, G.; Gerald, A. B.; Pathak, M. A., and Fitzpatrick, T. B.: The ultrastructure of racial color differences in man; in Riley Pigmentation: its genesis and biologic control, pp. 23–41 (Appleton Century Crofts, New York 1972).

5 Sagebiel, R. W. and Odland, G. F.: Ultrastructural identification of melanocytes in early human embryos; in Riley Pigmentation: its genesis and biologic control, pp. 43–50 (Appleton Century Crofts, New York 1972).

6 Toda, K.; Pathak, M. A.; Fitzpatrick, T. B.; Quevedo, W. C., jr.; Morikawa, F., and Nakayama, Y.: Skin color: its ultrastructure and its determining mechanism; in McGovern, Russell and Riley Pigment Cell, vol. 1, pp. 66–81 (Karger, Basel 1973).

7 Toda, K.; Pathak, M. A.; Parrish, J. A., and Fitzpatrick, T. B.: Alteration of racial differences in melanosome distribution in human epidermis after exposure to ultraviolet light. Nature new Biol. 236: 143–145 (1972).

8 Toda, K. and Fitzpatrick, T. B.: The origin of melanosomes; in Kawamura, Fitzpatrick and Seiji Biology of normal and abnormal melanocytes, pp. 265–278 (University of Tokyo Press, Tokyo 1971).

9 Walsh, R. J.: Variation in the melanin content of the skin of New Guinea natives at different ages. J. invest. Derm. 42: 261–265 (1964).

10 Wolff, K. and Konrad, K.: Phagocytosis of latex beads by epidermal keratinocytes in vivo. J. Ultrastruct. Res. 39: 262–280 (1972).

11 Zimmerman, A. A. and Becker, S. W.: Melanoblasts and melanocytes in fetal Negro skin; in Ill. Monogr. Med. Sci., vol. 6, pp. 1–59 (University of Illinois Press, Urbana 1959).

12 Zimmerman, A. A.: Die Entwicklung der Hautfarbe beim Neger vor der Geburt. Mitt. Thurgauischen naturforschenden Ges. Sonderabdruck 37: 33–71 (1954).

Dr. I. Rosdahl, Hudkliniken, Sahlgrenska sjukhuset, S–41345 Göteborg (Sweden)

Pigment Cell, vol. 3, pp. 13–32 (Karger, Basel 1976)

Cytoplasmic Filaments in Melanocytes

Their Nature and Role in Melanin Pigmentation[1]

Kowichi Jimbow, Peter F. Davison, Madhu A. Pathak and
Thomas B. Fitzpatrick

Department of Dermatology, Harvard Medical School, Massachusetts General
Hospital, and Department of Fine Structure Research, Harvard Medical School,
Boston, Mass.

Introduction

Evidence has been accumulated to indicate that three types of cytoplasmic filaments exist in a variety of cells: (1) thin (50–70 Å in diameter);
(2) intermediate (90–100 Å in diameter), and (3) thick (150–220 Å in diameter)
filaments. Thin filaments are found to be related to cellular morphogenesis
and mobility, and composed of actin-like protein, as indicated by the capacity to bind anti-F-actin sera and to form ATP-dissociable arrowhead
structures when complexed with heavy meromyosin [1–12]. Thick filaments
are found in amebas, and are related to ameboid movement and primarily
composed of myosin protein [7, 9, 10, 12]. Little, however, is known about
the intermediate filaments.

Previously, we reported that these intermediate filaments are characteristically present in the melanocytes of human skin. They resemble the
neurofilaments in nerve cells, and appear to be related to melanin pigmentation [13]. In this study, we examined: (1) the fine structure and arrangement of the intermediate (100 Å) filaments in epidermal melanocytes of
human skin and retinal pigment cells of chick eyes before and after exposures
in vivo and *in vitro* to light and chemical agents, and (2) the electrophoretic
mobilities of the proteins of these filaments in the epidermal melanocytes and
retinal pigment cells after dissociating the proteins in SDS (sodium dodecyl
sulfate).

1   This study was supported by UPHSS Grants R01 CA12108, CA13651, CA05003,
P91 DE01766, GB36796, and RR05711.

Materials and Methods

Exposure of Pigment Cells in vivo to Light
Epidermal Melanocytes Exposed to Ultraviolet Light
Areas of skin of 21 adult volunteers (9 Caucasoids, 6 Mongoloids, and 6 Negroids) were exposed to ultraviolet (UV) lights to induce melanin pigmentation (immediate and delayed reactions). UV exposures were carried out on the least-exposed skin of the buttocks and the habitually exposed skin of the forearm. The immediate tanning reaction (ITR) was induced by either a Xenon arc lamp (340–400 nm), a USHIO 500-W light ($\lambda = 365$ nm), or filtered sunlight ($\lambda > 340$ nm). Skin biopsies of the unexposed (control) and exposed regions were obtained at 0 min and 24 h. A delayed tanning reaction (DTR) was induced by natural sunlight (whole spectrum), a Hanovia hot-quartz lamp with a filter (290–320 nm), or a Westinghouse fluorescent sunlamp (290–320 nm). Skin biopsies of unexposed (control) and exposed regions were obtained at days 5 and 10.

Retinal Pigment Cells Exposed to Visible Light
Eyes of 18 chicks, 2–3 days old, were exposed to visible light (light adaptation). These chicks included 12 White Leghorns with black eyes, 4 chicks with sex-linked imperfect albinism with dark-red eyes, and 2 chicks with autosomal albinism with bright-red eyes [14, 15] (Dr. R. G. Somes, University of Connecticut, Storrs, Conn., kindly supplied the albino chicks). Light adaptation was induced by exposing the chick eyes for 1 h to the pinpoint light emitted by a 15-W bulb and passed through the optic condenser of a Zeiss light microscope. Control specimens of dark-adapted eyes were obtained by placing the chicks in a dark-room, free from any kind of visible light, for 3 h.

Exposure of Pigment Cells in vitro to Chemical Agents
Epidermal Melanocytes Exposed to Cytochalasin-B and Vincristine Sulfate
Specimens of human skin (irradiated and nonirradiated) were obtained from buttock skin by Thiersch's biopsy, by which an entire epidermis and subpapillary corium may be obtained. The skin was sliced approximately 10 mm in width and placed in a tissue-culture medium made of Pucks' N-16 medium (Grand Island Biological Company), fetal calf serum, and gentamycin. The pieces of skin were then treated separately with either cytochalasin B (cyto-B) or vincristine sulfate (VCR), 5–10 µg per ml of culture medium, for 3 h at 37°C (cyto-B was kindly supplied by Dr. A. Krishan of the Children's Cancer Research Foundation and the Department of Pathology, Harvard Medical School, Boston, Mass.).

Retinal Pigment Cells Exposed to Cytochalasin B and Vincristine Sulfate
Sheets of retinal pigment cells were isolated from 8-day-old White Leghorn chick embryos (Spafas Inc., Norwich, Conn.). Whole eyes were placed in trypsin-EDTA solution (Grand Island Biological Company) for 20 min at 37°C. The choroid and scleral layers were peeled off readily, leaving the pigment layer, which is more resistant to trypsin treatment [16], exposed and free of extraneous cells. The retinal pigment cells were dissociated by trituration after another 5 min incubation with trypsin-EDTA solution. They were then placed in the plastic culture plates and cultured in the Nutrient Mixture F-10 (Grand Island Biological Company), fetal calf serum, and gentamycin, with the ratio of 2.5×10^4 cells

per ml of medium. At days 7–14 after primary culture, the retinal pigment cells were exposed to either cyto-B (5–10 μg/ml) or VCR (5–10 μg/ml) for 3 h at 37°C.

Light and Electron Microscopy

The *in vivo* and *in vitro* tissues exposed to physical lights and chemical agents were prefixed with 2.5% formaldehyde-2.5% glutaraldehyde mixture in 0.1 M cacodylate buffer, pH 7.2, for 2 h at room temperature and postfixed with 2% osmium tetroxide in 0.1 M cacodylate buffer, pH 7.2, for another 2 h at room temperature. They were then stained *en bloc* with saturated uranyl acetate in 0.1 M Veronal buffer, pH 7.0, for 20 min at room temperature, dehydrated by ethyl alcohols and embedded in epoxy resins. The epoxy-embedded tissues were sectioned by a LKB ultratome and stained with Mallory's Azur II-methylene blue solutions for light microscopy and with uranyl acetate and lead citrate for electron microscopy. Electron microscopic observations were made with a Siemens Elmiskop I.

For histochemical identification of whole melanocytes, some of the human skins were directly immersed into 2 N NaBr for 2–3 h at 37°C and split into epidermal sheets and dermis. Epidermal sheets were then incubated with 1% 3,4-dihydroxyphenylalanine in 0.1 M phosphate buffer, pH 7.4 for 4 h, fixed with 10% formalin in 0.1 M phosphate buffer, pH 7.0, dehydrated by alcohol solutions, and mounted on glass slides.

Filaments from chick pigment epithelial cells were examined in negatively stained dispersions by washing a concentrate of the cultured cells with a glass homogenizer in water, saline or deuterium oxide. The dispersion was applied to a carbon-filmed grid, stained with 1% uranyl acetate and examined in a Philips EM300 microscope.

Preliminary Investigations of Proteins Comprizing the 100-Å Filaments
Epidermal Melanocytes

Human skin was obtained from autopsy subjects (6 Caucasoids and 2 Negroids) by Thiersch's operation. The sheets of epidermis were split by incubating the skin pieces in trypsin-EDTA solution for 30 min at 37°C, and transferred into glass Petri dishes containing chicken serum. The epidermal melanocytes and keratinocytes in the basal layer were scraped off and collected.

Retinal Pigment Cells

Chick retinal pigment cells were prepared in culture and were obtained from White Leghorn chick embryos (8 days old). At days 10–14 after primary culture, these cultured cells were scraped off the culture dishes in 0.14 M NaCl or glycerol-MES (see below) with a rubber policeman.

The cells were concentrated by centrifugation at low speed and then dissolved with heating in 1% SDS (sodium dodecyl sulfate), 0.01 M mercaptoethanol, 0.01 M phosphate buffer, pH 7.5, in preparation for disc electrophoresis.

Zone sedimentation through a discontinuous sucrose gradient was employed in order to concentrate filamentous subcellular components. This procedure was most effective with cultured cells, e. g. the chick pigment epithelial cells. The cells were washed from culture flasks in physiological saline or (if microtubules were to be preserved intact) 4 M glycerol, 0.1 M MES buffer, 0.5 mM ATP, 0.5 mM magnesium chloride, pH 6.4 [33], and then concentrated by low speed centrifugation. The packed mass of cells was ground in a test tube homogenizer and the homogenate, freed of intact cells by low speed centrifugation, was applied to a discontinuous gradient containing layers of 10, 20, and 30% sucrose in the glycerol buffer. After centrifugation for 1 h at 35,000 rpm (Spinco model L. rotor SW50) the material at the successive interfaces and at the bottom of the tube were separately collected. The solutions were diluted with water and the particulates were sedimented by a further centrifugation run and finally each pellet was redissolved in 1% SDS, 0.01 M phosphate, pH 7, 0.01 M mercaptoethanol (brief heating to 100° was used to accelerate dissolution); the solutions were then made denser by the addition of 1/10th volume glycerol and applied to a polyacrylamide gel slab.

The total cell proteins, or the particulate fractions obtained by zone sedimentation were dissolved in the SDS-mercaptoethanol buffer and subjected to electrophoresis in 10% polyacrylamide gel slabs after the procedure of LAEMMLI [49]. Urea was added to the gel formulation to promote the resolution of the α and β units of tubulin [50]. After electrophoresis, the proteins were fixed by immersing the gels in 15% trichloracetic acid solutions and the gels were subsequently washed, stained in 0.1% Coomassie blue in 50% methanol, and finally destained in water-methanol-acetic acid (7:3:1).

For internal comparison tubulin, actin and neurofilament proteins from chick optic nerve or human brain were run on the same gel. The stained gels were scanned with a Joyce-Loeb 1 densitometer.

Results

Melanosomes and Filaments in Pigment Cells after Exposure to Light
Epidermal Melanocytes Exposed to UV Light

Human epidermal melanocytes contain a large population of cytoplasmic filaments that are 114±(SD) 27.1 Å (100 Å) in diameter, quite distinct from the thin (50–70 Å) filaments commonly seen in other cells. They occur characteristically in the perinuclear area in the melanocytes of unirradiated skin, intermingling closely with each other and forming bundles. They are usually absent in the dendrites [18].

These 100-Å filaments in human epidermal melanocytes changed their distribution directly following an ITR at 0 min evoked by exposure to UV light. They, together with the melanosomes, were then found in the dendritic processes, which were extended. At 24 h after exposure, when the ITR subsided, light microscopy showed that the elongated dendrites were less extended (probably due to contraction). At this stage, under the electron microscope, melanosomes and 100-Å filaments were hardly seen in the dendritic processes. The 100-Å filaments were present in the perinuclear area and were densely aggregated. The melanosomes in the melanocytes were less visible than they had been at 0 min.

During a delayed tanning reaction (DTR), in which melanin pigmen-

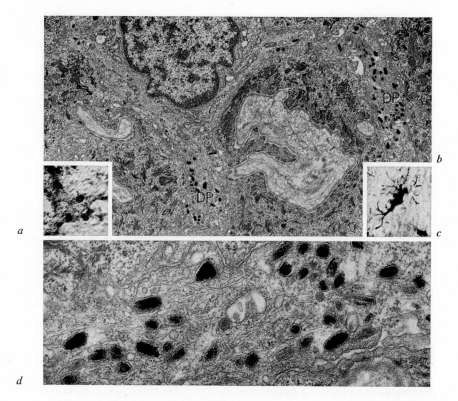

Fig. 1. The effect of exposure to UV light *in vivo* on the melanocytic dendrites and filaments during DTR. (a) Before exposure. Light micrograph of the melanocyte in the least-exposed skin of a Caucasoid. (b) At day 5 after exposure. The melanocytic filaments are aggregated, together with melanosomes, in the tip of the well-developed dendrite (DP). The specimen was obtained from Caucasoid buttock skin at day 5 after exposure. × 7,600. (c) At day 5 after exposure. Note a marked elongation of melanocytic dendrites. (d) A high-power view of the melanocytic dendrite. Melanocytic filaments and melanosomes intermingle closely. × 51,000.

tation occurs owing to an increase in the synthesis of new melanosomes and in the transference of these newly synthesized melanosomes to the keratinocytes, there was a distinct change in the distribution of 100-Å filaments. At day 5 during DTR, the split-dopa preparation showed marked elongation and arborization of the dendritic processes and hypertrophy of the perikaryon of the melanocytes. The 100-Å filaments and melanosomes were diffusely scattered in both dendrites and perikaryon after DTR. In the perikaryon, the 100-Å filaments, running mostly in short courses, were seen

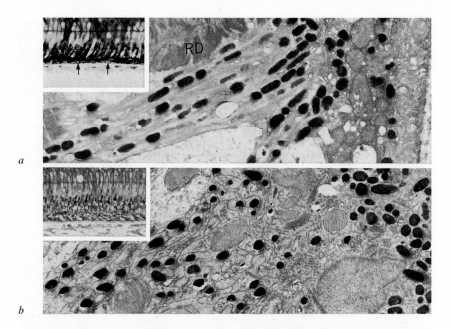

Fig. 2. Effects *in vivo* of visible light on the melanocytic filaments in the retinal pigment cells of black eyes (White Leghorn). (a) Light-adapted eye. The light-micrograph insert shows a linear arrangement of melanosomes in the processes of retinal pigment cells (arrows). Under the electron microscope, this arrangement of melanosomes becomes more obvious. The melanosomes are less visible in the perikaryon than in the processes. RD = Rods of receptor cells. × 8,800. (b) Dark-adapted eye. Both the light (insert) and the electron micrograph show the diffuse distribution of melanosomes in both the perikaryon and the processes. Melanosomes are less visible in the processes than in perikaryon. There is no obvious linear arrangement of melanosomes in the processes. × 8,800.

either forming bundles or scattered randomly around the melanosomes in various developmental stages. In the dendrites, there were bundles of 100-Å filaments running in long or short courses (fig. 1). At day 10 during a DTR, when new melanogenesis subsided gradually, the perikaryon and dendritic processes of the melanocytes became less prominent than at day 5. Most of the melanocytes contained diffusely scattered 100-Å filaments, microtubules, and melanosomes throughout the entire perikaryon. The dispersal of the melanosomes in the bundles of 100-Å filaments was not prominent in the dendrites. Most of the melanocytes, however, still contained a larger number of melanosomes than they did before exposure.

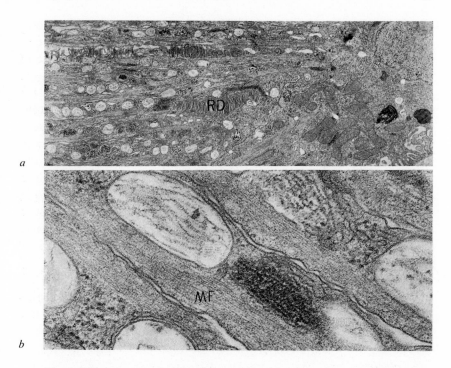

Fig. 3. Effects *in vivo* of visible light on the melanocytic filaments in the retinal pigment cells of red eyes (chicks with sex-linked recessive albinism). (a) A low-power view of a light-adapted eye. Note an aggregate of unmelanized melanosomes along the well-developed processes of the retinal pigment cells. RD = Rods of receptor cells. × 6,600. (b) A high-power view of *a*. Well-developed processes are aggregated with an abundance of melanocytic filaments intermingled with melanosomes. These filaments (MF), however, are more parallel and straighter than the filaments in epidermal melanocytes of human skin. There is no microtubule in the processes. × 76,000.

Retinal Pigment Cells Exposed to Visible Light

Figure 2a and b clearly show changes in the distribution pattern of melanosomes in the retinal pigment cells after exposure to visible light. In the dark-adapted cells, the melanosomes were primarily located in the center of cytoplasm, with only a few in the dendritic processes (fig. 2b). After exposure to visible light, the melanosomes were seen predominantly in the processes that extended among the photoreceptor cells of the retina. These melanosomes were characteristically arranged in a row after exposure (fig. 2a). The linear alignment of melanosomes in the cytoplasmic processes of the retinal pigment cells could be seen both in the black and in the red eyes of the chicks. In the red eyes, along the row of unmelanized melanosomes, one could see the 100-Å filaments closely intermingled or running as parallel lines (fig. 3a, b). In the dark-adapted cells, such an aggregate of 100-Å filaments and melanosomes in the processes could be hardly seen. Thus, one could presume that the 100-Å filaments had some role in the translocation of melanosomes into the processes of retinal pigment cells after exposure to visible light. Although these 100-Å filaments could be seen in the perikaryon of the retinal pigment cells before exposure, they were markedly less numerous than they were in the human epidermal melanocytes. Again, as in human epidermal melanocytes, there were more 100-Å filaments than microtubules in the retinal pigment cells (fig. 3b). The microtubules could, however, occasionally be seen in the processes after exposure. There was no topographic finding that suggested an incorporation of endoplasmic reticulum in the linear arrangement of melanosomes in the processes of retinal pigment cells [19].

Retinal pigment cells *in vivo* also contained a few thin (50–70 Å) filaments. These filaments were in close contact with the junctional complexes between the neighboring retinal pigment cells. These thin filaments did not change their distribution pattern nor was there evidence of any morphologic interaction with 100-Å filaments during light exposure.

Melanosomes and Filaments in Pigment Cells after Exposure to Chemical Agents
Epidermal Melanocytes Exposed to Cytochalasin B and
Vincristine Sulfate
In tissues incubated with cyto-B (5–10 μg/ml), there were no obvious changes in the fine structure and distribution pattern of the 100-Å filaments. Most of the UV-irradiated melanocytes still revealed an elongation of the long dendritic processes in which the central parts were laden with aggregates, or bundles, of 100-Å filaments with an ultrastructure and distr bution pattern that are the same as those seen in the UV-irradiated, cyto-B-free specimens. A characteristic was the swelling and partial disruption of the cytoplasmic membrane. Although this membranous swelling is often seen in any kind of experiments *in vitro*, these changes in the cyto-B-treated tissue appeared to be significant, inasmuch as there was apparently little swelling of the membrane in the control specimen of nontreated tissues. The membranous swelling and disruption were, however, seen both in the melanocytes and in the keratinocytes.

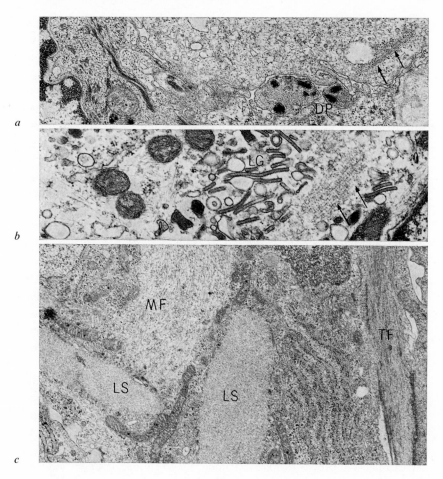

Fig. 4. Effects of chemicals on the melanocytic filaments in Caucasoid buttock skin *in vitro*. (a) Effect of VCR on the melanocyte. There are lattice-like structures in the melanocyte (arrows). There is, however, no fine-structure change indicative of an interconnection between these lattice structures and melanocytic filaments. DP indicates a cross-section view of melanocytic dendrites aggregated with melanocytic filaments and melanosomes. × 12,300. (b) Effect of VCR on an epidermal Langerhans cell. Note Langerhans granules (LG) and lattice-like structures (arrows). × 26,200. (c) Effect of 10 μg/ml of VCR on retinal pigment cells in monolayer culture (White Leghorn chick embryo). Note three aggregates of lattice-like structures (LS). These aggregates do not have any morphologic interconnection with intermediate filaments, melanocytic filaments (MF), and thin filaments (TF). × 5,700.

In contrast to cyto-B treatment, VCR-treated tissues showed crystal-like and lattice-like aggregates (fig. 4a). Although the aggregates were often seen close to the bundles of 100-Å filaments, there was not any interconnection between these aggregates and the 100-Å filament bundles. These aggregates appeared to correspond to the doses of VCR applied; the tissues treated with 5 μg/ml of VCR showed lattice-like aggregates, whereas tissues treated with 10 μg/ml of VCR showed crystal-like aggregates similar in ultrastructure to those of 'VCR' crystals reported in other tissues [20]. The aggregates, however, were seen not only in melanocytes but also in keratinocytes, Langerhans cells, and fibroblasts (fig. 4b). The presence of a VCR-induced lattice structure in the cells free of the 100-Å filaments indicates that VCR does not directly affect the 100-Å filaments.

Retinal Pigment Cells Exposed to Cytochalasin B and
Vincristine Sulfate

Retinal pigment cells in the culture conditions *in vitro* contained two distinct filamentous units: 50–70-Å (thin) filaments and 100-Å (intermediate) filaments. These filamentous units revealed fine structure and distribution patterns characteristic to each. Thin filaments were located in the periphery of the cells and formed aggregates parallel to each other, with dense zones similar to the bands of actin filaments (fig. 4c) [7, 10, 21].

The 100-Å filaments were in the center of the cells, did not run parallel, and did not have dense bands of actin filaments. They were distributed randomly or formed bundles of filaments, often encircling melanosomes. Interestingly enough, when the cultured cells were confluent, these two filamentous units ran short courses, whereas when the cells were dispersed and the cytoplasmic processes were extended, they ran long courses, indicating some role of these units for cytomorphosis.

When the retinal pigment cells were treated with cyto-B, there were no obvious morphological changes in the 100-Å filaments, whereas the thin, 50-Å filaments were slightly altered in their distribution pattern, though they still remained parallel. A distinctive change was that the sheets of the parallel 50-Å filaments and plasma membrane were dissociated and that 50-Å filaments attached to the plasma membrane appeared to be disrupted. This indicates that an alteration of the 50-Å filaments after cyto-B treatment was not related to the alteration of the filaments themselves, but related to the alteration of contacts between the plasma membrane and 50-Å filaments.

When the cultured cells were treated with VCR, they formed an aggregate of crystalloid or lattice structures, and were seen in the center of the cells. They did not, however, have any interconnection with an aggregate of either 50- or 100-Å filaments (fig. 4c). The number and fine structure of these two filaments were similar to those of untreated control specimens. This may again indicate that 100-Å filaments do not have structural units that are similar to microtubules.

Characteristics of Pigment Cell Proteins in Cell Homogenates and Comparison with Neurofilaments

Homogenates of chick pigment epithelial cells in D_2O when negatively stained and viewed in the electron microscope showed masses of 100-Å

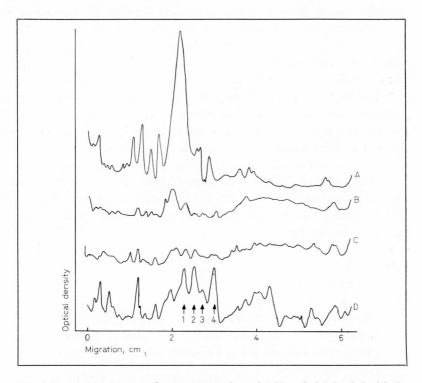

Fig. 5. Densitometric traces from a 10% polyacrylamide gel slab loaded with the SDS-solubilized particulates recovered from the: (A) 10%; (B) 20%; (C) 30% sucrose layers, and (D) base of the tube after gradient centrifugation of a homogenate from cultured chick retinal pigment epithelial cells. The interface between the spaces and running gels is at 0, and the discontinuous buffer front was at 6.3 cm. The usual positions of α- and β-tubulin (1 and 2), neurofilaments (3), and actin (4) are indicated by arrows. These positions were pinpointed by appropriate samples run on the same gel.

filaments as well as melanosomes, other particulates and a few microtubules. The fine morphology of the filaments was very similar to that of neurofilaments [51]. To compare these cell components more objectively, the proteins in the cells were studied by disc gel electrophoresis. Extracts from neurons were run for comparison: the electrophoretic characteristics of neurofilament protein will be reported elsewhere [DAVISON, in preparation].

Extracts from epidermis after gel electrophoresis showed prominent bands attributable to actin and smaller levels of α- and β-tubulin but no protein corresponding to neurofilaments. The chick pigment epithelial cells did show a band in the position of neurofilament protein, but it was markedly fainter than the bands of tubulin or actin. Experience has shown that at low protein concentrations and with prolonged staining, the Coomassie blue densitometry gives a semiquantitative correlation with the amounts of protein in the gel. By this criterion, we can conclude that while there may be neurofilament protein in the pigment cells, it is present at too low a level to account for the numbers of filaments seen in the cells.

For further clarification the zone sedimentation experiments were performed. Neurofilaments and microtubules were recovered from a nerve homogenate in the 30% sucrose layer and at the base of the cell. Figure 5 shows that there is only a minor band of protein in the neurofilament position in the C and D samples. On the other hand, a large single band in the position of α-tubulin is seen in the material from the 10% sucrose interface. A similar band was seen in the extracts from epidermis, but not from dermis. The possibility that this protein is the subunit of the 100-Å filaments is under investigation (fig. 5).

Discussion

Characterization of 100-Å Filaments in Melanocytes
1. Fine-Structure Characterization of Melanocytic Filaments in Comparison with the 100-Å Filaments in Other Cell Systems
in vivo and *in vitro*

The present study clearly indicates that pigment cells of the skin and retina *in vivo* and *in vitro* contain intermediate, or 100-Å, filaments. The fine structure (i.e. size, distribution in cells and, probably, electron density) of these melanocytic filaments is different from that of the thin, or 50–70-Å filaments reported in frog melanocytes [22] and also from thick, or 150–220-Å, myosin filaments of ameboid cells [7, 9, 12, 21]. Nerve cells, however, contain specific filaments, neurofilaments, with a dimension similar to that of melanocytic filaments. Several investigators reported finding 'side arms' of 40–70-Å in width and up to 150 Å in length in these neurofilaments [23–25]. Melanocytic filaments do not appear to have these side arms. The distribution and aggregation pattern of these two filaments, however, appear to be similar; neurofilaments run in swathes in the perikaryon and extend from the center of the cell toward the axonal tip in a way similar to that seen by us in the processes of the melanocytes and retinal pigment cells. As with 100-Å filaments of retinal pigment cells, the neurofilaments aggregate in a straighter and more-parallel fashion, whereas 100-Å filaments in epidermal melanocytes aggregate in a closely intermingling fashion.

In ganglion cells *in vitro*, YAMADA *et al.* [26] found an aggregate of neurofilaments and a network of thin filaments (40–60 Å) just beneath the plasma membrane in the growth-cone periphery and in the processes arising from it. These thin filaments showed periodic densities of Z-bands similar in ultrastructure and distribution pattern to those seen in smooth-muscle cells [10]. We did not find any thin filaments in melanocytes. *In vitro*, however, the retinal pigment cells had thin filaments beneath the plasma membrane that were particularly abundant on the side that sticks to the culture-glass surface, but could hardly be seen *in vivo*. Perhaps, *in vitro*, these thin filaments, which are found also in nerve cells, are necessary to maintain the attachment of the melanocytes to the surface of the culture-glass and to cause locomotion of the melanocytes. Furthermore, in experiments *in vitro*, WIKSWO and SZABO [27] found both thin (30–70 Å) and intermediate (60–110 Å) filaments in guinea pig skin melanocytes, which contain, *in vivo*, only intermediate filaments [personal commun.].

Pigment cells and nerve cells have many similarities in addition to having ultrastructurally similar cytoplasmic filaments. Embryonically, the epidermal melanocytes and the nerve cells both originate from the neural crest [28], and the retinal pigment cells originate from the optic-nerve cup [29]. Metabolically, the pigment cells and nerve cells both possess 'tyrosine hydroxylase', which catalyzes the oxidation of tyrosine to dopa as the initiation of the dopa-quinone-melanin pathway in the epidermal melanocytes and retinal pigment cells, and also catalyzes the oxidation of tyrosine to dopa as the initiation of the dopa quinone-melanin pathway in the epidermal melanocytes and retinal pigment cells, and also catalyzes the oxidation of tyrosine to dopa as the initiation of the dopa-amine-epinephrine pathway in the nerve cells. Functionally, both the epidermal melanocytes and the retinal pigment cells are controlled by the nerve cells. On the basis of all these similarities, studies were done to determine whether melanocytic filaments and neurofilaments are built from similar proteins.

Comparison of Melanocytic Filaments with the Neurofilaments, Microtubules and the 100-Å Filaments in Other Cell Systems *in vivo* and *in vitro*

The physicochemical properties of 100-Å filaments in many cells are still a matter for speculation except for those of tonofilaments in keratinizing cells [30], glial filaments [50], and of neurofilaments [17, 31]. Contrary to our findings in human epidermal melanocytes and chick retinal pigment cells, the studies of frog epidermal melanocytes by MOELLMANN *et al.* [32] showed that cytoplasmic areas normally occupied with 100-Å filaments are replaced by vincristine crystals, i.e. reorganized proteinaceous material of microtubules. KRISHAN and HSU [20] also found that cultured fibroblasts contain large aggregates of cytochalasin-insensitive filaments that are in intimate contact with vincristine crystals. BUNGE and BUNGE [34] presented evidence of changes similar to those in neurons after treatment with colchicine, and suggested that microtubules and neurofilaments may be interconvertible and comprise a common protein subunit. PETERS and VAUGHN [35] proposed, in a study of developing neurons, that microtubules may progressively give rise to neurofilaments, and DANIELS [36] suggested that neurofilaments can take the place of microtubules after treatment with colchicine. Also, an increase in the number of 80–100-Å filaments, accompanied by a disappearance of microtubules, was reported after treatment with colchicine in virus-induced syncytium, in interphase HeLa cells, and in osteoclasts [37–39].

Recently, however, DALES *et al.* [40] demonstrated that antisera made to vincristine-induced crystals specifically bind to the microtubules, but do not bind to any of the 100-Å filaments in HeLa and L cells. HUNEEUS and DAVISON [17] characterized biochemically, using the giant axon from the squid, a presumptive neurofilament subunit with a molecular weight of 80,000; the composition was similar to that of actin and tubulin, but lacked the colchicine- and nucleotide-binding activities of microtubules. DAVISON and WINSLOW [51] showed that mammalian tubulin and neurofilament protein can be distinguished by gel electrophoresis. SHELANSKI *et al.* [31] also characterized neurofilaments isolated from mammalian brain. They found that the neurofilament subunit in mammals had a molecular weight of 60,000 and that its protein did not conjugate with microtubule protein and did not bind to colchicine and nucleotides. From these findings and our studies of chemical treatment *in vitro*, we conclude that the melanocytic filaments are not related to those of microtubules or neurofilaments, although the fine structure of the latter is similar. A question of whether chemical properties of melanocytic filaments are unique or similar to those of other types of 100-Å filaments in fibroblasts, osteoclasts, and muscle cells must await further study.

Role of 100-Å Filaments in Melanocytes
Melanocytic Filaments in Cytomorphosis during Melanin Pigmentation

The function of 100-Å filaments in cultured cells (macrophages, fibroblasts, and muscle cells) is still unknown. In nerve cells, however, the 100-Å filaments (neurofilaments) are known to constitute a cytoskeletal system that is involved in axoplasmic transport or the elongation and contraction of the dendrites of the nerve cells, or axons [4]. Microtubules participate in the development or maintenance, or both, of the cell shape and dendrites in various locomotive cells (see review of Ciba Foundation Symposium) [41]. YAMADA et al. [26] suggested that both microtubules and neurofilaments are necessary for the cytoskeleton and that none of them alone can be sufficient for axonal elongation. Although melanocytic filaments and neurofilaments may have different physicochemical properties, these two filaments could constitute a similar functional unit, inasmuch as the nerve cells and pigment cells possess many similarities in tissue origin, metabolism, function, and cell morphology, including the fine structure of the cytoplasmic filaments. In melanocytes, the filaments are abundant, and the microtubules, although scarce, were often present in the protruding area of the cytoplasm, indicating that they could be involved in cytomorphosis. It is therefore likely that both melanocytic filaments and microtubules participate in a cytoskeleton for elongation and contraction of melanocytic dendrites during melanin pigmentation.

Melanocytic Filaments for Movement of Melanosomes within
Melanocytes during Melanin Pigmentation

The mechanism by which the melanosomes move inside the pigment cells and their dendritic processes (from the perinuclear and endoplasmic regions toward the tip of the dendrites) and are transferred into the surrounding epithelial cells is still not ascertained. Although the mechanisms in the movement of the melanosomes have been extensively studied in the chromatophores, melanophores, and melanocytes in fish and frog skin in relation to the effect of the MSH (see review of BAGNARA and HADLEY [42]), studies of mammalian systems have been limited. Light microscopic studies of these fish and frog tissues indicated that there are three possibilities that might account for the movement of the melanosomes: (1) a change in the intracellular current flow caused by a local difference in membrane potentials between the central and peripheral parts of the cell (the electrophoresis theory) [43], (2) the ionic release or ionic exchange of the membrane-bound ions, thus initiating the intracellular movement of the melanosomes (the ion-exchange theory) [44], and (3) solation and gelation transformation, causing changes in the hydrostatic pressures of the cytoplasm (the sol-gel transformation theory) [45]. Ultrastructural studies of these tissues, however, indicated that movement of the melanosomes could be mediated through the channels surrounded by microtubules (the microtubule theory) [46, 47].

McGUIRE and MOELLMANN [22] reported that melanocytes in frog skin contained cytochalasin-sensitive filaments (65–75 Å) that occupied an intermediary position between MSH-dependent activation of adenyl cyclase and dispersion of the melanosomes. They found that cytochalasin: (1) prevented the dispersion of melanosomes by MSH, and (2) caused the aggregation of pigment granules in frog melanocytes that had been treated with MSH. MALAWISTA [47] also found that colchicine and vincristine inhibited translocation of the melanosomes. In contrast to these findings, ROBINSON and CHARLTON [48] found that shrimp chromatophores contained abundant microtubules and cytochalasin-insensitive filaments in their dendrites. During the translocation of pigment granules mediated through the process of coat discoloration (i.e. 'physiological' color change), they found that pretreatment with either colchicine or vincristine did not inhibit the translocation of pigment granules, even though the vincristine-elicited production of crystalline complexes of microtubular proteins in place of the normal bundles of microtubules. They also found a reversible inhibition of pigment aggregation by cytochalasin, with no apparent loss or disruption of chromatophore filaments.

We presume that melanocytic filaments are involved not only in the elongation of the dendrites, but also in the movement of the melanosomes. We do not, however, think that microtubules are directly involved in the melanosome movement. This presumption is based on our present findings in epidermal melanocytes and retinal pigment cells that: (1) melanocytic filaments changed their location reversibly, after exposure to UV and visible light; (2) the melanosomes also changed their location, being shifted from the perinuclear and endoplasmic region to the tip of the dendrites and, in human skin, this translocation of melanosomes resulted in an increase in the number of melanosomes transferred into the keratinocytes; (3) those melanosomes in the dendrites were embedded in the bundles, or clusters, of the melanocytic filaments, some of which actually encircled the melanosomes; (4) there was no morphologic interconnection between microtubules and melanosomes whatsoever, and (5) the microtubules were very rarely seen in the dendrites. ROBINSON and CHARLTON [48] found that: (1) neither cytochalasin nor vincristine inhibits the movement of melanosomes, which correlates with our assumption that the melanocytic filaments are unaffected by these chemicals, and (2) that each chemical partly inhibits the development of dendrites, which correlates with our presumption that both microtubules and melanocytic filaments are involved in the development of melanocytic dendrites, and correlates also with the findings of our present study and of EVERHART and RUBIN [8] that the primary site for the effect of cytochalasin is the surface of the plasma membrane, not the thin filaments. Still undetermined, however, is whether these melanocytic filaments are directly involved in the transfer of melanosomes from melanocytes to keratinocytes, even though there is an increase in the number of melanosomes transferred to the keratinocytes during tanning reactions [13]. Also undetermined is the initial trigger for translocation of melanocytic filaments; it is not clear whether UV and visible light affect melanocytic filaments directly or whether UV and visible light first affect the other photoreceptor cells, e. g. keratinocytes in the skin and cones and rods in the retina, which then send the message for the shifting of melanocytic filaments by changing the membranous or cellular potentials or ionic strength.

Summary

Ultrastructural and biochemical characterization of the nature and role of melanocytic filaments (intermediate, or 100-Å, filaments) was carried out on the pigment cells in human skin and chick eyes. To compare the chemical effects on melanocytic filaments with those on other types of cytoplasmic filaments, epidermal melanocytes and retinal pigment cells were exposed *in vitro* to cytochalasin B and vincristine sulfate. Electrophoretic mobilities of melanocytic filaments isolated from human melanocytes and retinal pigment cells were compared with known mobilities of neurofilaments in humans and chicks. To examine the role of melanocytic filaments in melanin pigmentation, human skin and chick eyes were exposed *in vivo* to UV and visible light.

We found that the structural units of melanocytic filaments are unique and different from those of thin filaments, and microtubules. Although melanocytic filaments possess an ultrastructure similar to that of neurofilaments, melanocytic filaments do not show physicochemical properties comparable to those of neurofilaments. These melanocytic filaments are related to the development of the dendrites and the intracellular movement of melanosomes after exposure to physical light. In human skin, they are also involved in the transfer of melanosomes from melanocytes to epithelial cells.

References

1 GOLDMAN, R. D. and FOLETT, E. A. L.: The fine structure of the major cell processes of isolated BHK-21 fibroblasts. Expl Cell Res. *57:* 263 (1969).

2 MCNUTT, N. S.; CALP, L. A., and BLACK, P. H.: Contact-inhibited revertant cell lines isolated from SV-40-transformed cells. J. Cell Biol. *50:* 691 (1971).

3 PERDUE, J. F.: The distribution, ultrastructure, and chemistry of microfilaments in cultured chick embryo fibroblasts. J. Cell Biol. *58:* 265 (1973).

4 SPOONER, B. S.; YAMADA, K. M., and WESSELS, N. K.: Microfilaments and cell locomotion. J. Cell Biol. *49:* 595 (1971).

5 SUTTON, J. S. and WEISS, L.: Transformation of monocytes in tissue culture into macrophages, epitheloid cells and multinucleated giant cells. J. Cell Biol. *28:* 103 (1966).

6 PROTLEY, J. N. and MCQUILLEN, N. K.: The role of microfilaments in frog skin ion transport. J. Cell Biol. *56:* 850 (1973).

7 POLLARD, T. D.; SHELTON, S.; WEIBING, R. R., and KOVIN, E. D.: Ultrastructural characterization of F-actin isolated from *Acanthamoeba castellanii* and identification of cytoplasmic filaments as F-actin by reaction with rabbit heavy meromyosin. J. molec. Biol. *50:* 91 (1970).

8 EVERHART, L. P. and RUBIN, R. W.: Cyclic changes in the cell surface. II. The effect of cytochalasin B on the surface morphology of synchronized Chinese hamster ovary cells. J. Cell Biol. *60:* 442 (1974).

9 COMLY, L. T.: Microfilaments in *Chaos carolinensis;* membrane association, distribution, and heavy meromyosin binding in the glycerinated cell. J. Cell Biol. *58:* 230 (1973).

10 ISHIKAWA, H.; BISCHOFF, R., and HOLTZER, H.: Formation of arrowhead complexes with heavy meromyosin in a variety of cell types. J. Cell Biol. *43:* 312 (1969).

11 MCNUTT, N. S.; CULP, L. A., and BLACK, P. H.: Contact-inhibited revertant cell lines isolated from SV-40-transformed cells. IV. Microfilament distribution and cell shape in untransformed, transformed, and revertant Balb/c 3T3 cells. J. Cell Biol. *56:* 412 (1973).

12 NACHMIAS, V. T.: Further electron microscope studies on the fibrillar organization of the ground cytoplasm of *Chaos chaos*. J. Cell Biol. *38:* 40 (1968).

13 JIMBOW, K.; PATHAK, M. A., and FITZPATRICK, T. B.: Effect of ultraviolet on the distribution pattern of microfilaments and microtubules and on the nucleus in human melanocytes. Yale J. Biol. Med. *46:* 411 (1973).

14 WARREN, D. C.: Inheritance of albinism in domestic fowl. J. Hered. *24:* 379 (1933).

15 MUELLER, C. B. and HUTT, F. B.: Genetics of the fowl; sex- linked imperfect albinism. J. Hered. *32:* 71 (1941).

16 TRINKAUS, J. P.: Behavior of dissociated retinal pigment cells in heterotypic cell aggregates. Ann. N.Y. Acad. Sci. *100:* 413 (1963).

17 HUNEEUS, F. C. and DAVISON, P. F.: Fibrilar proteins from squid axons. I. Neuro-filament protein. J. molec. Biol. *52:* 415 (1970).

18 JIMBOW, K.; PATHAK, M. A.; SZABO, G., and FITZPATRICK, T. B.: Ultrastructural changes in human melanocytes after ultraviolet radiation; in PATHAK et al. Sunlight and man, p. 195 (Tokyo University Press, Tokyo 1974).

19 PORTER, K. R. and YAMADA, E.: Studies on the endoplasmic reticulum. V. Its form and differentiation in pigment epithelial cells of the frog retina. J. biophys. biochem. Cytol. 8: 181 (1960).

20 KRISHAN, A. and HSU, D.: Observations on the association of helical polyribosomes and filaments with vincristine-induced crystals in Earle's L-cell fibroblasts. J. Cell Biol. 43: 553 (1969).

21 WOLPERT, L.: Cytoplasmic streaming and amoeboid movement. Symp. Soc. gen. Microbiol. 15: 270 (1965).

22 McGUIRE, J. and MOELLMANN, G.: Cytochalasin B. Effects on microfilaments and movement of melanin granules within melanocytes. Science 175: 642 (1972).

23 BERTOLINI, B.; MONAGO, G., and ROSSI, R.: Ultrastructure of a regular arrangement of microtubules and neurofilaments. J. Ultrastruct. Res. 33: 173 (1970).

24 GUILLERY, R. W.; SOBKOWICZ, H. M., and SCOTT, G. L.: Relationship between glial and neuronal elements in the development of long-term cultures of the spinal cord of the fetal mouse. J. comp. Neurol. 140: 1 (1970).

25 WUEKER, R. B. and PALAY, S. L.: Neurofilaments and microtubules in anterior born cells of the rat. Tissue Cell 1: 387 (1969).

26 YAMADA, K. M.; SPOONER, B. S., and WESSELLS, N. F.: Ultrastructure and function of growth cones and axons of cultured nerve cells. J. Cell Biol. 49: 614 (1971).

27 WIKSWO, M. A. and SZABO, G.: Effects of cytochalasin B on mammalian melanocytes and keratinocytes. J. invest. Derm. 59: 163 (1972).

28 RAWLES, M. E.: Origin of melanophores and their role in development of color patterns in vertebrates. Physiol. Rev. 20: 383 (1948).

29 WESTON, J. A.: Neural crest cell migration and differentiation. UCLA Forum med. Sci. 14: 1 (1971).

30 TEZUKA, T. and FREEDBERG, I. M.: Epidermal structural proteins. II. Isolation and purification of newborn rats. Biochem. biophys. Acta 263: 382 (1972).

31 SHELANSKI, M. L.; ALBERT, S.; DEVRIES, G. H., and NORTON, W. T.: Isolation of filaments from brain. Science 174: 1242 (1972).

32 MOELLMANN, G.; McGUIRE, J., and LERNER, A. B.: Intracellular dynamics and the fine structure of melanocytes. Yale J. Biol. Med. 46: 337 (1973).

33 GASKIN, F.; KRAMER, S. B.; CANTOR, C. R.; ADELSTEIN, R., and SHELANSKI, M. L.: A dynein-like protein associated with neurotubules. Fed. Eur. Biol. Soc. 40: 281 (1974).

34 BUNGE, R. and BUNGE, M.: Electron microscopic observations on colchicine-induced change in neuronal cytoplasm. Anat. Rec. 160: 323 (1968).

35 PETERS, A. and VAUGHN, J. E.: Microtubules and filaments in the axons and astrocytes of early postnatal rat optic nerve. J. Cell Biol. 32: 113 (1967).

36 DANIELS, M. P.: Fine structural changes in neurons and nerve fibers associated with colchicine inhibition of nerve fiber formation in vitro. J. Cell Biol. 58: 463 (1973).

37 HOLMES, K. V. and CHOPPINO, D. W.: On the role of microtubules in movement and alignment of nuclei in virus-induced syncytia. J. Cell Biol. 39: 526 (1968).

38   ROBBINS, E. and GONATAS, N. K.: Histochemical and ultrastructural studies of HeLa cell cultures exposed to spindle inhibitors with special reference to interphase cell. J. Histochem. Cytochem. *12:* 704 (1964).

39   HOLTROP, M. E.; RAISG, L. G., and SIMMONS, H. A.: The effects of parathyroid hormone, colchicine, and calcitonin on the ultrastructure of osteoclasts in organ culture. J. Cell Biol. *60:* 346 (1974).

40   DALES, S.; HSU, K. C., and NAKAYAMA, A.: The fine structure and immunological labelling of the achromatic mitotic apparatus after disruption of cell membrane. J. Cell Biol. *59:* 643 (1973).

41   Ciba Foundation Symposium: Locomotion of tissue cells (Elsevier, Excerpta Medica, North Holland, Amsterdam 1973).

42   BAGNARA, J. T. and HADLEY, M. E.: Theories on the mechanism of pigment granule movement; in BAGNARA and HADLEY Chromatophores and color change, pp. 144–159 (Prentice Hall, New Jersey 1973).

43   KINOSHITA, H.: Electrophoretic theory of pigment migration within fish melanophore. Ann. N.Y. Acad. Sci. *100:* 992 (1963).

44   NOVALES, R. R. and NOVALES, B. J.: The effects of osmotic pressure and calcium deficiency on the response of tissue-cultured melanophores to melanocyte-stimulating hormone. Gen. comp. Endocr. *5:* 568 (1965).

45   MARSLAND, D. and MEISNER, D.: Effects of D_2O on the mechanism of pigment dispersal in the melanocytes of *Fundulus heroditus*. A pressure-temperature analysis. J. Cell Physiol. *70:* 209 (1967).

46   GREEN, L.: Mechanism of movement of granules in melanocytes of *Fundulus heteroditus*. Proc. natn. Acad. Sci. USA *59:* 1179 (1968).

47   MALAWISTA, S. E.: The melanocyte model. Colchicine-like effects of other anti-mitotic agents. J. Cell Biol. *49:* 848 (1971).

48   ROBINSON, W. T. and CHARLTON, J. S.: Microtubules, microfilaments, and pigment movement in the chromatophores of *Palaemontes vulgaris* (crustacea). J. exp. Zool. *186:* 279 (1973).

49   LAEMMLI, U. K.: Cleavage of structural proteins during the assembly of the head of bacteriophage T4. Nature, Lond. *227:* 680 (1970).

50   BRYAN, J.: Biochemical properties of microtubules. Fed. Proc. Fed. Am. Socs exp. Biol. *32:* 152 (1974).

51   DAVISON, P. S. and WINSLOW, B.: The protein subunit of calf brain neurofilament. J. Neurobiol. *5:* 119 (1974).

K. JIMBOW, MD, PhD, Department of Dermatology, Sapporo Medical College, Sapporo, Minami 1, *Nishi 16* (Japan)

Pigment Cell, vol. 3, pp. 33–45 (Karger, Basel 1976)

The Role of Multivesicular Bodies in Melanosome Formation[1]

WILLIAM A. TURNER, jr., JOHN D. TAYLOR and T. T. TCHEN

Department of Biology, and Department of Chemistry,
Wayne State University, Detroit, Mich.

Introduction

A number of studies have supported the theory of melanosome origin from the Golgi complex based on the proximity of premelanosomes to Golgi complexes and the cytochemical localization of tyrosinase within Golgi complexes and premelanosomes [1, 5–8, 18, 25–28].

Some recent studies have suggested an alternative theory of origin and formation [2, 3, 14, 15, 20, 22]. Not all lamellar premelanosomes possess tyrosinase activity. Tyrosinase-positive vesicles have been found free and fusing with tyrosinase-negative premelanosomes [15, 21]. It has been postulated that premelanosomes form from dilations of endoplasmic reticulum inside of which a lamellar structural protein matrix is established. Tyrosinase is synthesized on ribosomes, transferred to a Golgi complex, and packaged in small vesicles which fuse with premelanosomes.

The ultrastructure of melanosome formation during melanocytogenesis has not been investigated in fishes. This study demonstrates a previously undescribed premelanosome, namely a multivesicular body, and attempts to determine, morphologically and cytochemically, the origin and assembly of premelanosome components and subsequent melanization within differentiating melanophores of the xanthic goldfish, *Carassius auratus* L.

1   This study was supported by Grants GB-16329 from the National Science Foundation and AM 13724 and AM 5384 from the USPHS. Part of this work is presented in greater detail elsewhere [29].

Materials and Methods

In order to study melanosome formation, preadapted xanthic goldfish adults free of visual melanophores were stressed by placing them in a 0.9% NaCl solution as described by CHAVIN [4].

In addition to standard electron microscopy techniques, two cytochemical procedures were utilized: (1) L-dopa for the localization of tyrosinase. Cacodylate buffer was used in order to prevent dopa autoxidation [24] and diethyldithiocarbamide, an inhibitor of tyrosinase, was also used [23]. (2) The other procedure was Friend's technique [10] of tissue incubation in osmium tetroxide at 40 °C for 48 h. Osmium tetroxide is chiefly reduced by compounds containing aliphatic double bonds, and sulfhydryl groups, which accounts for its characteristic oxidation of unsaturated lipids, lipoproteins, alcohols, and certain amino acids. Friend's technique does not indicate the location of any specific chemical moiety, but rather shows a close relationship and common origins of cellular components as reflected in their affinities for osmium reduction.

Results

Melanocytogenesis of fish exposed to the salt solution was observable in 3–5 days at the distal portions of the dorsal, pectoral, and caudal fins. Cellular boundaries of differentiating melanophores are smooth and regular showing no intedigitations or other relationships with adjacent cells; however, the plasmalemma does show numerous micropinocytotic vesicles. RER, some SER, and numerous polyribosomes and mitochondria are found. Scattered throughout the cytoplasm are numerous Golgi complexes with associated small vesicles. In addition to melanosomes, vesicles 0.4–0.5 μm are found apparently free and attached to RER (fig. 1).

Melanophores in early stages of melanocytogenesis contain numerous multivesicular bodies. These are approximately 0.4–0.5 μm in diameter and contain a variable number of small internal vesicles (fig. 2). These multivesicular bodies appear to originate from two different sources within the pigment cells. The larger outer vesicle arises from RER. The smaller vesicles found within the multivesicular bodies are similar in size and morphology to the small vesicles associated with the

---

Fig. 1. Melanophore undergoing melanocytogenesis. Among maturing melanosomes (PM), vesicles are found free (V) and connected to RER. ×40,000.

Fig. 2. Multivesicular bodies (MB) are found associated with the Golgi complex (GC) and Golgi-derived vesicles (GV). ×37,500.

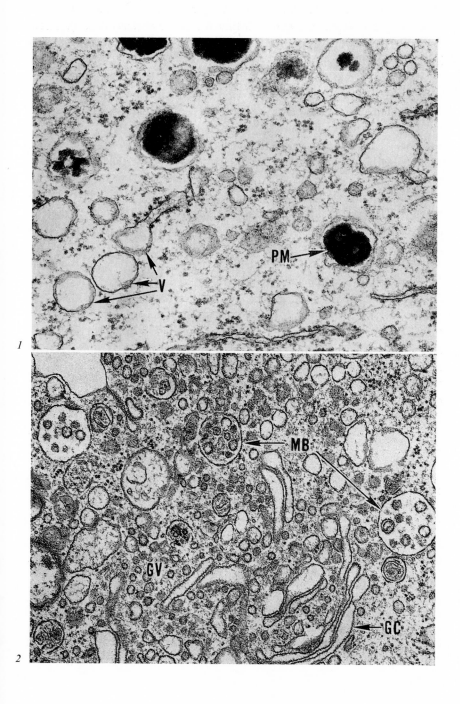

Golgi complexes. The small vesicles appear to fuse with the membrane of the larger vesicles and reform within the larger vesicles (fig. 3). These multivesicular bodies represent the premelanosomes of the differentiating melanophores.

Melanization of the premelanosomes is seen first around the periphery of the internal vesicles (fig. 4). The electron-opaque melanin matrix gradually surrounds these vesicles and expands into the intervesicular spaces. Partially melanized premelanosomes take on a 'waffle' appearance, having holes within the melanin matrix. The holes represent the lumens of the internal vesicles. Upon maturation, the internal vesicles are filled in by melanin. The fully melanized melanosomes are spherical, highly electron-opaque and approximately 0.4–0.5 μm in diameter. They are limited by a single membrane which in some cases, is connected to SER (fig. 5). A distinct space exists between the limiting membrane and the internal matrix.

Caudal fins from stressed adults incubated in osmium exhibit a positive osmophilic reaction within developing melanophores. It is specific for the maturing face of the Golgi complex, associated vesicles, and many vesicles free in the cytoplasm. Within premelanosomes, many internal vesicles are also found to have osmium deposits (fig. 6). Small vesicles, both inside and outside the large vesicles, usually exhibit a faint reaction product near the outer periphery. Other organelles within the melanophores did not exhibit a positive osmophilic reaction with the exception of some maturing melanosomes (fig. 7). Here, the osmium deposition is found along the inner surface of the limiting membrane

---

Fig. 3. (a) Small and large vesicle fusion. ×102,500. (b) Inversion (arrow). ×95,000.

Fig. 4. Melanization around peripheries of internal vesicles (arrows) of multivesicular bodies (premelanosomes). ×86,000.

Fig. 5. Melanosome conected to SER (arrow). ×110,000.

Fig. 6. Positive Friend's reaction in the maturing face of the Golgi complex (FMF), associated vesicles (V) and internal vesicles (IV) of multivesicular body. ×75,000.

Fig. 7. Positive Friend's reaction within the internal vesicles (IV), inner surfaces of the limiting membranes and the peripheries of the melanin matrix (arrows) of melanosomes. ×81,000.

Fig. 8. Dopa-melanin on the peripheries of internal vesicles (arrows) of a multivesicular body (premelanosome). Dopa-melanin within a small vesicle fusing with a large vesicle (V). ×130,000.

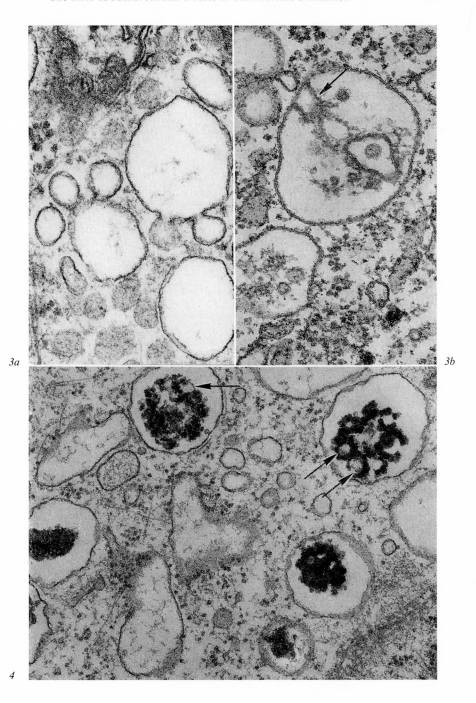

3a

3b

4

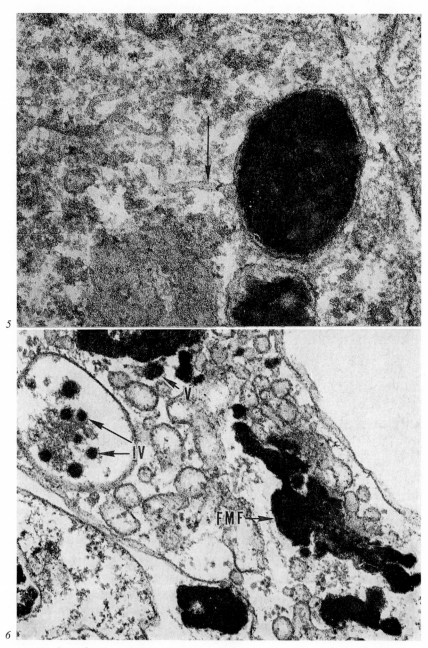

For legends, see p. 36.

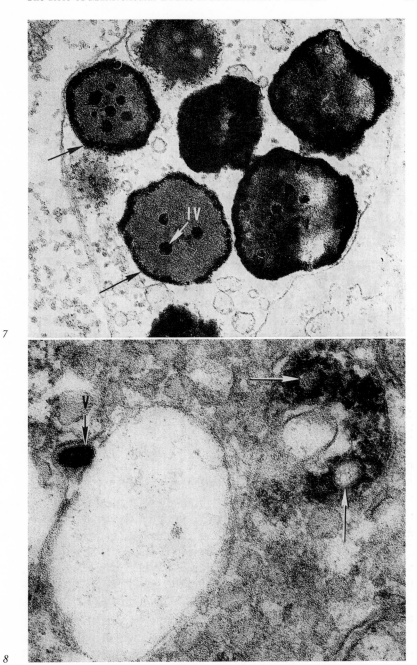

7

8

For legends, see p. 36.

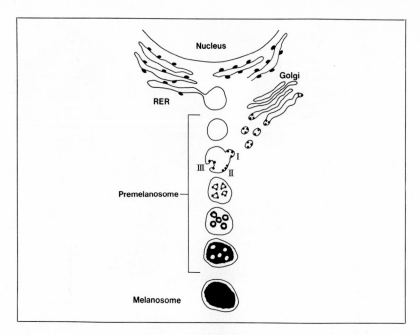

Fig. 9. Schematic interpretation of goldfish melanosome formation. Description in text.

and periphery of the melanin matrix. The inner vesicles or holes are also filled with osmium.

In caudal fins, incubated 4–6 h, dopa-melanin is restricted to melanophores. It is found in the maturing faces of Golgi complexes, inside many small vesicles associated with the maturing faces and inside many small vesicles scattered throughout the cytoplasm. Unlike the cytoplasmic small vesicles, small vesicles inside the premelanosomes demonstrate a faint reaction product around their peripheries, but not their insides (fig. 8). Unstained sections revealed that the electron-opaque depositions are not the result of heavy metal stains. Control tissues incubated in dopa-free media show no evidence of a dopa-melanin reaction. Tissues preincubated in diethyldithiocarbamide (DDC), a tyrosinase inhibitor, and then exposed to the dopa are also free of any such reaction product.

Figure 9 represents a schematic interpretation of goldfish melanosome formation. Large dilations are blebbed from RER while small vesicles, containing tyrosinase, are blebbed from the cisternae of the Golgi complex. These vesicles fuse with the membrane of the large vesicle (I) and are incorporated into it (II). The small vesicles invert and reform within the large vesicle (III) exposing tyrosinase. Melanin is synthesized around the periphery of the inverted vesicles and eventually fills the intervesicular spaces and finally the internal vesicles.

Some small cytoplasmic vesicles and some internal vesicles did not respond to the dopa or Friend's technique. Inasmuch as melanophores displayed numerous micropinocytotic vesicles, it seems reasonable that these are the vesicles which gave the negative responses to the cytochemical techniques. The possible role of micropinocytotic vesicles in the cytoplasm and/or in the premelanosomes is not clear.

The multivesicular body which serves as the premelanosome in melanophores of goldfish is similar in appearance to multivesicular bodies in other cell types. Many investigations have attempted to elucidate the function and origin of these cellular organelles [10]. It is believed that multivesicular bodies function as digestive vacuoles or 'autolysosomes' for endogenous and exogenous proteins. NOVIKOFF *et al.* [22] and GORDON *et al.* [11] have suggested that multivesicular bodies are formed by the penetration of small cytoplasmic vesicles through the membrane of the large vesicle. A second hypothesis proposes the enclosure of clusters of small vesicles by a smooth-membraned cisternae [10, 13]. A third hypothesis encompasses portions of the first two. FRIEND and FARQUHAR [9] and HIRSCH *et al.* [12] suggested that there are two types of small vesicles within multivesicular bodies: one type is engulfed in clusters and are of Golgi origin, the other is added later as a result of membrane inversion with cytoplasm incorporation. In this study, small Golgi-derived vesicles were seen fusing with and invaginating into the larger vesicles forming multivesicular bodies (premelanosomes). An understanding of the pattern of melanin synthesis within these premelanosomes allows further speculation of the mechanism of their assembly.

Melanin synthesis first begins on the periphery of the small internal vesicles once they are inside the large vesicle. This suggests release of the enzyme; however, the small vesicles appear to remain intact during melanin synthesis. Results of the L-dopa incubation demonstrate that tyrosinase is localized and mediates the formation of dopa-melanin inside the small vesicles before they fuse with the large vesicle. Once inside, the formation of tyrosine-melanin always occurs on the outside of the small vesicles. Tyrosinase does not penetrate the membranes of cytoplasmic small vesicles to react with L-dopa on their outer surfaces. It seems unlikely that the enzyme can penetrate small vesicle membranes to mediate tyrosine-melanin synthesis while inside the premelanosomes. A logical explanation is that the incorporation of small vesicles into the large involves a fusion, incorporation, and inversion of the small vesicle. The outside of the internal vesicle now would be the site of enzyme attachment as it was the original inner surface of the vesicle while in the cytoplasm.

The hypothesis of membrane inversion during the passage of small vesicles into the large vesicles would explain satifactorily the localization of tyrosinase. However, the Friend's staining results are in apparent contradiction with this hypothesis in that the interior of the small vesicles are stained whether these vesicles are inside or outside of the large vesicles. We believe that this can be explained in the following manner.

The small vesicle produces osmophilic substances on both sides of the membrane. The substance produced inside the vesicles would be present in high concentration, resulting in greater electron density. The substance produced outside of the vesicles would be greatly diluted by diffusion and therefore not show up by osmium staining. Indeed, close examination of the small vesicles inside and outside of the large vesicles show the following osmium staining properties: (1) The small vesicles, both inside and outside of the large vesicles, are almost always accompanied by a faint stained material near their outer peripheries. (2) Among the small vesicles in the large vesicles, one finds a gradation of the degree of osmophilicity in the interior of these vesicles. This would be expected if during the passage into the large vesicles, the small vesicles empty out the internal content and would proceed to accumulate the osmophilic substance after vesicle reformation. In general, there appears to be good correlation between the osmophilicity of the interior of the small vesicles with an amount of fuzzy dense material in the large vesicles but outside of the small vesicles. (3) As melanization proceeds, one finds that the melanin appears to force the osmophilic substance towards the membrane of the large vesicle and also to confine it to the interior of the small vesicle. When melanization is completed, there is, next to the membrane of the large vesicle, an unmelanized zone which is highly osmophilic in addition to the small vesicle interior which is also highly osmophilic. These observations are in accord with the postulate stated earlier and provide a reasonable explanation for the gradual build-up of osmophilic substance inside and outside the small vesicles while in the large vesicles. It is also in accord with the hypothesis of membrane inversion during the passage of the small vesicles into the large vesicles. Finally, this investigation does not identify the osmium-reducing substance. Whether it is complexed to or only associated with the tyrosinase by being in the same vesicle is not known.

Unlike premelanosomes found in mammals, fowl, reptiles and amphibians, no internal lamellar matrix forms within the goldfish premelanosomes. In higher vertebrates, melanization takes place on the lamellar matrix. Inasmuch as internal lamellae are not present in goldfish premelanosomes, the incorporation of small vesicles not only provides the enzyme for melanin synthesis, but serves as the structural foundation for melanin synthesis. Whether multivesicular bodies serve as premelanosomes in most species of fish awaits further investigation; however, lamellar melanosomes have been reported in lungfish and in coelacanth [16, 17]. In summary, Golgi-derived vesicle incorporation and inversion into RER-derived vesicle appears to be the mechanism of premelanosome formation in goldfish. Whether inversion of Golgi-derived vesicles play a role in lamellar melanosome formation in higher vertebrates awaits further investigation. However, vesicles have been found in this type of melanosome [19].

Summary

Melanosome formation in differentiating melanophores of embryonic and adult xanthic goldfish was studied by cytochemical methods at the ultrastructural level. Large vesicles (0.4–0.5 μm) are blebbed from rough endoplasmic reticulum. Golgi-derived small vesicles, containing the enzyme tyrosinase, fuse with the membrane of the large vesicle, invert and reform within the large vesicle exposing the tyrosinase. This multivesicular body represents the premelanosome. Melanin synthesis begins around the periphery of the inverted vesicles and eventually fills the intervesicular spaces and finally the inverted vesicles. Inasmuch as an internal lamellar matrix is not characteristic of goldfish premelanosomes, the incorporation of Golgi-derived vesicles not only provides tyrosinase for melanin synthesis, but serves as the structural foundation for melanin synthesis.

References

1 BARNCOT, N. A. and CUCKOW, F. W.: The electron microscopy of human hair pigments. Ann. hum. Genet. *19:* 231–249 (1955).
2 BRUMBAUGH, J.: The ultrastructural effects of the I and S loci upon black-red melanin differentiation in the fowl. Devl Biol. *24:* 392–412 (1971).

3 BRUMBAUGH, J.; BOWERS, R. R., and CHATTERJEE, G. E.: Genotype-substrate interactions altering Golgi development during melanogenesis; in RILEY Pigment Cell, vol. 1, pp. 47–54 (Karger, Basel 1973).

4 CHAVIN, W.: Pituitary-adrenal controls of melanization in goldfish, *Carassius Auratus* L. J. exp. Zool. *133:* 1–46 (1956).

5 DALTON, A. J. and FELIX, M. D.: Phase contrast and electron microscopy of the Cloudman S91 mouse melanoma; in GORDON Pigment cell growth, pp. 267–274 (Academic Press, New York 1953).

6 DROCHMANS, P.: Ultrastructure of melanin granules. Advances in biology of skin, vol. 8, pp. 169–177 (1967).

7 FITZPATRICK, T. B. and SZABO, G.: The melanocyte cytology and cytochemistry. J. invest. Derm. *32:* 197–209 (1959).

8 FITZPATRICK, T. B.; SEIJI, S. M., and McGUGAN, A. D.: Melanin pigmentation. New Engl. J. Med. *266:* 328–333 (1961).

9 FRIEND, D. S. and FARQUHAR, M. G.: Function of coated vesicles during protein adsorption in the rat vas deferens. J. Cell Biol. *35:* 357–376 (1967).

10 FRIEND, D. S.: Cytochemical staining of multivesicular body and Golgi vesicles. J. Cell Biol. *41:* 269–279 (1969).

11 GORDON, G. B.; MILLER, L. R., and BENSCH, K. G.: Studies on the intracellular digestive process in mammalian tissue culture cells. J. Cell Biol. *25:* 41–56 (1965).

12 HIRSCH, J. G.; FEDORKO, M. E., and COHN, Z. A.: Vesicle fusion and formation at the surface of pinocyte vacuoles in macrophages. J. Cell Biol. *38:* 629–635 (1968).

13 HOLTZMAN, E.; NOVIKOFF, A. B., and VILLAVERDE, H.: Lysosomes and GERL in normal and chromatolytic neurons of the rat ganglion. J. Cell Biol. *33:* 419–435 (1967).

14 HORI, Y.; TODA, K.; PATHAK, M. A.; CLARK, W. H., and FITZPATRICK, T. B.: A fine structure study of the human melanosome complex and acid phosphatase activity. J. Ultrastruct. Res. *25:* 109–120 (1968).

15 IDE, C.: The development of melanosomes in the pigment epithelium of the chick embryo. Z. Zellforsch. *131:* 171–186 (1972).

16 IMAKI, H. and CHAVIN, W.: Ultrastructure of lungfish integumental melanophores. Am. Zoologist *12:* 732 (1972).

17 IMAKI, H. and CHAVIN, W.: Ultrastructure of integumental melanophores in the coelacanth. Am. Zoologist *13:* 521 (1973).

18 JIMBOW, K. and KUKITA, A.: Fine structure of pigment granules in the human bulb; in KAWAMURA, FITZPATRICK and SEIJI Biology of normal and abnormal melanocytes, pp. 171–193 (University Park Press, Baltimore 1971).

19 JIMBOW, K. and FITZPATRICK, T. B.: Characterization of a new melanosomal structural component – the vesiculo globular body – by conventional transmission, high-voltage and scanning electron microscopy. J. Ultrastruct. Res. *48:* 269–283 (1973).

20 MAUL, G. G.: Golgi-melanosome relationship in human melanoma *in vitro*. J. Ultrastruct. Res. *26:* 163–176 (1969).

21 MAUL, G. G. and BRUMBAUGH, J. A.: On the possible function of coated vesicles in melanogenesis of the regenerating fowl feather. J. Cell Biol. *48:* 41–48 (1971).

22 NOVIKOFF, A. B.; ALBALA, A., and BIEMPICA, L.: Ultrastructural and cyto-chemical observations on B-16 and Harding-Passey mouse melanomas. J. His-tochem. Cytochem. *16:* 299–319 (1968).

23 OKUN, M. R.; EDELSTEIN, L. M.; OR, N.; HAMADA, G.; DONNELLAN, B., and IEVER, W. F.: Histochemical differentiation of peroxidase-mediated from ty-rosinase-mediated melanin formation in mammalian tissues. Histochemie *23:* 295–309 (1970).

24 RODRIGUEZ, H. A. and McGAVRAN, M. H.: A modified dopa reaction for the diagnosis and investigation of pigment cells. Am. J. clin. Path. *52:* 219–227 (1969).

25 SEIJI, M. and FITZPATRICK, T. B.: The reciprocal relationship between melani-zation and tyrosinase activity in melanosomes (melanin granules). J. Biochem. *49:* 700–706 (1961).

26 SEIJI, M.; ITAKURA, H., and MIYAZAKI, K.: The membrane system and melanin formation in melanocytes; in KAWAMURA, FITZPATRICK and SEIJI Biology of normal and abnormal melanocytes, pp. 221–239 (University Press, Baltimore 1971).

27 TODA, T. and FITZPATRICK, T. B.: The origin of melanosomes; in KAWAMURA, FITZPATRICK and SEIJI The biology of normal and abnormal melanocytes, pp. 265–278 (University Park Press, Baltimore 1971).

28 ZELICKSON, A. S. and HARTMANN, F.: The fine structure of the melanocyte and melanin granule. J. invest. Derm. *43:* 23–27 (1960).

29 TURNER, W. A.; TAYLOR, J. D., and TCHEN, T. T.: Melanosome formation in the goldfish: the role of multivesicular bodies. J. Ultrastruct. Res. *51:* 16–31 (1975).

Dr. WILLIAM A. TURNER, jr., Department of Biology, Wayne State University, *Detroit, MI 48202* (USA)

Pigment Cell, vol. 3, pp. 46–52 (Karger, Basel 1976)

Serial Sections of Dopa-Positive Nuclei in Two Vertebrate Species [1]

HARRIET M. MCCURDY

Department of Biology, The University of Victoria, Victoria, British Columbia

Introduction

Colouration in vertebrates is provided by cells differentiated for that purpose in early embryology. Melanocytes specifically produce black and brown melanins. Normally, melanocytes are colourless until the appearance of the black or brown melanin granules (melanosomes).[2] These melanin granules, the end-point of melanogenesis, are impervious to water, alcohols, clearing hydrocarbons, and so make the melanocyte a self-marking cell, even in prepared slides.

In 1917, BLOCH announced a specific reaction for 'actively functioning melanoblasts' (i.e. melanocyte) [LAIDLAW, 1932]. The enzyme synthesized by the melanocyte, specifically for melanin production, could combine with exogenous dopa to give diffuse, visible melanin while the enzyme was free in the cytoplasm, prior to its incorporation into the melanin granules. This melanin is also impervious to water, alcohols and clearing hydrocarbons. BLOCH [1927] called this discovery the 'dopa reaction' (3,4-dioxyphenylalanine was abbreviated to 'dopa'). Its application revealed that many melanocytes could be colourless (without melanized granules) but the enzyme could be present in the cytoplasm and would combine with exogenous dopa, giving diffuse melanin, to identify the cells as melanocytes.

1   Supported in part by a Grant-in-Aid from Sigma Delta Epsilon and the Victoria Medical Research Foundation.
2   EPPIG and DUMONT [1971] showed that the pigment granules (melanosomes) present in the egg and the developing embryo prior to the appearance of the melanophore, are of oocyte origin. These melanin granules are present in the cells of the blastula and gastrula stages in amphibian embryology.

This discovery was used in expertly plotting the similar course of melanogenesis in the adult melanocyte of mammals and in the adult melanophore of amphibians. The amphibian melanophore has the ability to aggregate or disperse its melanin granules (melanosomes) to conform with its
background or to the light intensity. The mammalian melanocyte lacks this
ability. When melanogenesis begins, the enzyme is located proximal to the
endothelial reticulum in the cytoplasm. Its course could be from the nucleus,
through the endothelial reticulum to its functional position in the adult cell.

DuShane's [1934] transplantations of *Taricha torosa* neural crest
showed that the site of origin for the melanoblast, the precursor of the
melanophore, was the neural crest. This is a transitory tissue formed in
the area between the dorsum of the recently formed neural tube and the
overlying ectoderm. Twitty [1945], Niu [1947] and Algard [1953] by
tissue cultures were able to give eye-witness accounts of the outgrowth of
melanoblasts from sections of the neural crest. With no labelling, the cer-
tainty of the melanophore origin in these tissue cultures could not be established until the melanin granules apeared in the cytoplasm. The melanoblast as a cell could not be identified.

Twitty [1945] and Niu [1947], working independently, had also
shown that the neural crest grown in tissue cultures with coelomic fluid
medium, gave 100% melanophores. They felt that cells other than melanophores had been transformed into melanophores.

Model and Dalton [1968], using ³H-dopa, identified the melanoblast
in tissue cultures of *Ambystoma mexicanum* neural crest. They noted silver grains over the nucleus of the melanoblast and stated that: 'The appearance of silver grains in the emulsion over the nucleus does not necessarily indicate that this organelle has incorporated the label ... it is likely that
the label has been concentrated in the cytoplasm of the differentiating cells
and not in the nucleus.' This observation was made on tissue cultures.

The dopa reaction had revealed Bloch's dopa oxidase in the cytoplasm of the melanoblast; cautiously, the above comment had been added
anent its appearance in the nuclear region. In tissue cultures, the relation
of the label to the nucleus could not be resolved.

This paper is concerned not with melanogenesis (that process occurs in
the adult melanocyte or melanophore), but with the appearance of the
dopa reaction in the nucleus of the melanoblast and in nuclei generally in
urodele embryos, preceding the formation of the medullary (neural) tube
and the neural crest. Again, was the nuclear dopa reaction adsorbed on
the nuclear membrane, or did it occur within the nucleus?

Materials and Methods

One series of *Taricha torosa* embryos was treated from the two-cell stage until hatching, with exogenous dopa (3,4-dioxyphenylalanine) and serial sections were cut at 8–10 nm. A parallel series was used as controls, only omitting the dopa treatment. Several series were made, over a period of ten years' collecting. A dopa series and a control series was made for each year of five years, of an allied species, *Taricha granulosa*. Tissue cultures of *Taricha torosa* neural crests from the medullary plate stage (stage 15 of TWITTY and BODENSTEIN's [1962] table) from four collections of eggs in 1966, through the closure of the medullary tube, were prepared. Dopa-treated cultures and control cultures were studied.

The details of preparation for the serial sections and the tissue cultures are described in an earlier paper [MᶜCURDY, 1969]. In serial sections of whole embryos of *Taricha torosa* and *Taricha granulosa*, close adherence to BLOCH's dopa-reaction technique, as described by LAIDLAW [1932], rewarded with the latter's 'browns, blacks, and grays of a correct dopa reaction' that 'form an extremely delicate picture'. Control embryos gave no such reaction.

The dopa reaction in figures 1–10 and 21 was incubated at 37 °C. The same reaction occurs at room temperature, but at a more precise, slower rate. Figures 11–15, 16–20 and 22–25 were incubated at room temperature.

Results

In tissue cultures of *Taricha torosa* at the same stages as those of MODEL and DALTON, nuclei of every cell gave a dopa reaction. There was no cytoplasmic reaction in the earlier neural crest cultures. In the later ones, the cytoplasm of only melanoblast and branching melanophores gave a dopa reaction [MᶜCURDY, 1969].

Fig. 1–5. Serial sections of a nuclear dopa reaction in the ectodermal cell of a *Taricha torosa* embryo at the late blastula stage. × 170.

Fig. 6–10. Serial sections of a nuclear dopa reaction in a *T. torosa* entodermal cell at the late blastula stage. × 170.

Fig. 11–15. Serial sections of a nuclear dopa reaction in a *T. torosa* melanoblast of the neurula stage, migrating toward the epidermis. × 170.

Fig. 16–20. Two melanoblasts of *Taricha granulosa* in serial sections, showing the nuclear dopa reaction throughout the nuclei. × 170.

Fig. 21. *T. torosa* blastula mitosis (anaphase) of an ectodermal cell with dopa-positive chromosomes. × 400.

Fig. 22–25. *T. torosa.* Neurula stage. Serial sections of a resting melanoblast and one in anaphase. The former shows a dopa reaction throughout the nucleus. The latter shows that the chromosomes alone give a dopa reaction. Mirsky filter. × 400.

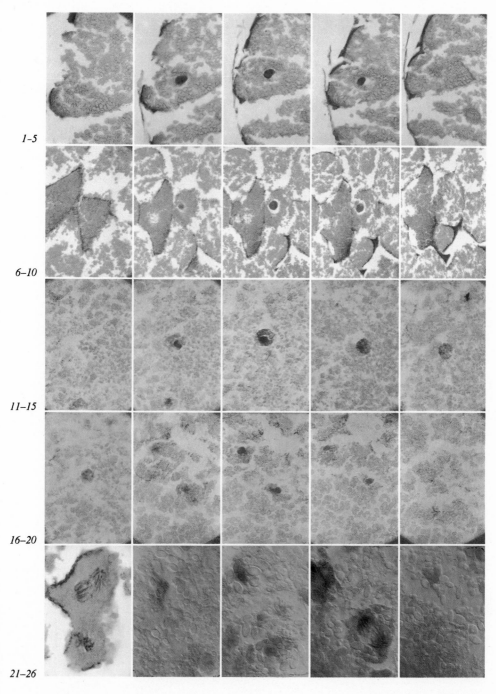

The crucial test for nuclear enzyme location, as rendered by the dopa reaction, lay in the sequence of the serial sections through the nuclei.

In early embryonic development, *Taricha torosa* and *T. granulosa* cells are large. The nucleus will occupy three, sometimes four, serial sections.

Serial sections of whole embryos from the two-cell stage show no dopa reaction until late blastula stages. Then, increasing numbers of cells showed a nuclear dopa reaction, as embryonic development proceeded, until all nuclei of the embryo showed a dopa reaction [McCurdy, 1969].

Figures 1–5 show serial sections in the cells of the ectoderm of a late blastula embryo *(Taricha torosa)*. One cell is followed to show that the nuclear dopa reaction occurs throughout the nucleus. There is no cytoplasmic response.

Figures 6–10 show serial sections of a nucleus with a dopa reaction, within the entoderm of a late blastula embryo *(Taricha torosa)*.

Figures 11–15 show serial sections of a *Taricha torosa* melanoblast during the neurula stage when the melanoblast is migrating to the region beneath the epidermis. The dopa reaction occurs throughout the nucleus of the melanoblast.

Figures 16–20 show two melanoblasts of *Taricha granulosa* migrating to the region beneath the epidermis. Here, also, the serial sections show a dopa reaction throughout the nuclei. Figure 21 shows a *Taricha torosa* blastula with a cell in anaphase mitosis, where the chromosomes show a dopa reaction. There is, of course, no nuclear membrane. The cytoplasm shows no dopa reaction, only the chromosomes.

Figures 22–25 show the anaphase of a melanoblast in the neurula stage of the embryo of *Taricha torosa*, in serial sections. Here, the dopa reaction is confined to the chromosomes. The dopa reaction in the accompanying resting nucleus of another melanoblast is diffuse and throughout the nucleus. In this series, a Mirsky filter was used.

The results were consistent for all collections. The nuclei from the late blastula stages through neurulation gave a dopa reaction. On the formation of the neural crest, some cells in this region gave a cytoplasmic dopa reaction. These were the melanoblasts, the only cells to give a cytoplasmic dopa reaction. As development of the embryo proceeded, the nuclear reaction faded from all but the melanoblasts. As the latter developed into melanophores, the nuclear reaction faded; the cytoplasmic reaction persisted until the melanin granules were plentiful, then here, also, the dopa reaction ceased. When the melanophore had synthesized its quota of melanosomes, there was no dopa reaction in either nucleus or cytoplasm [McCURDY, 1969]. It might be noted that the melanosomes line the dendritic cytoplasmic membrane of the melanophore. There is a lumen in each dendrite and that lumen in the adult melanophore is colourless. It gives no gray or black dopa reaction [McCURDY, 1972].

Discussion

Pigmentation in vertebrates occurs not only because the pigment cells are present, but also because the environment of the cell is favourable to pigment production in that cell at that time. This has been proven so for melanin-forming pigment cells in particular. TWITTY [1945] and NIU [1947] found that neural crest tissue cultures of *T. torosa* and *T. rivularis* responded consistently to their media. Those tissues grown in Holtfreter's standard salt solution average 10–15% chromatophores (melanophores) of the total number of cells. In coelomic fluid (from spawning females), 'the corresponding figure would probably approach 50% and in individual cases, the proportion may be considerably higher' [NIU, 1947]. NIU states that: 'In coelomic fluid media, not uncommonly, individual cultures are composed exclusively of pigment cells (melanophores). It is strongly indicated, therefore, that under the influence of coelomic fluid, cells normally destined for other fates are caused to develop as chromatophores.' It might well be that the coelomic media favoured the release, at this stage, of the melanin-forming enzyme from the nucleus into the cytoplasm with the consequent formation of melanophores from still multipotential cells. Normally, the dopa reaction appearing in all nuclei of the embryo of the late gastrula and neurula stages, fades as development proceeds and only the potential melanophores retain the nuclear reaction that fades as the cytoplasm gives a dopa reaction.

MODEL and DALTON [1968] noted the labelling silver grains over the nuclei of their recognized melanoblasts in their ³H-dopa-treated tissue cultures of *Ambystoma mexicanum*, but cautiously refrained from implicating the nucleus in a dopa reaction. In tissue cultures, they could not discern whether the dopa reaction was adsorbed on the cytoplasmic side of the nuclear membrane, or actually within the nucleus of the melanoblast.

Serial sections of *Taricha torosa* and *Taricha granulosa* embryos, in which melanoblasts could be identified, showed that the dopa reaction was within and throughout the nucleus.

During a ten-year period, a study has been made of other urodeles and anurans in their early embryology, using the dopa reaction and also control embryos of the same stages. At species-specific stages in the early embryonic development of *Ambystoma gracile, Rana aurora* and *Hyla regilla,* all nuclei of these species have shown a dopa reaction. Furthermore, the location of the dopa reaction in the *T. torosa* and *T. granulosa* serial sections of both the resting nuclei and the mitotic divisions, i.e. the close adherence of the dopa reaction to the dispersed chromatin and to the chromosomes, follows the criteria of SIEBERT and HUMPHREY [1965] for the properties and location of an enzyme synthesized in the nucleus.

These authors write that the enzyme DPN (diphosphopyridine nucleotide) pyrophosphorylase is of exclusive nuclear origin and that it is firmly bound to chromatin material in the chromatin space. SIEBERT and HUMPHREY define the chromatin space as a 'nuclear region where enzymes are tightly bound to nucleoproteins, presumably to chromosome material'. 'It is expected that *in vivo* enzymes belonging to the chromatin space also act in their bound state.... Only the substrates of these enzymes can be expected to move around and give rise to an impact which may lead eventually to the formation of an enzyme-substrate complex; the enzyme itself will not move. Furthermore, since the chromatin-bound enzymes are not soluble, there will be a lowered substrate concentration only in the close vicinity of the enzymes and not in more remote regions.' A co-enzyme known to be formed in the nucleus is DPN. It is exported to the cytoplasm, seeks the mitochondria and is incorporated therein.

The series of slides here presented makes it reasonable to look to the nucleus of these urodele embryos as the site of synthesis of the melanin-forming enzyme. Further experimentation could be expected to extend this property of nuclear synthesis of this enzyme to vertebrates in general.

Summary

In vertebrate melanogenesis, the essential enzyme, tyrosinase, or dopa oxidase, has been identified in the cytoplasm by Bloch's dopa reaction. This same technique shows that a nuclear response precedes the cytoplasmic response in the melanoblasts of *Taricha torosa,* the California newt. In specific earlier stages in the embryonic development of the urodeles *T. torosa* and *T. granulosa,* the nuclear response occurs in all three tissue layers. This nuclear response follows the description of Siebert and Humphrey for the *in situ* reaction of a nuclear enzyme to an introduced substrate. This suggests an embryonic nuclear origin for the enzyme tyrosinase

(Bloch's dopa oxidase) that could migrate through the endothelial reticulum to its functional position in the adult, melanin-forming cell.

Acknowledgements

Grateful acknowledgement is made of valued consultations with Dr. VERNON RILEY, of the photography of Mr. TOM GORE and of the grants-in-aid from Sigma Delta Epsilon and the Victoria Medical Research Foundation.

References

ALGARD, F. T.: Morphology and migratory behaviour of embryonic pigment cells studied by phase microscopy. J. exp. Zool. *123:* 499–522 (1953).

BLOCH, B.: Das Pigment; in JADASSOHN Handbuch der Haut- und Geschlechts-krankheiten (Springer, Berlin 1927).

DuSHANE, G. P.: The origin of pigment cells in amphibia. Science *80:* 620–621 (1934).

EPPIG, J. J., jr. and DUMONT, J. N.: The distribution of melanosomes in larvae reared from normal and from pigmentless eggs of *Xenopus laevis*. J. exp. Zool. *177:* 79–88 (1971).

LAIDLAW, G. F.: The dopa reaction in normal histology. Anat. Rec. *53:* 399–413 (1932).

McCURDY, H. M.: Enzyme localization during melanogenesis. J. Cell Biol. *43:* 220–228 (1969).

McCURDY, H. M.: Dopa-positive nuclei and melanogenesis; in RILEY Pigmentation: its genesis and biologic control (Appleton Century Crofts, New York 1972).

MODEL, P. G. and DALTON, H. C.: The uptake and localization of radioactive DOPA by amphibian melanoblasts *in vitro*. Devl Biol. *17:* 245–271 (1968).

NIU, M. C.: The axial organization of the neural crest, studied with particular reference to its pigmentary component. J. exp. Zool. *105:* 79–114 (1947).

SIEBERT, G. and HUMPHREY, G. B.: The enzymology of the nucleus. Advances in enzymology and related subjects of biochemistry, vol. 27, pp. 239–288 (Interscience, New York 1965).

TWITTY, V. C.: The developmental analysis of specific pigment patterns. J. exp. Zool. *100:* 141–178 (1945).

TWITTY, V. C. and BODENSTEIN, D.: Staging of amphibian embryos. *Triturus torosus;* in RUGH Experimental embryology (Burgess Publishing, Minneapolis 1962).

H. M. McCURDY, PhD, Department of Biology, University of Victoria, *Victoria, B.C. V8W 2Y2* (Canada)

Pigment Cell, vol. 3, pp. 53–63 (Karger, Basel 1976)

The Comparative Biology of a
New Melanophore Pigment from Leaf Frogs

JOSEPH T. BAGNARA, WAYNE FERRIS and JOHN D. TAYLOR

Department of Cellular and Developmental Biology, University of Arizona, Tucson, Ariz. and Department of Biology, Wayne State University, Detroit, Mich.

Introduction

Comparisons of the composition and ultrastructure of melanosomes found throughout the vertebrate classes have revealed the existence of a striking uniformity. Eumelanin is the principal pigmentary component of most melanosomes whose appearance as a uniformly electron-dense ellipsoid of approximately 0.5 μm in diameter holds for most melanophores (cytes) [3]. A deviation from this pattern occurs in those species which utilize phaeomelanin as a melanophore pigment. However, even this red or yellow pigment is found in a melanosome that is apparently much like those that contain eumelanin [6] and its synthesis, at least in the initial steps, is identical to that of eumelanin.

As far as current knowledge holds, the only major deviation from the typical vertebrate melanin system is that which was originally shown in *Agalychnis dacnicolor,* a leaf frog from Mexico [8, 9]. In adults of this species, it was discovered that melanosomes are unusually large, usually over 1 μm in diameter. Moreover, it was demonstrated that these organelles are red in color and are composed of a dense kernel that is surrounded by a fibrous matrix. Subsequent investigation [5] revealed that the red pigment is unique and that it is present in several other species of leaf frogs (sub-family Phyllomedusinae). Tentatively, it has been designated *rhodomelanochrome* [BAGNARA and PROTA, unpublished].

In the present presentation, it is our aim to provide a detailed description of the ultrastructural relations of melanophores that contain this unusual pigment and its organelle. In addition, we shall discuss the current status of the chemistry and biology of this pigment.

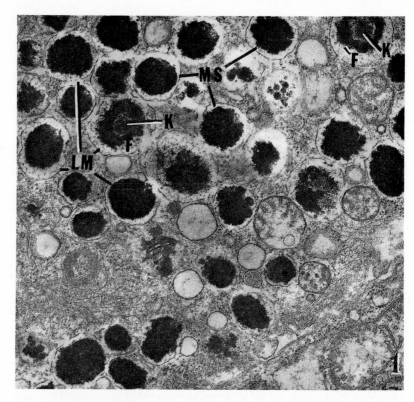

Fig. 1. Portion of a dermal melanophore from an adult *Agalychnis dacnicolor* showing melanosomes (MS). At the center of the melanosome an electron-dense kernel (K) surrounded by a fibrous cortex (F) that is separated from the limiting membranes (LM) by a space. × 11,000.

Phyllomedusine Melanosomes and Dermal Chromatophore Units

Since their original discovery, the melanosomes of adult *A. dacnicolor* have been studied a great deal and a knowledge of their morphology has provided a frame of reference that can be utilized in understanding the structure of melanosomes of related species. As is shown in figure 1, the *A. dacnicolor* melanosome consists of an electron-dense core (kernel) which is surrounded by a thin halo and a large concentric mass of dense fibers. The whole organelle is surrounded by a space which is often quite large. This melanosome is larger than the usual vertebrate melanosome and may possess a diameter as great as 1.02 μm. Despite the fact that the

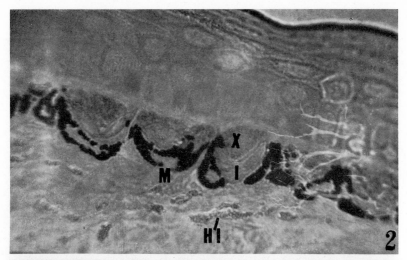

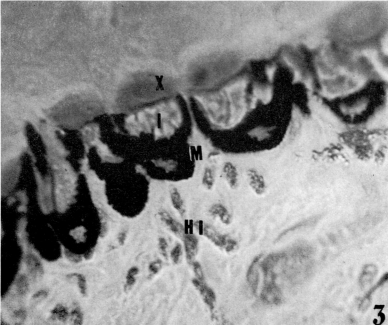

Fig. 2. Thick section of dorsal skin of an adult *Phyllomedusa iherengi* showing a dermal chromatophore unit consisting of a melanophore (M), iridophore (I), and xanthophore (X). The wedgeshaped xanthophore beneath the basal lamina is accommodated by a cup-like iridophore. Hypodermal iridophores (HI) are also visible. × 500.

Fig. 3. Thick section of dorsal skin of adult *P. sauvagii* showing a similar dermal chromatophore unit. × 1000.

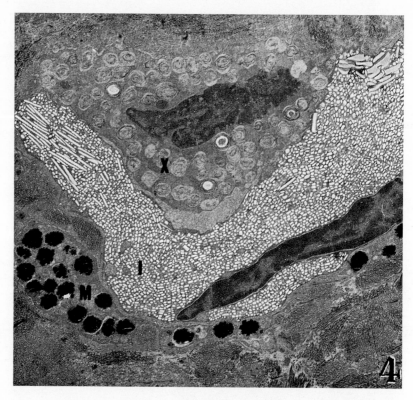

Fig. 4. Dermal chromatophore unit of *P. iherengi.* The wedge-shaped xanthophore (X) is heavily laden with pterinosomes, the pteridine-containing organelles
typical of such cells. The iridophore (I) is cup-shaped and contains rounded reflecting
platelets except at the edges of the cell where longer platelets are encountered. A
portion of a melanophore (M) containing phyllomedusine melanosomes is visible beneath the iridophore. × 7,500.

Agalychnis melanosome has an unusual morphology and contains a distinctive red pigment that is neither eumelanin nor phaeomelanin [5], there
can be no doubt that this organelle is present in a cell that is truly a melanophore. It occupies the appropriate position in the dermal chromatophore unit of this species and functions as a typical melanophore [4].

In the course of an examination of two other members of the genus,
A callidryas and *A. moreleti,* it was discovered that they, too, contain the
new red pigment, rhodomelanochrome [5]. Moreover, an examination of
the *A. callidryas* melanosome with the electron microscope revealed that

its form was much like that of the *A. dacnicolor* melanosome. The question arose of whether this unusual melanosome is typical of the Phyllomedusinae, a sub-family of the hylids. Accordingly, we have studied skin preparations of the genus *Phyllomedusa,* another member of this family. These have included *P. sauvagii, P. iherengi, P. hypochondrialis,* and *P. trinitatus.* A cursory examination of these preparations has revealed the presence of both the large unusual melanosome and rhodomelanochrome [2]. The following is a more detailed examination of these melanosomes and of the melanophore type in which they are found. Usual electron micrcscopic techniques, such as we have employed previously, were utilized in this study [1, 2, 9].

In the adult skin of all species studied, typical dermal chromatophore units were observed. The melanophore cell body is found beneath an iridophore, and processes from it extend upward to enclose the iridophore (fig. 2–5). If the melanophore is in a dispersed state, melanosomes may fill processes that extend over the top of the iridophore. These processes, filled with melanosomes, are clearly seen between the upper surface of the iridophore and the overlying xanthophore (fig. 5). Often, especially in *P. iherengi,* the iridophore is cupshaped and accommodates a xanthophore that is in the form of a wedge (fig. 2–4).

The pigmentary organelles in xanthophores and iridophores of these phyllomedusine species are much like those described for other frogs [9]. Xanthophores contain many pterinosomes that are interspersed between carotenoid vesicles. Iridophore reflecting platelets, for the most part, present rounded profiles; however, at the upper edges of the iridophore, longer platelets are frequently encountered (fig. 4). These long platelets more closely resemble those seen in iridophores of other frogs [4]. They are also similar to the platelets found in dermal iridophores that are not part of the dermal chromatophore unit. For example, in the dermis, scattered at various depths, iridophores that appear white with reflected light are often found. They contain long and thick reflecting platelets (fig. 4). Iridophores of this type are prevalent at the base of the collagen layers in the hypodermis and are especially prevalent in *P. sauvagii.* Iridophores of the dermal chromatophore units of these frogs appear bluish with reflected light and this is undoubtedly a structural color resulting from the ordered distribution of the rounded reflecting platelets. These platelets seem to be aligned in rows that are chain-like in appearance and are best seen in *P. sauvagii* (fig. 7). In many ways, the alignment of these reflecting platelets resembles that described for the lizard, *Anolis* [7, 10].

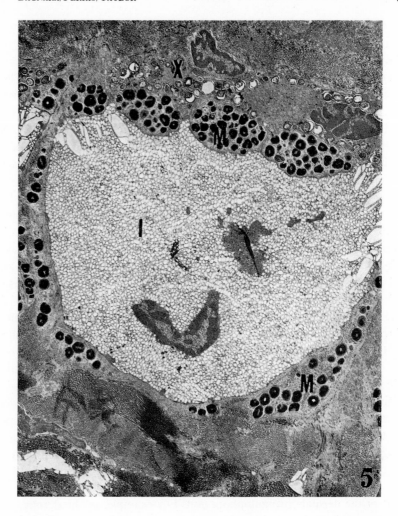

Fig. 5. Dermal chromatophore unit of *P. hypochondrialis* showing a typically flattened xanthophore (X), an iridophore (I) laden with rounded reflecting platelets, and a melanophore (M) in which the finger-like pocresses that overlay the iridophore are filled with melanosomes. Note how they indent the upper surface of the irido-phore to produce a scalloped effect. × 4,000.

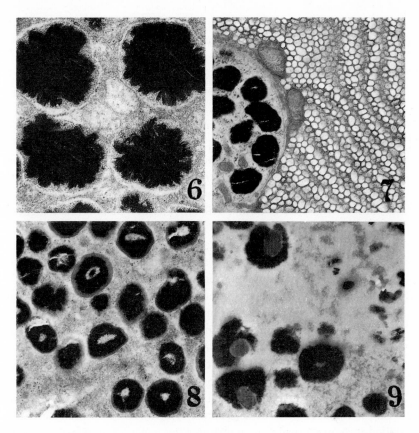

Fig. 6. Melanosomes of *P. iherengi* showing typical irregular profiles. No kernels are visible within the dense fibrous matrix. A distinctive limiting membrane encloses each melanosome and it is separated from the pigmented mass by a granular substance. × 19,500.

Fig. 7. Adjacent melanophore and iridophore of *P. sauvagii.* Melanosomes are quite electron-dense, seem to lack kernels, and are not separated from the limiting membrane by a space. The rounded reflecting platelets of the iridophore are strikingly oriented in the form of long rows of chains. × 9,000.

Fig. 8. Melanosomes of *P. hypochondrialis* showing rounded profiles, few distinctive kernels, and a halo of less electron-dense material around the main pigmented mass. × 11,000.

Fig. 9. Melanosomes of *Litoria caerulea* showing typical phyllomedusine characteristics including an obvious core and a surrounding electron-dense mass of pigment. × 13,000.

While melanosomes of all the phyllomedusine species so far studied bear a general resemblance to one another, each possesses distinctive characteristics. Those of *P. iherengi* (fig. 6) have rather irregular profiles, seem strongly electron-dense, and show little evidence of the presence of a kernel in the fully formed organelle. A limiting membrane is discernible, and the space between it and the pigment mass is filled with a granular material. Similarly, melanosomes of *P. sauvagii* are quite electron-dense and lack kernels. However, they present more rounded profiles and the limiting membrane seems closely apposed to the surface of the pigmented area (fig. 7). Melanosomes of *P. trinitatus* resemble those of *P. sauvagii*, although kernels are more prevalent. The most distinctive melanosomes are those of *P. hypochondrialis* (fig. 8). These organelles have a rounded appearance, and while no electron-dense kernel is visible, the core region of these melanosomes stands out as a light area that, in some cases, resembles the kernel of unstained preparations of *A. dacnicolor*. Between the limiting membrane and the pigmented mass of the melanosome is a wide zone of granular material much denser than that seen in *P. iherengi*. This gives the melanosome the appearance of having a halo. While these species differences between melanosomes are to be noted, the general characteristics of phyllomedusine melanosome ultrastructure must be emphasized as a distinctive feature. For example, it is likely that all members of the Phyllomedusinae possess this characteristic melanosome type and that its presence together with the occurrence of rhodomelanochrome serve as evidence of close taxonomic relatedness. This premise is exemplified in figure 9, which demonstrates the appearance of melanosomes in *Litoria caerulea,* a hylid frog from Australia. According to current taxonomic classification, this frog is not closely related to the Phyllomedusinae; however, it can be clearly seen, even in this preparation, taken from a fixed museum specimen subsequently prepared for electron microscopy, that the melanosomes are like those of the phyllomedusine frogs discussed above. Moreover, the presence of rhodomelanochrome in this and other species from Australia has led us to conclude that these frogs are more closely related to South American hylids than was previously believed [2].

Discussion

The importance of the discovery of this unique pigment, rhodomelanochrome, and the unusual melanosome in which it is found, in a not widely known group of frogs, in a sense seems obscure. However, in view of the remarkable consistency of melanosome composition and form among most other vertebrates, this departure from such a conservative scheme is provocative and poses many questions. It is not the function of this presentation to investigate these questions in depth, however, we wish to consider them briefly in the light of the descriptive material presented in this paper.

First of all, it should be emphasized that rhodomelanochrome is clearly different from any other melanophore pigment. Its unique solubility characteristics and ultraviolet absorption spectrum indicate that it is neither eumelanin nor phaeomelanin [5]. It is possible, however, that its pathway of synthesis is related to that of the melanins for when skins of *A. dacnicolor* are incubated in ^{14}C-labeled amino acids, the labels from dopa or tyrosine are taken up specifically. Rhodomelanochrome is readily soluble in alkali; however, it is quickly converted to a yellow reaction product, and this property has rendered chemical elucidation difficult.

We have taken advantage of the solubility of rhodomelanochrome in alkali for several purposes. To detect the presence of the pigment, one merely needs to place a skin sample, fresh or fixed, dry or wet, in a small volume of NaOH and in a matter of moments, a bright red pigment is leached out into the medium. The red color disappears gradually as it is converted to its reaction product. Through the use of this test, we have shown rhodomelanochrome to be present in all of 14 species of phyllomedusine frogs that were tested and in two of five species of hylid frogs from Australia [2]. It was also possible to use the NaOH test both in studying the ontogeny of the *A. dacnicolor* melanosome and in learning the precise localization of rhodomelanochrome in the melanosome.

In a study in progress [BAGNARA *et al.*, unpublished], we have found that dermal melanophores of *A. dacnicolor* tadpoles contain neither rhodomelanochrome nor the adult type of melanosome. Larval melanosomes resemble the typical eumelanin-containing melanosome except that they are much smaller in size. As metamorphosis approaches, their number increases dramatically; moreover, there is a striking elevation of the melanosome-limiting membrane, so that at metamorphic climax a large space exists between the membrane and the pigmented mass. At a stage when all vestiges of the tail are gone, the presence of rhodomelanochrome is revealed for the first time, and during the ensuing week of development the rhodomelanochrome content of the skin becomes richer. These observations become increasingly significant in light of a study which involved electron microscopic observations either of adult skin that had been placed in NaOH or of skin sections that were similarly treated. We found that the fibrous component of the melanosome was markedly diminished in density and often had lost large areas, whereas, the kernel appeared relatively unchanged [1]. It seems possible, therefore, that the kernel of the adult *A. dacnicolor* melanosome is composed of eumelanin and that it is derived from the small larval melanosome which, during the first week after metamorphosis, begins to acquire a coating of rhodomelanochrome that becomes thicker until the adult melanosome type is formed. This, of course, is highly speculative and has important implications; however, it seems to be the most reasonable explanation of our present data. If this tentative hypothesis is correct, many questions are raised. Perhaps the most important one concerns the mechanism by which the eumelanin-containing organelle suddenly acquires the ability to synthesize or at least to deposit a new and different pigment. Another question concerns the origin of new melanosomes in the adult which lacks the small melanosome typical of the larva. In this regard, we are reminded that not all melanosomes of adult melanophores contain a kernel, especially in *P. iherengi* What does this mean? Obviously, we are dealing with an important and intriguing system that offers many questions answerable only by continued experimentation.

Summary

The presence of an unusual melanosome and a new red pigment in melanophores of various species of leaf frogs (Phyllomedusinae) is disclosed. Comparative aspects of the ultrastructure of this melanosome are presented and selected details of other chromatophores in the dermal chromatophore unit of those species are considered. Various biological implications about the red pigment and its melanosome are discussed. These range from biochemical and developmental considerations to those of taxonomy and evolution.

Acknowledgments

We are grateful to Vaughn Shoemaker, William E. Duellman, J. S. Kenny, Richard Wassersug, David Wake, Mike Robinson, Richard Nishioka, and Giuseppe Prota for providing material or advice used in this study. We acknowledge financial support from National Science Foundation Grant GB-27639 and Grant GB-16329.

References

1 BAGNARA, J. T. and FERRIS, W.: Localization of rhodomelanochrome in mela-nosomes of leaf frogs. J. exp. Zool. *190:* 367–372 (1974).
2 BAGNARA, J. T. and FERRIS, W.: The presence of phyllomedusine melanosomes and pigments in Australian hylids. Copeia, 592–595 (1975).
3 BAGNARA, J. T. and HADLEY, M. E.: Chromatophores and color change (Prentice-Hall, Englewood Cliffs 1973).
4 BAGNARA, J. T.; TAYLOR, J. D., and HADLEY, M. E.: The dermal chromatophore unit. J. Cell Biol. *38:* 67–79 (1968).
5 BAGNARA, J. T.; TAYLOR, J. D., and PROTA, G.: Color changes, unusual melano-somes, and a new pigment from leaf frogs. Science *182:* 1034–1035 (1973).
6 GESCHWIND, I. I.; HUSEBY, R. A., and NISHIOKA, R.: The effect of melanocyte-stimulating hormone on coat color in the mouse. Recent Prog. Horm. Res. *28:* 91–130 (1972).
7 ROHRLICH, S. T. and PORTER, K.: Fine structural observations relating to the production of color by the iridophores of a lizard, *Anolis carolinensis*. J. Cell Biol. *53:* 38–52 (1972).
8 TAYLOR, J. D. and BAGNARA, J. T.: Melanosomes of the Mexican tree frog *Agalychnis dacnicolor*. J. Ultrastruct. Res. *29:* 323–333 (1969).
9 TAYLOR, J. D. and BAGNARA, J. T.: Dermal chromatophores. Am. Zoologist *12:* 43–62 (1972).
10 TAYLOR, J. D. and HADLEY, M. E.: Chromatophores and color change in the lizard, *Anolis carolinensis*. Z. Zellforsch. *104:* 282–294 (1970).

Dr. JOSEPH T. BAGNARA, Department of Cellular and Developmental Biology, University of Arizona, *Tucson, AZ 85721* (USA)

Pigment Cell, vol. 3, pp. 64–68 (Karger, Basel 1976)

Spatial Structure of Melanins

Y. T. Thathachari[1]

University of California, San Francisco, Calif., and
Indian Institute of Technology, Madras

Introduction

The following model of melanin structure is suggested by the studies of several investigators: in particular Hempel [1], Nicolaus [2], Binns *et al.* [3], Blois *et al.* [4] and their associates. Any melanin, whatever its source or method of preparation, is made up of not one, but several different types of monomers, and the sequence of the monomers may not follow any simple pattern. The polymer chains may not all have the same structure in any melanin, Also, the same types of monomers may not be linked by the same types of bonds throughout a polymer chain. For instance, in melanoma melanin, an indolequinone may be linked to an adjacent monomer through the carbons at the third, fourth or seventh position of the indole ring. The chemical structure being so random, there is likely to be little order in the spatial structure of the polymer.

Spatial Order in Melanin Structure

Another aspect of the melanin structure emerges from our X-ray diffraction studies on a large number of natural and synthetic melanins [5–7]. There may be uncertainties regarding the types of monomers present in a particular melanin and how the monomers are linked. However,

1   I thank Dr. M. S. Blois for his interest, Dr. T. E. Hopkins for assistance in collecting some of the X-ray data, and Mrs. M. Thathachari for assistance in computation. This research was supported by NIH Grant CA 12043-3.

there is little doubt that the monomers are either planar molecules like catechol or indolequinone, or molecules like dopa or dopa quinone which
contain planar portions. The X-ray data show unequivocally that in most
melanins, whatever their source or method of preparation, the planar
groups tend to align in a parallel fashion, with an interlayer separation of
about 3.4 Å.

This tendency – which I will refer to as *parallel stacking* – is found to
extend throughout the polymeric structure. In other words, a monomer
chosen anywhere at random in any melanin is likely to be flanked by one
or more parallel layers with an average interlayer spacing of about 3.4 Å.
The spatial order present in melanins is not as extensive as in crystalline
materials. The average thickness of the stack, a statistical parameter estimated from the diffraction data, is a rough measure of the extent of order
present in the sample studied. For example, in one of the melanins studied, the average thickness was estimated to be about 14 Å. This means
that the parallel stack contains on an average about five parallel layers. It
also implies that, for separations much larger than 14 Å, a pair of monomers can be expected to assume completely random orientations. The
diffraction data show that the parallel layers in a stack may not be exactly
overhead, but may be displaced laterally. This lateral displacement between adjacent parallel layers is much smaller than the size of the layers.

Parallel Stacking in Other Known Structures

It has often been claimed that this observed short range order in the
spatial structure of melanins does not represent any significant new information. It is argued that it is only natural for the planar molecules in any
structure to align parallel. Since the 'van der Waals thickness' of an organic layer is about 3.4 Å, the parallel layers will also be 3.4 Å apart. Recently, we made a systematic survey of the environments of the planar
molecules in all known structures – polymers as well as smaller molecules. This survey demonstrates that the presence of planar molecules in a
structure does not necessarily lead to their parallel association unless certain other conditions are also met.

In figure 1, the arrangement of planar molecules in four typical compounds has been sketched. In each case, adjacent molecules are sketched.
One of them, drawn in solid lines, is in the plane of the figure. The other
molecule is drawn in dotted lines. In the terphenyl structure sketched in

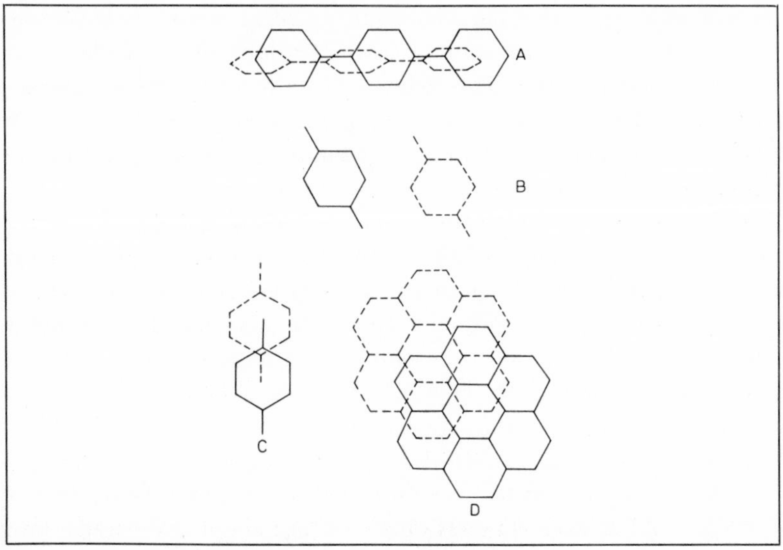

Fig. 1. Arrangement of planar molecules in organic structures. Two molecules are sketched for each of the four typical arrangements. The molecule drawn in full lines is in the plane of the figure. The second molecule is drawn in dotted lines. *A* Terphenyl. The adjacent molecules are considerably inclined – about 120°. *B para-*Benzoquinone. The adjacent molecules are parallel but have practically no overlap. *C* Charge transfer complex – quinhydrone. *D* Coronene. In *B*, the second molecule is about 3 Å from the plane of the first. In *C* and *D*, the second molecule is about 3.4 Å from the plane of the first. In *C* and *D,* there is considerable overlap in the projections of the two adjacent parallel molecules.

'A', the adjacent molecules are at considerable inclination, about 120°. Similar arrangements are found in a large number of unsubstituted hydrocarbons like benzene, quarterphenyl, anthracene, pentacene, etc., with ring structures extending in *one* dimension. In a number of small layer structures like *para*-benzoquinone sketched in 'B', the adjacent layers are parallel, but have little or no overlap. In 'B', the second molecule is at a height of about 3 Å from the plane of the first molecule. In charge transfer complexes like quinhydrone sketched in 'C', and in molecules with ring structures extending in two dimensions like coronene, sketched in 'D', the adjacent layers are parallel and have significant overlap. In both 'C' and 'D', the second molecule is about 3.4 Å from the plane of the first molecule.

Parallel Stacking in Polymers

The planar molecules in polymers have even more constraints than in simpler compounds. As such additional conditions must be met for parallel stacking to occur, few polymers containing planar molecules are in fact found to show parallel stacking. For instance, no parallel stacking occurs in polyaromatics like polystyrene, polyvinylnaphthalene, etc. On the other hand, in the highly regular DNA structure, the planar bases are stacked parallel and about 3.4 Å apart. In graphite and other carbonaceous structures, the layers are large and the parallel stacking is a principal feature of their structure.

Conclusions

Simple model building experiments show that the observed short range order in the spatial structure of melanins, i.e. the observed parallel stacking, does imply certain order in their chemical structure as well. It is not possible at present to determine precisely the nature of this chemical order. It may, for instance, mean that: (a) in each melanin, certain monomer sequences may occur more often than others – certain bonding sites may be more common than others in linking similar types of monomers; (b) charge transfer complexes as in quinhydrone may be present, and (a) the conjugation between adjacent monomers in the same polymer chain may force them into near planarity. The polymer will then contain layers effectively larger than the constituent monomers like catechol or indolequinone.

To explain away the parallel stacking in melanins, a colleague suggested the following analogy. When a large number of disks are thrown as a heap, a considerable fraction will pile up naturally as parallel stacks. However, this analogy has more implications than would seem apparent at first sight. For one thing, to represent polymer chains, the disks must be linked. More importantly, however, this question arises: What *is* a disk? The tacit assumption is that the diameter is much larger than the thickness. For instance, coronene will be more of a disk than catechol. One may also imagine the surfaces of the disks to be sticky – a situation similar to charge transfer complexes.

As pointed our earlier [7], the parallel stacking in melanin accounts for the high density of melanins (over 1.5). This in turn accounts for the high contrast of melanosomes in the electron micrographs of even unstained tissues. Calculation show that heavy atoms like copper and zinc (present only in trace concentrations) cannot account for the observed 'electron density' of melanins, contrary to the belief of earlier investigators.

In conclusion, X-ray diffraction studies furnish significant new information on melanin structure not revealed by any other technique. These studies may lead to a better understanding of some of the known properties of melanins in health and in disease.

Summary

Melanins are polymers believed to be disordered in all levels of organization. However, as a class they seem to share some physical and chemical features, e.g. their color (usually brown or black) and their affinity for a variety of chemical compounds including a number of drugs. While there may be uncertainties about the structure of constituent monomers and how they are linked, there is no doubt that the monomers in melanins are either planar molecules like catechol and indole quinone or molecules like dopa having planar portions. X-Ray diffraction data show that the monomers in melanins are either planar molecules like catechol and indole tendency is extensive and not limited to isolated domains. A careful survey of the literature will show that: (a) apart from carbons like graphite and coal, few materials exhibit this kind of spatial order, and (b) the presence of planar units in a structure does not necessarily imply their parallel alignment. The observed parallel alignment of monomeric layers in melanins suggest in turn other short range order in their structure: e.g. limited conjugation of adjacent monomers, π complexing of parallel layers or preference of certain monomer sequences. These features of melanin structure may provide clues to a better understanding of their known or suspected roles in health and in disease and of their biosynthesis.

References

1 HEMPEL, K.: in DELLA PORTA and MUHLBOCK Structure and control of the melanocyte, p. 162 (Springer, Berlin 1966).
2 NICOLAUS, R. A.: Melanin, p. 96 (Herman, Paris 1970).
3 BINNS, F.; CHAPMAN, R. F.; ROBSON, N. C.; SWAN, G. A., and WAGGOT, A.: J Chem. Soc. 1128 (1970).
4 BLOIS, M. S.; ZAHLAN, A. B., and MALING, J. E.: Biophys. J. 4: 405 (1964).
5 THATHACHARI, Y. T. and BLOIS, M. S.: Biophys. J. 9: 77 (1969).
6 THATHACHARI, Y. T.: J. Sci. Ind. Res. 30: 529 (1971).
7 THATHACHARI, Y. T.: Pigment Cell, p. 158 (Karger, Basel 1972).

Dr. Y. T. THATHACHARI, University of California, *San Francisco, CA 94145* (USA)

Pigment Cell, vol. 3, pp. 69–81 (Karger, Basel 1976)

Electron Transfer Properties of Melanin and Melanoproteins

I. A. MENON, E. V. GAN and H. F. HABERMAN

Clinical Science Division, Section of Dermatology University of Toronto, Toronto, Ont.

Introduction

It has been reported that melanin is a stable free radical [1–8]. MASON et al. [3] suggested that due to this property melanin could possibly function as an electron transfer agent. PULLMAN and PULLMAN [9] have pointed out that dopa-melanin could exist in more than one oxidation-reduction state. LONGUET-HIGGINS [4] and ALLEN and INGRAM [10] have suggested that melanin could act as a one-dimensional semiconductor, with bound protons producing electron traps in the system. On these bases and on the basis of molecular orbital calculations, PULLMAN and PULLMAN postulated that melanin should be an extremely good electron acceptor. More recent experiments, however, have shown that although under some circumstances *in vitro* melanins show a kind of semiconduction, they are not really semiconductors [11]. The experimental evidence suggesting that melanin may function as an electron transfer agent was provided by VAN WOERT [12, 13] who reported that melanin could oxidize NADH, molecular oxygen being simultaneously reduced to H_2O_2. Recent reports from our laboratory [14, 15] showed that although in agreement with VAN WOERT's observation, melanin synthesized by the action of mushroom tyrosinase on dopa could oxidize NADH, this property could not be detected in melanin isolated from B16 melanoma. This paper describes our findings regarding the activities of several types of melanin as oxidizing and reducing agents in various oxidation-reduction systems.

Materials and Methods

Preparation of Melanins and Melanoproteins

Melanins were synthesized *in vitro* by (a) the autoxidation of the specified pre-cursors at pH 8.0 according to SWAN [16] and, (b) enzymically by the action of purified mushroom tyrosinase upon the particular substrates as previously described [12, 13, 15]. Since H_2O_2 is known to be formed during the melanin synthesis *in vitro,* in one set of experiments catalase was employed to remove the H_2O_2 that may be formed *in situ.* The melanin formed was isolated as described previously. In the experiments with hydroquinone, adrenaline and adrenochrome, the melanin was precipitated by adding the reaction mixture to 4 volumes of 0.5 NHCl and the precipitate was washed with 0.01 NHCl, suspended in H_2O and dialyzed against H_2O. Melanin from B16 melanoma was isolated as previously described [15].

The proteins bound to melanins were hydrolyzed by treatment with HCl as described previously [15].

Reduction of cytochrome *c*: Cytochrome *c* (35.0 mg) was dissolved in 2.0 ml 0.1 M phosphate buffer, pH 7.2. The solution was reduced with 5 mg potassium as-corbate [17]. Excess ascorbate was then removed by dialysis against 0.1 M phosphate buffer pH 7.2 for 20 h with 2 changes of buffer.

Reduction of 2,6-dichlorophenol-indophenol (DCPIP): DCPIP (0.4 mg) was dissolved in 1.0 ml 0.1 M phosphate buffer pH 7.2. The solution was then reduced with 2.7 mg sodium dithionite. Excess dithionite was oxidized by bubbling air through the solution for 5–10 min.

Oxidizing properties: The ability of melanin to oxidize the reduced components of a number of reduction-oxidation systems was determined spectrophotometrically using a suitable wavelength having the maximum difference between the reduced and oxidized components. The reduction-oxidation systems and the appropriate wavelengths included phenylalanine/dihydroxyphenylalanine (285 nm), ferrocyanide/ferricyanide (420 nm), cytochrome *c* Fe^{++}/Fe^{+++} (550 nm), DCPIP red/ox (600 nm), hydroquinone/quinone (275 nm), NADH/NAD (340 nm), NADPH/NADP (340 nm), and glutathione red/ox (260 nm). The standard reaction mixture contained 0.1 ml melanin suspension, 0.3 ml of the reduced component and 1.8 ml 0.1 M phosphate buffer, pH 7.2, in a total volume of 3.0 ml. All reactions were monitored contin-uously at room temperature using a Gilford 2400 recording spectrophotometer with the appropriate controls.

Reducing properties: The reducing properties of melanin were studied using the oxidized components of a few selected systems, namely ferricyanide/ferrocyanide, DCPIP ox/red, and cytochrome *c* Fe^{+++}/Fe^{++}; changes in the absorb-ance at the wavelengths mentioned above were determined.

Electron-transfer properties: The electron-transfer properties of melanin were investigated in the presence of NADH and a suitable artificial electron acceptor such as ferricyanide. The NADH-melanin-ferricyanide reaction was studied by si-multaneous determination of the absorbances at 340 and 420 nm. The reaction mix-ture consisted of 0.1 ml melanin suspension, 0.3 ml 1.28 mM NADH, 0.3 ml ferri-cyanide and 1.5 ml 0.1 M phosphate buffer, pH 7.2, in a total volume of 3.0 ml. The change in the absorbance at 340 nm produced by the reduction of ferricyanide was taken into account in calculating the amount of NADH oxidized.

Calculation of data and reproducibility of results: The rates of the reactions were determined from initial period when the reaction proceeded linearly with time. The readings for the zero time were calculated by addition of the absorbance values of the appropriate controls. By using the molar extinction coefficients, the amounts of the compounds oxidized or reduced were calculated. The results are expressed in terms of nmoles of the particular compound oxidized or reduced per min per mg melanin, except in table III where the total amounts oxidized or reduced during the entire reaction period are given.

Each experiment was carried out at least three times. Closely similar results were obtained in all cases. The results of one set of experiments are included in this paper.

Results

Oxidizing and Reducing Properties of Dopa-Melanin and Melanoma-Melanin

Table I summarizes the properties of dopa-melanin and melanoma-melanin as oxidizing and reducing agents in a number of oxidation-reduction systems. In agreement with previous reports [12, 13], dopa-melanin was found to oxidize NADH. The dopa-melanin was also found to oxidize NADPH although to a much smaller extent. The melanin did not

Table I. Oxidizing and reducing properties of melanin

Oxidation–reduction systems	nmoles oxidized or reduced/mg melanin	
	dopa–melanin	melanoma–melanin
Oxidizing properties		
Phenylalanine/dihydroxyphenylalanine	nil	nil
Ferrocyanide/ferricyanide	nil	nil
Cytochrome c Fe^{++}/Fe^{+++}	nil	nil
DCPIP red/ox	nil	nil
Hydroquinone/quinone	nil	nil
NADH/NAD	411	nil
NADPH/NADP	96	nil
Glutathione red/ox	nil	nil
Reducing properties		
Ferricyanide/ferrocyanide	1,725	93
Cytochrome c Fe^{+++}/Fe^{++}	228	nil
DCPIP ox/red	57	6

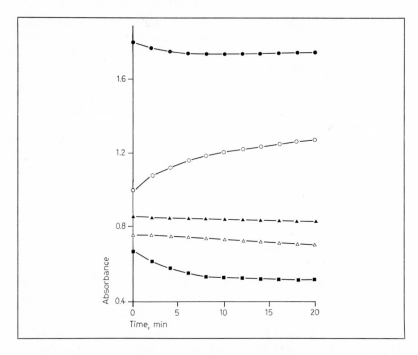

Fig. 1. Oxidizing and reducing properties of melanin. The concentration of the components added was NADH = 128 μM; NADPH = 156 μM; ferricyanide = 640 μM; DCPIP = 128 μM; cytochrome c Fe^{+++} = 128 μM. Melanin was present in all tubes. Oxidation: $\triangle$ = NADH; $\blacktriangle$ = NADPH. Reduction: $\blacksquare$ = ferricyanide; $\bullet$ = DCPIP; $\circ$ = cytochrome c.

have any effect on the other systems studied. The melanoma melanin did not show oxidizing activity in any of the systems studied. A comparison of the reducing properties of the melanins showed that dopa-melanin reduced to a considerable extent ferricyanide, oxidized form of cytochrome c and DCPIP. The melanoma-melanin reduced ferricyanide and DCPIP to a very small extent; it did not have any effect on cytochrome c.

A comparison of the kinetics of the oxidizing and reducing properties of dopa-melanin is shown in figure 1. The oxidation of NADH in the presence of melanin was linear up to 60 min. On the other hand, the reduction of ferricyanide, cytochrome c and DCPIP were initially very fast, tended to slow down after 10 min, and subsequently, came to a stop. When an additional amount of melanin was added, the reaction proceeded at approximately the same rate and to the same extent as previously.

When dopa-melanin was employed, the oxidation of NADH was proportional to the amount of melanin when the amount of melanin added was in the range of 0-50 μg per ml reaction mixture. The reduction of ferricyanide was not always strictly proportional to the amount of melanin; however, the reaction was approximately proportional to the amount of melanin when the melanin added was less than 20 μg per ml reaction mixture.

Coupled Oxidation and Reduction in Presence of Dopa-Melanin

The possibility that the oxidation of NADH in the presence of melanin could be coupled to the reduction of ferricyanide was next investigated. In the first series of experiments, the oxidation of NADH and the reduction of ferricyanide were determined in their mutual presence with and without melanin (table II). It was found that the amount of NADH oxidized when all three compounds were present was higher than the combined amounts of NADH oxidized in the presence of melanin alone and ferricyanide alone. Similarly, the amount of ferricyanide reduced in the presence of NADH and melanin was higher than the total of ferricyanide reduced in presence of NADH alone and in the presence of melanin alone. Attempts were made to calculate the relationship between the amount of NADH oxidized and that of ferricyanide reduced. In the system containing NADH and ferricyanide only, the amount of ferricyanide reduced, in molar concentrations, was approximately twice the amount of NADH oxidized. In order to calculate the amount of oxidized NADH coupled to the reduction of ferricyanide in the presence of melanin, it was assumed that the interactions between these three compounds were independent of one another under the experimental conditions. The amount of oxidized NADH coupled to the reduction of ferricyanide was calculated as the difference between the amount of NADH oxidized in their combined presence and the sum of the amounts of NADH oxidized in presence of melanin and in presence of ferricyanide alone. A similar formula was used to calculate the reduction of ferricyanide coupled to the oxidation of NADH. It was found that the value for the amount of ferricyanide reduced was approximately twice that of NADH oxidized.

When melanoma-melanin was added to a mixture of NADH and ferricyanide, NADH was not oxidized and ferricyanide not reduced.

The relationship between the oxidation of NADH and the reduction of ferricyanide was further investigated as follows. In this experiment, the reaction was allowed to proceed to completion and the amounts of ferri-

Table II. Oxidation of NADH and reduction of ferricyanide in the presence of dopa-melanin

Reaction system	nmoles oxidized or reduced	
	NAHD oxidized	ferricyanide reduced
1. NADH+melanin	9.3 (46.5)	
2. NADH+ferricyanide	43.8	90.0
3. Ferricyanide+melanin		345.0 (1,725)
4. NADH+ferricyanide+melanin	289.5 (1,446)	891.0 (4,455)
5. 1+2+3 (calculated)	53.1	345.0
6. 4–5 (calculated)	236.4 (1,182)	456.0 (2,280)

The numbers in parentheses represent nmoles oxidized or reduced per mg melanin.

Table III. Effect of NADH on the reduction of ferricyanide

Reaction system: melanin added, μg	Ferricyanide: ferricyanide reduced, nmol	NADH+ferricyanide	
		NADH oxidized, nmol	ferricyanide reduced, nmol
25	192	371	726
50	276	373	759
100	519	369	785
200	873	365	779
400	1,407	207	317

The reduction of ferricyanide by melanin was allowed to proceed to completion. Then NADH was added and the oxidation of NADH and reduction of ferricyanide were measured. Ferricyanide added = 384 nmol. NADH added = 1,920 nmol.

cyanide reduced during the entire period were calculated. The reduction of ferricyanide by varying amounts of melanin was determined (table III). Increasing amounts of ferricyanide reduced per mg melanin was calculated for each amount of melanin added. The mean of these values was found to be 10,500 nmol/mg melanin. When NADH was added to the reaction system after the reduction of ferricyanide ceased to proceed, both the reduction of ferricyanide and the oxidation of NADH proceeded at a fast rate and eventually came to a stop when either NADH or ferricyanide was used up. In each case, except at the highest concentration (200 μg) of melanin, the amounts of NADH oxidized and ferricyanide reduced were approximately equal, irrespective of the amount of melanin, and the ratio of ferricyanide reduced to NADH oxidized was approximately 2:1. When 200 μg of melanin was employed, the extent of the coupled reaction was less, presumably because of the increased amount of ferricyanide reduced before the addition of NADH.

Effect of Hydrolysis of Protein Bound to Melanin on the Oxidation of NADH

The possibility that the inability of the melanoma-melanin to oxidize NADH may be because the active sites are blocked by proteins bound to the melanin was investigated. The question was explored by the hydrolysis of protein by acid and then determining the oxidation of NADH by the melanin obtained after the treatment. The amount of protein hydrolyzed increased as the period of hydrolysis was increased (fig. 2). After the hydrolysis procedure, the melanoma-melanin was found to oxidize NADH. The ability to oxidize NADH gradually increased as the hydrolysis was prolonged, and followed a pattern similar to the amounts of protein hydrolyzed. There was a considerably smaller amount of protein hydrolyzed from dopa-melanin. Similarly, the oxidation of NADH also was enhanced to a relatively lesser extent.

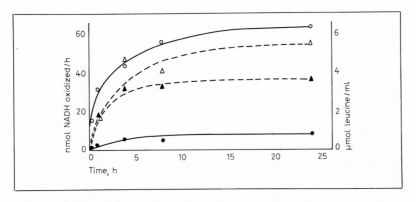

Fig. 2. Oxidation of NADH by melanin and hydrolysis of melanin-bound protein by treatment with acid. ○ = NADH oxidized by dopa-melanin; △ = NADH oxidized by melanoma-melanin; ● = amino acids (leucine equivalents) from dopa-melanin; ▲ = amino acids from tumor-melanin.

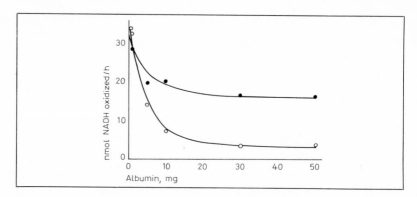

Fig. 3. Effect of albumin on the oxidation of NADH by dopa-melanin ○ = Albumin added during the synthesis of melanin; ● = albumin added after melanin was synthesized and isolated.

Effect of Addition of Albumin upon the Oxidation of NADH by Dopa-Melanin

The above results indicated that the hydrolysis of protein bound to melanin increased the ability of the melanin to oxidize NADH. The question whether addition of protein to melanin would decrease this activity was next examined. The results are given in figure 3. When varying amounts of albumin were added to the melanin-synthesizing system, the oxidation of NADH was decreased. Similarly, experiments where albumin was added to melanin which had already been synthesized showed that addition of increasing amounts of albumin decreased the oxidation of NADH.

Effects of Polyamino Acids on the Oxidation of NADH by Melanin

The effects of acidic and basic polyamino acids upon the oxidation of NADH by melanin were next investigated. In the first series of experiments, the polyamino acids were added during the melanin synthesis. As seen from figure 4, polyglutamate and polyaspartate did not have any significant effect on the NADH oxidation. On the other hand, polylysine and polyarginine produced a considerable decrease in the oxidation of NADH. The addition of polyglutamate and polyaspartate to melanin already prepared did not have any significant effect on the oxidation of NADH. Addition of polylysine or polyarginine to the melanin suspension resulted in aggregation of the melanin and rapid sedimentation of the particles. Probably these polypeptides form cross-linkages between the me-

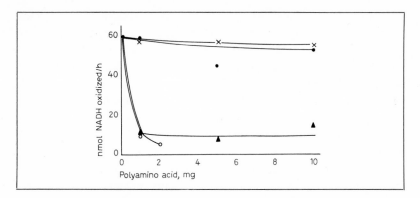

Fig. 4. Effects of addition of polyamino acids during the synthesis of melanin on the oxidation of NADH by melanin. × = Polyaspartate; ● = polyglutamate; ▲ = polylysine; ○ = polyarginine.

lanin granules causing the aggregation. Therefore, the effects of these substances under these conditions could not be studied.

Oxidation-Reduction Properties of Various Melanins

The properties of melanins prepared from various precursors were studied. Dopa-melanin was prepared enzymically employing tyrosinase and by autoxidation. Melanins were also prepared from dopamine, adrenaline, adrenochrome and hydroquinone. Preliminary experiments have shown that all these melanins are active in the above oxidation-reduction reactions.

Discussion

The above results indicate that melanin has a remarkable specificity in its oxidizing properties. Among a series of oxidation/reduction systems studied, NADH was oxidized most efficiently; the rate of oxidation of NADPH was considerably lower than that of NADH. Other systems studied were not significantly oxidized in the presence of melanin. However, such a distinct specificity was not observed in the reducing properties of melanin. Melanin was found to reduce ferricyanide, cytochrome *c* and DCPIP. It was interesting to observe that while melanin reduced the oxidized forms of these compounds, it did not oxidize the corresponding reduced forms. The finding that reduced cytochrome *c* is not oxidized by melanin indicates that the high rate of oxygen uptake by homogenates of melanotic melanoma in presence of reduced cytochrome c as reported by RILEY [13] is not likely due to the action of melanin in these homogenates. When both NADH and ferricyanide were added, the ratio of the amount of NADH oxidized to that of ferricyanide reduced was found to be 1:2. This stoichiometric proportion is in agreement with the values expected if the oxidation of NADH is coupled to the reduction of ferricyanide, i.e. the electrons are transferred from NADH to ferricyanide. It appears that when ferricyanide alone was present, the melanin was completely oxidized and further reduction of ferricyanide could take place only when NADH was added. These results indicate that melanin is reversibly oxidized by ferricyanide and reduced by NADH as shown below:

1. Melanin (reduced) + $2Fe(CN)_6{}^{---}$ $\longrightarrow$
   melanin (oxidized) + $2Fe(CN)_6{}^{----}$.

2. Melanin (oxidized) + NADH + H^+ $\longrightarrow$
   melanin (reduced) + NAD^+.

The melanin from melanoma did not oxidize NADH. When the melanoma melanin was subjected to acid hydrolysis under conditions routinely employed for the hydrolysis of proteins, the resulting product had considerable NADH-oxidizing activity. When bovine serum albumin was added to the melanin-synthesizing system or to melanin already synthesized, the NADH-oxidizing activity was decreased. These results show that when proteins are bound to melanin, the resulting melanoproteins have lower NADH-oxidizing activity. It may be concluded from these results that melanin as isolated from the melanoma is present as melanoprotein. The proteins are presumably bound to melanin in such a manner that the free radical sites on the melanin are blocked.

Studies on the effects of the synthetic polypeptides of known composition showed that polyglutamate and polyaspartate had no effect on the oxidation of NADH while polylysine and polyarginine produced a marked inhibition. These results show that basic polypeptides are more effective in decreasing the NADH-oxidizing activity and may also form complexes with melanin more effectively. Analysis of the amino acid composition of the proteins in the melanosomes showed that there was no obvious abundance of either the basic or acidic groups of amino acids [15]. It is possible that specific regions of proteins having concentrations of basic amino acids may be responsible for the binding to melanin.

It is not possible to make definite conclusions regarding the biologi-

cal significance of the present results. However, we would like to postulate the following probable role for melanoproteins. It has been proposed
that the free radical structure of melanin may be important in its protective role against radiation and toxic free radicals [8, 18]. It has also been
postulated that melanin may act as a biological electron exchange polymer and may protect cells and tissues against oxidizing and reducing conditions which would have harmful effects on cellular structure and metabolism [3]. Our observations on the presence of melanin in the melanoma
as melanoproteins not capable of electron transfer may have relevance in
these functions of melanin. This may represent the state in which melanin
may be stored within the cell. Our results showing that removal of proteins bound to melanin could produce melanin active in electron transfer
could lead to the postulate that similar mechanisms for 'activation' of melanin may be prevalent in cells. For example, it may be proposed that
high energy photons may dissociate the melanoproteins and thereby produce free melanin active as a free radical. The storage of melanin as relatively inactive melanoproteins would eliminate the possible side effects
which may be caused by the presence of active melanin within the cells all
the time. Thus, by this means, it may be possible to preserve a potentially
active defense mechanism to be utilized only when the conditions demand
its function.

The data that we have is far from adequate to examine the contribution of melanin to the oxidation-reduction processes within melanin-containing cells. However, a comparison of these aspects seems to be interesting. Determination of the oxygen utilization by a number of normal
and malignant tissues *in vitro* shows that the oxygen uptake by many tissues is of the order of 10 nmol O_2/min/mg dry weight tissue [19]. The activity of the coupled reduction of ferricyanide and oxidation of NADH
(from pyruvate) by brain and liver mitochondria has been reported to be
approximately 16 nmol ferricyanide reduced/min/mitochondria from
1.0 mg dry weight brain and liver [20] and 0.03 nmol/min/mitochondria
from 1 mg dry weight liver [21]. Our data with melanin show that
760 nmol ferricyanide are reduced/min/mg melanin. Since our preliminary
results show that 5–10 μg melanin could be isolated from 1.0 mg dry
weight B16 melanoma, the amount of ferricyanide reduced *in vitro* by
melanin from 1.0 mg dry weight melanoma would be of the order of
3–8 nmol/min. Although these comparisons cannot be taken accurately,
nevertheless, these data suggest strongly that quantitatively the electron
transfer properties of melanin are of a fairly high rate.

Summary

The melanin synthesized by the action of monophenol mono-oxygenase (EC 1/4.18.1) on 3,4-dihydroxyphenylalanine (dopa-melanin) was found to oxidize NADH and to a much smaller extent NADPH. This melanin reduced potassium ferricyanide, 2,6-dichlorophenol indophenol (DCPIP) and cytochrome c. A coupled oxidation-reduction reaction in which NADH was oxidized and ferricyanide was reduced also proceeded at a fast rate in presence of dopa-melanin. Melanin isolated from B16 melanoma was found to reduce ferricyanide, but did not oxidize NADH or NADPH or catalyze the coupled oxidation of NADH and reduction of ferricyanide. The reduction of ferricyanide by dopa-melanin was approximately proportional to the amount of melanin added and the reaction ceased to proceed after 10–15 min; the reduction of ferricyanide proceeded further when more melanin was added to the reaction system. When the proteins present in the melanin preparation from melanoma were hydrolyzed the resulting product oxidized NADH at a high rate. When bovine serum albumin, polylysine or polyarginine was added to dopa-melanin, the NADH-oxidizing activity was decreased. The results indicate that basic components of the proteins bound to melanin may be blocking the active sites of melanin involved in the oxidation of NADH. It is postulated that the electron transfer properties of melanin may be important in its protective role against radiation and toxic free radicals and that the inactive melanoprotein, as it occurs in the cell, may be converted to active melanin upon dissociation or degradation of the protein by agents such as radiation. Melanins synthesized from dopamine, adrenalin, adrenochrome, and hydroquinone also had electron transfer properties similar to dopa-melanin. The results seem to indicate that melanin may be reversibly oxidized by ferricyanide and reduced by NADH and the oxidized and reduced forms of melanin may participate in the electron transfer reactions of melanin.

Acknowledgements

We would like to acknowledge the excellent technical assistance of Kok-May Lam. The authors wish to acknowledge the Medical Research Council of Canada for a grant (MA-5043) and a fellowship to E. V. Gan, and Ontario Geriatric Society and Ontario Cancer Treatment and Research Foundation for grants. H. F. Haberman is an Associate of Ontario Cancer Treatment and Research Foundation.

References

1   Commoner, B.; Townsend, J., and Pake, G. E.: Free radicals in biological materials. Nature, Lond. *174:* 689–691 (1954).
2   Adams, M.; Blois, M. S., and Sands, R. H.: Paramagnetic resonance spectra of some semiquinone free radicals. J. Chem. Phys. *28:* 774–776 (1958).

3 MASON, H. S.; INGRAM, D. J. E., and ALLEN, B.: The free radical property of melanins. Archs Biochem. Biophys. 83: 225–230 (1960).
4 LONGUET-HIGGINS, H. C.: On the origin of the free radical property of melanins. Archs Biochem. Biophys. 86: 231–232 (1960)
5 COPE, F. W.; SEUER, R. J., and POLIS, B. D.: Reversible free radical generation in the melanin granules of the eye by visible light. Archs Biochem. Biophys. 100: 171–177 (1963).
6 MULAY, I. L. and MULAY, L. N.: Magnetic susceptibility and electron spin resonance absorption spectra of mouse melanomas S91 and S91A. J. natn. Cancer Inst. 39: 735–743 (1967).
7 BLOIS, M. S.: Biological free radicals and the melanins; in WYARD Solid state biophys., pp. 245–262 (McGraw Hill, New York 1969).
8 EDELSTEIN, L. M.: Melanin. A unique biopolymer. Pathobiology Ann. 1: 309–324 (1971).
9 PULLMAN, A. and PULLMAN, B.: The band structure of melanins. Biochim. biophys. Acta 54: 384–385 (1961).
10 ALLEN, B. T. and INGRAM, D. J. E.: The investigation of the unpaired electron concentrations produced in large molecules by ultraviolet irradiation; in BLOIS, BROWN, LEMMON, LINDBLOM and WEISSBLUTH Free radicals in biological systems, pp. 215–225 (Academic Press, New York 1961).
11 BORG, D.: Biochemistry of neuromelanins. Adv. Neurol. 5: 232–233 (1964).
12 WOERT, M. H. VAN: Oxidation of reduced nicotinamide adenine dinucleotide by melanin. Life Sci. 6: 2605–2612 (1967).
13 WOERT, M. H. VAN: Reduced nicotinamide-adenine dinucleotide oxidation by melanin: inhibition by phenothiazines. Proc. Soc. exp. Biol. Med. 129: 165–171 (1968).
14 GAN, E. V.; HABERMAN, H. F., and MENON, I. A.: Oxidation of NADH by melanin and melanoproteins. Proc. Can. Fed. Biol. Soc. 17: 20 (1974).
15 GAN, E. V.; HABERMAN, H. F., and MENON, I. A.: Oxidation of NADH by melanin and melanoproteins. Biochim. biophys. Acta 370: 62–69 (1974).
16 SWAN, G. A.: Current knowledge of melanin structure; in McGOVERN and RUSSELL Pigment Cell, vol. 1, pp. 151–157 (Karger, Basel 1973).
17 WHARTON, D. C. and TZAGOLOFF, A.: Cytochrome oxidase from beef heart mitochondria; in ESTABROOK, PULLMAN, COLOWICK and KAPLAN (Meth. Enzym., vol. 10, pp. 245–250 (Academic Press, New York 1967).
18 PATHAK, M. A.: Photobiology of melanogenesis: biophysical aspects; in MONTAGNA and HU Adv. Biol. Skin, vol. 8, pp. 397–420 (Pergamon Press, Oxford
19 WEINHOUSE, S.: Oxidative metabolism of neoplastic tissues. Adv. Cancer Res. 3: 269–325 (1955).
20 ARAVINDAKSHAM, I. and BRAGANCA, B. M.: Preferential inhibition of phosphorylation in different parts of the respiratory chain in mitochondria obtained from animal injected with cobra venom. Biochem. J. 79: 80–84 (1961).
21 COPENHAVER, J. H. and LARDY, H. A.: Oxidative phosphorylations. Pathways and yield in mitochondrial preparations. J. biol. Chem. 195: 225–238 (1952).

Dr. I. A. MENON, Clinical Science Division, Section of Dermatology, University of Toronto, Medical Sciences Building, *Toronto, Ont. M5S 1A8* (Canada)

Pigment Cell, vol. 3, pp. 82–88 (Karger, Basel 1976)

The Bifunctional Role of Mammalian, Avian and Amphibian Tyrosinases in Melanogenesis

JOHN J. EPPIG, jr. and VINCENT J. HEARING

Biology Department, Brooklyn College, CUNY, Brooklyn, N.Y. and Dermatology Branch, National Cancer Institute, National Institutes of Health, Bethesda, Md.

Introduction

There has been considerable controversy in recent years concerning the generally accepted bifunctional role of tyrosinase in converting tyrosine to dihydroxyphenylalanine (dopa), and dopa to dopaquinone. It has been suggested that mammalian tyrosinase cannot catalyze the initial step, tyrosine to dopa, in melanin synthesis. It was proposed that peroxidase carries out this conversion and that tyrosinase, really only a dopa oxidase, catalyzes the dopa to dopaquinone step [7–9]. Indeed, small amounts of peroxidase are present in crude homogenates of melanogenic tissues [10], and peroxidase alone can oxidize tyrosine to dopa [2, 5, 6]. The salient questions, however, are: (1) Can tyrosinase utilize tyrosine as a substrate? (2) Does peroxidase function in melanogenesis *in vivo*?

The experiments presented here indicate that tyrosinase isolated from purified melanin granule fractions of a variety of melanogenic tissues does convert tyrosine to melanin, or an immediate acid-insoluble precursor. Further, these enzyme preparations, containing considerable tyrosine-oxidizing capacity, contain no demonstrable peroxidase activity. Therefore, since there is no demonstrable peroxidase at the major site of melanin synthesis, the melanin granule [13, 14], it is not likely that peroxidase plays a role in melanogenesis *in vivo*.

Materials and Methods

Melanogenic Tissues

Melanin granules were isolated from the eyes of 5-day newborn C57BL black mice, S-91 Cloudman melanoma, the eyes of 15-day White Leghorn chick embryos, and from stage III and IV oocytes of the African clawed frog, *Xenopus laevis*, 2–3 days after injecting the frog with 1,000 IU of human chorionic gonadotropin (HCG). HCG injection of the frog greatly increases melanogenesis in oocytes of these stages [3].

Isolation of Melanin Granules

Tissues were homogenized in ice-cold 0.1 M sodium phosphate buffer, pH 7.4, and centrifuged at 1,000 *g* for 5 min to remove cellular debris and unbroken cells. The supernatant was layered on a continuous sucrose gradient ranging from 0.24 to 2.0 M and centrifuged in a Beckman SW 27 rotor at 82,500 *g* for 90 min. The resulting melanin granule pellet was resuspended in the phosphate buffer.

Solubilization of Melanogenic Enzyme

Triton X-100 (TX-100) was added to the isolated melanin granules to a final concentration of 1%. After incubation at 4 °C for 18 h, the melanin granules were pelleted by centrifugation at 10,000 *g* for 15 min. This TX-100 treatment solubilizes 75–95% of the melanogenic enzyme activity from the melanin granules.

Enzyme Assays

For most experiments, a modification of the assay used by ACHAZI and YAMADA [1], which measures the conversion of ^{14}C-tyrosine to ^{14}C-melanin, or an immediate acid-insoluble melanin precursor was used. The incubation mixture contained in final concentrations: 0.05 mM L-tyrosine (specific activity 100 mCi/mM), 0.005 mM L-dopa, 200 U/ml penicillin G, 0.20 mg/ml chloramphenicol, and 0.25 mg/ml cycloheximide in 0.1 M sodium phosphate buffer, pH 7.4. The assays are prepared by mixing 12 μl of sample, 12 μl of assay reagents, and 6 μl of buffer, or additions such as diethyldithiocarbamate (DDC) or H_2O_2. The mixtures were incubated for 1 h at 37 °C and then 20 μl were spotted on Whatman 3MM filter disks and processed according to the method of ACHAZI and YAMADA [1].

Other assays used were the tyrosine hydroxylation assay of POMERANTZ [11], and the dopa oxidase spectrophotometric assay of FLING *et al.* [4]. Peroxidase activity was determined by the spectrophotometric assay described in the Worthington Enzyme Manual (Worthington Biochemical Corporation, Freehold, New Jersey) using *o*-dianisidine as substrate.

Polyacrylamide Gel Electrophoresis

Samples dialyzed against stacking gel buffer were run on 7.5% gels utilizing system A as described by RODBARD and CHRAMBACH [12]. For analysis, gels were either incubated in 0.2% L-dopa for 1 h to localize dopa oxidase, in 0.05% 3,3'-diaminobenzidine or *o*-dianisidine plus 0.001% H_2O_2 for peroxidase, or sectioned into 1-mm slices and incubated in the ^{14}C-tyrosine mixture described above for determination of ability to convert tyrosine to melanin. Samples of Sigma type II peroxidase were also run on the gels as a control for the demonstration of peroxidase activity.

Results and Discussion

Since the melanin granule is the major site of melanogenesis, our efforts have been focused on the melanogenic enzymes localized in this organelle. Our previous studies [in preparation] demonstrated that 75–95% of the melanogenic enzyme activity of the melanin granule can be solubilized by TX-100 treatment; hence, most of the experiments reported here utilize the TX-100-solubilized enzyme. These samples, although containing considerable melanogenic activity (from about 30 to 200 nM tyrosine converted/h/mg), contained no peroxidase activity as assayed by the very sensitive o-dianisidine technique (fig. 1). When the melanogenic enzymes were run on polyacrylamide gels, again no peroxidase activity was demonstrable, even though dopa oxidase activity was present in several bands.

It has been argued that mammalian tyrosinase is unable to utilize tyrosine as a substrate; rather, it was suggested that tyrosinase can catalyze only the oxidation of dopa and thus should be referred to only as a dopa oxidase [10]. Analysis of TX-100-solubilized melanin granule proteins, separated on polyacrylamide gels, and which contained no demonstrable peroxidase activity, shows that most bands which can utilize dopa can also convert tyrosine to an acid-insoluble product (fig. 2). Additional evidence that the melanin granule enzyme which converts tyrosine to melanin is tyrosinase rather than peroxidase is presented in table I. When compared to control tubes (group 1), it is seen that the addition of catalytic amounts of H_2O_2 (group 2) increased melanogenic activity by only 5% or less. Also, the addition of catalase, in order to eliminate contaminating endogenous H_2O_2, had no inhibiting effect on melanogenic activity [5]. H_2O_2 is an essential substrate for peroxidase, but not for tyrosinase. Further evidence against a possible role of peroxidase in the melanin granule is the fact that pretreatment of granule melanogenic enzyme samples with DDC results in the irreversible inhibition of enzyme activity. DDC-pretreated samples were dialyzed extensively to remove the DDC, but activity was not restored. To ensure that unbound DDC was reduced to noninhibitory levels by the dialysis, fresh enzyme (6 μl) was added to the DDC-pretreated dialyzed sample (group 8). The resultant enzyme activity was comparable to that of a similar amount of enzyme added to a non-

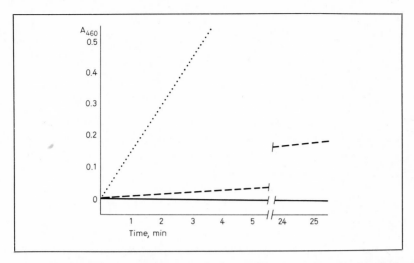

Fig. 1. Comparison of peroxidase activity in crude homogenates and melanin granules of S-91 melanoma. ..... = 1 U horseradish peroxidase; ------ = crude melanoma homogenate; ——— = coincident baseline plots of soluble and insoluble melanosome TX-100 extract.

DDC-pretreated sample (group 3). This is further evidence in favor of tyrosinase as the sole melanogenic enzyme in melanin granules, since it has been shown that DDC binds irreversibly to the copper-containing enzyme tyrosinase, but reversibly to the iron-containing enzyme peroxidase.

The results shown in table II indicate that the data obtained using the ^{14}C-tyrosine assay can be duplicated employing the other two commonly used assays for melanogenic activity: the ^{3}H-tyrosine assay of POMERANTZ [11] and the spectrophotometric assay of FLING *et al.* [4]. Each of these assays measures a different facet of melanin biosynthesis. The ^{3}H-tyrosine assay measures the hydroxylation of tyrosine to dopa, while the spectrophotometric assay measures the conversion of dopa to dopachrome. The ^{14}C-tyrosine assay measures the conversion of tyrosine to melanin, or an intermediate acid-insoluble precursor. Therefore, these various assays measure all the enzyme-dependent oxidative steps required for melanin biosynthesis from tyrosine.

In conclusion, we do not contest that peroxidase can convert tyrosine to melanin, or that peroxidase is present in crude homogenates of melanogenic tissues. However, our data shows that: (1) peroxidase is not demonstrable in melanin granules, the primary site of melanogenesis, and (2) tyrosinase is a bifunctional enzyme which can catalyze both the conversion

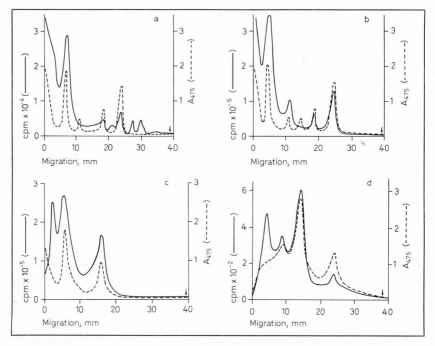

Fig. 2. Electropherograms of TX-100 solubilized melanosomal proteins from: (a) C57BL eye; (b) S-91 murine melanoma; (c) chick eye, (d) *Xenopus* oocytes. Graphs illustrate that most bands which are dopa-positive are also capable of converting tyrosine to acid-insoluble melanin precursors. No reaction was seen in these samples after DAB or *o*-dianisidine incubation, indicating lack of peroxidase activity.

of tyrosine to dopa, and dopa to dopaquinone. This is not only the case for mammalian tyrosinase, but also for tyrosinase from chick and amphibian sources.

Summary

In view of the recent controversy regarding the enzymes responsible for melanin synthesis, we studied the possible roles of tyrosinase and peroxidase in melanin formation in a variety of pigmented tissues. Melanin granules were isolated from S-91 murine melanomas, choroid and retina of newborn black mice and embryonic chicks, and from developing oocytes of the frog, *Xenopus laevis*. Melanogenic enzymes were solubilized from the purified melanin granules by 1% Triton X-100, and were then subjected to analysis by polyacrylamide gel electrophoresis, and agents

Table I. Effects of DDC[a] and H_2O_2[b] on melanogenic enzyme activity[c]

No.	Sample	Addition	Solibilized melanin granule enzymes				
			perox[d]	mouse	melanoma chick		amphibian
1	Control	buffer	00	26,395	10,692	3,268	1,886
2	Control	H_2O_2	15,174	27,666	10,655	3,743	1,669
3	Control	sample	n.d.	43,563	15,058	3,973	3,055
4	DDC-pretreated	buffer	00	442	381	442	00
5	DDC-pretreated	H_2O_2	7,281	328	375	69	228
6	DDC-dialyzed	buffer	00	541	507	217	235
7	DDC-dialyzed	H_2O_2	15,370	441	419	203	218
8	DDC-dialyzed	sample	n.d.	13,838	4,132	515	736

[a] DDC pretreatment concentration, 10 mM; final assay concentration, 4 mM.
[b] H_2O_2 final assay concentration, 10 mM.
[c] Counts per minute minus background.
[d] Horseradish peroxidase (Sigma, type II) final concentration 0.32 mg/ml.

Table II. Effects of DDC[a] and H_2O_2[b] on melanogenic enzyme activity of S-91 melanosomes assayed with various techniques

Sample	Addition	^{14}C-tyr[c]	^3H-tyr[c]	$\Delta A_{457}/h$
Control	buffer	10,692	4,486	0.450
Control	H_2O_2	10,655	4,682	0.490
Control	sample	15,058	5,710	0.710
DDC-pretreated	buffer	381	1,420	0.090
DDC-pretreated	H_2O_2	375	958	0.125
DDC-dialyzed	buffer	507	1,406	0.135
DDC-dialyzed	H_2O_2	419	1,020	0.132
DDC-dialyzed	sample	4,132	3,693	0.420

[a] DDC pretreatment concentration, 10 mM; final assay concentration, 4 mM.
[b] H_2O_2 final assay concentration, 10 mM.
[c] Counts per min.

known to affect tyrosinase and peroxidase activity. The results indicate that in the tissues studied, there was no peroxidase activity demonstrable in the melanosome (the major site of intracellular melanin formation) and that all of the observed tyrosine hydroxylation and dopa oxidation was tyrosinase-dependent. It is concluded from these data that in melanin granules isolated from a variety of animals and tissues, peroxidase had no visible function in melanogenesis; it was also evident from our radioactive precursor studies that tyrosinase *is* capable of tyrosine hydroxylation when provided with small amounts of dopa cofactor.

References

1   ACHAZI, R. and YAMADA, T.: Tyrosinase activity in the Wolffian lens regenerating system. Devl Biol. 27: 295–306 (1972).

2   BAYSE, G. S.; MICHAELS, A. W., and MORRISON, M.: The peroxidase-catalyzed oxidation of tyrosine. Biochim. biophys. Acta 284: 34–42 (1972).

3   EPPIG, J. J., jr. and DUMONT, J. N.: Oogenesis in Xenopus laevis (Daudin). II. The induction and subcellular localization of tyrosinase in developing oocytes. Devl Biol. 36: 330–342 (1974).

4   FLING, M.; HOROWITZ, N. H., and HEINEMANN, S. F.: The isolation and properties of crystalline tyrosinase from Neurospora. J. biol. Chem. 238: 2045–2053 (1963).

5   HEARING, V. J.: Mammalian melanogenesis. Tyrosinase versus peroxidase involvement, and activation mechanisms. Archs Biochem. Biophys. 158: 720–725 (1973).

6   MASON, H.; ONOPRIENKO, I., and BUHLER, D.: Hydroxylation: the activation of oxygen by peroxidase. Biochim. biophys. Acta 24: 225–231 (1957).

7   OKUN, M. R.; EDELSTEIN, L. M.; OR, N.; HAMADA, G.; DONNELLAN, B., and LEVER, W. F.: Histochemical differentiation of peroxidase-mediated from tyrosinase-mediated melanin formation in mammalian tissues. Histochemie 23: 295–309 (1970).

8   OKUN, M. R.; EDELSTEIN, L. M.; OR, N.; HAMADA, G., and DONNELLAN, B.: The role of peroxidase vs. the role of tyrosinase in enzymatic conversion of tyrosine to melanin in melanocytes, mast cells and eosinophils. J. invest. Derm. 55: 1–12 (1970).

9   PATEL, R. P.; OKUN, M. R.; YEE, W. A.; WILGRAM, G. F., and EDELSTEIN, L. M.: Inability of murine melanoma 'tyrosinase' (dopa oxidase) to oxidize tyrosine in the presence or absence of dopa or dihydroxyfumarate cofactor. J. invest. Derm. 61: 55–59 (1973).

10 PATEL, R. P.; OKUN, M. R.; EDELSTEIN, L. M., and CARIGLIA, N.: Peroxidatic oxidation of tyrosine to melanin in supernatant of crude mouse melanoma homogenates. Biochem. J. 142: 441–443 (1974).

11 POMERANTZ, S. H.: L-Tyrosine-3,5-^{3}H assay for tyrosinase development in skin of newborn hamsters. Science 164: 838–839 (1969).

12 RODBARD, D. and CHRAMBACH, A.: Estimation of molecular radius, free mobility, and valence using polyacrylamide gel electrophoresis. Analyt. Biochem. 40: 95–134 (1971).

13 SEIJI, M.; SHIMAO, K.; BIRBECK, M. S. C., and FITZPATRICK, T. B.: Subcellular localization of melanin biosynthesis. Ann. N.Y. Acad. Sci. 100: 497–533 (1963).

14 SEIJI, M. and IWASHITA, S.: Intracellular localization of tyrosinase and site of melanin formation in the melanocyte. J. invest. Derm. 45: 305–314 (1965).

Dr. JOHN J. EPPIG, jr., The Jackson Laboratory, Bar Harbor, ME 04609 (USA)

Pigment Cell, vol. 3, pp. 89–97 (Karger, Basel 1976)

Recent Experiments on the Roles of Aerobic Dopa Oxidase (Tyrosinase) and Peroxidase in Mammalian Melanogenesis[1]

Milton R. Okun, Ravindra P. Patel, Barbara Donnellan, Leon M. Edelstein and Nancy Cariglia

Department of Dermatology, Tufts University School of Medicine and Boston City Hospital, Boston, Mass., and Departments of Pathology and Medicine (Dermatology), University of Massachusetts School of Medicine and St. Vincent Hospital, Worcester, Mass.

Inability of Isolated Mammalian 'Tyrosinase' to Oxidize Tyrosine to Melanin [1]

A partially purified enzyme preparation was obtained from a heavily melanized line of Harding-Passey mouse melanoma, using a modification of the method of Brown and Ward [2]. This preparation contained no significant peroxidase activity. Assay of the ability of this 'tyrosinase' preparation to oxidize tyrosine was carried out with the following methods: (a) spectrophotometric recording of dopachrome formation, using dopa or dihydroxyfumaric acid as co-factor; (b) Raper lead acetate method [3] for quantitative determination of dopa; (c) determination of labeled dopa formation from labeled tyrosine with alumina gel column chromatography [4]; (d) polyacrylamide gel electrophoretic assay of melanogenic potential of enzyme bands.

With all methods cited, mammalian 'tyrosinase' was shown to be an active aerobic dopa oxidase with no ability to oxidize tyrosine.

Spectrophotometric assay showed no differential dopachrome formation with tyrosine plus dopa (fig. 1) as compared with dopa alone (using a wide spectrum of tyrosine:dopa ratios). With tyrosine alone or with dihy-

1 Supported by USPHS Grant T1 AM 5220 and by The Dermatopathology Foundation.

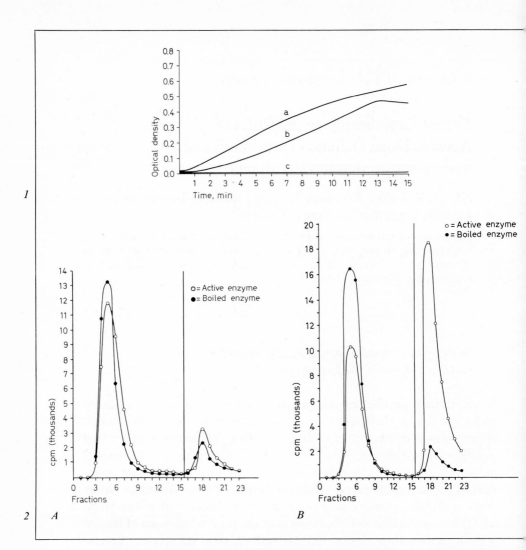

Fig. 1. Formation of dopachrome by the action of melanoma dopa oxidase ('tyrosinase') on (A) DL-dopa alone, (B) DL-dopa plus L-tyrosine in 1:4 molar ratio, and (C) L-tyrosine alone. Less dopachrome is formed in the presence of tyrosine, since the enzyme binds to the active site without being oxidized.

Fig. 2. A Radiolabeled tyrosine (segment a) and radiolabeled dopa (segment b) from alumina gel columns using reaction mixtures containing labeled tyrosine, unlabeled dopa, ascorbate and active or boiled melanoma dopa oxidase ('tyrosinase'). Tyrosine fractions were 10 times as dilute as the dopa fractions. No enzymatic conversion of tyrosine to dopa is observed. *B* Radiolabeled tyrosine (segment a) and dopa (segment b) when mushroom tyrosinase was substituted for melanoma dopa oxidase ('tyrosinase') in the reaction mixture cited in *A*, enzymatic conversion of tyrosine to dopa is observed.

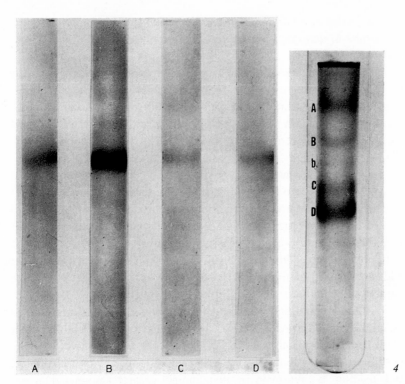

Fig. 3. Melanosomal dopa oxidase ('tyrosinase') band from trypsin-treated pellet from B16 mouse melanoma. A = Coomassie blue protein stain; B = melanin
band resulting from 0.15⁰/₀ dopa incubation; C = melanin band resulting from incubation in tyrosine and dopa, each in 0.2 mM concentration; D = melanin band resulting from incubation in 0.2 mM dopa without tyrosine. There is no visible enhancement of melanin formation in the presence of tyrosine.

Fig. 4. Enzyme bands from 100,000 *g* crude mouse melanoma supernatant after incubation in dopa. A = Catalase; B and b = peroxidase; C and D = dopa oxidase ('tyrosinase'). All of these enzymes oxidized dopa to melanin.

droxyfumaric acid as co-factor, no dopachrome was formed from tyrosine.

Similarly, neither the lead acetate method nor the alumina gel ra-
dioassay method (fig. 2) showed dopa formation from tyrosine.

Enzyme bands of aerobic dopa oxidase ('tyrosinase') visualized by
polyacrylamide gel electrophoresis showed no enhancement of melanin
formation when tyrosine and dopa were present as compared to dopa
alone. Similar results were obtained with aerobic dopa oxidase ('tyrosinase') solubilized from melanosomes (fig. 3) [5].

Biochemical Studies of Peroxidatic Melanogenesis in
Crude Melanoma Preparations [6]

100,000 g supernatant of a crude homogenate of a heavily melanized line of Harding-Passey mouse melanoma showed intense peroxidase activity (benzidine reaction) and catalase activity. Peroxidase, catalase and aerobic dopa oxidase ('tyrosinase') bands were demonstrated by acrylamide gel electrophoresis; all of these bands oxidized dopa to melanin (fig. 4).

When tyrosine was used as substrate for this supernatant (without added hydrogen peroxide), conversion to dopachrome was recorded with spectrophotometric assay after an initial lag period (fig. 5). With the addition of 10^{-2} M hydrogen peroxide, a curve of similar configuration was obtained having an absorption peak about 5 times as high as that of the initial curve (fig. 5). Ultimately, insoluble melanin formed with and without added hydrogen peroxide. With added hydrogen peroxide the greater amount of melanin formed was visually evident (fig. 6).

Although catalase and sulfhydryl compounds are effective as differential inhibitors of melanogenesis due to peroxidase and aerobic dopa oxidase in histochemical systems [7–9], they are not effective for this purpose in *in vitro* systems. In histochemical systems, catalase in the incubation medium is present in overwhelmingly greater amounts than peroxidase in tissue sections, and possible peroxidase activity of catalase in the incubation medium [10] would compete with rather than add to, peroxidase activity in tissue sections. The converse is true in *in vitro* systems. In our experiments, peroxidase activity was noted in the presence of catalase, a result similar to that of Knox [11].

Preincubation with sulfhydryl compounds followed by their total removal resulted in selective suppression of aerobic dopa oxidase ('tyrosinase') in histochemical systems [7–9]. However, in our *in vitro* system, a sufficient concentration of such compounds remained, even after repeated dialysis, to act as possible nonselective inhibitors of peroxidase.

Our study indicated that, unless preparations of melanocyte-bearing tissue are completely free of peroxidase activity, oxidation of tyrosine to melanin cannot be attributed to aerobic dopa oxidase ('tyrosinase'). In crude preparations, endogenous co-factor and hydrogen peroxide requirements for peroxidase activity are present. Our data support a peroxidase dependency for the initial step of melanogenesis (hydroxylation of tyrosine) mediated by the crude supernatant. The configuration of the do-

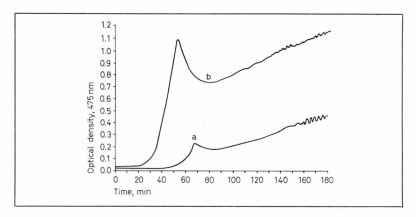

Fig. 5. The curves represent changes in OD$_{475}$ (dopachrome) by the action of crude mouse melanoma supernatant on L-tyrosine. Curve a = without added hydrogen peroxide; curve b = with added hydrogen peroxide. The wavy terminal portions of the curves are produced by a suspension of insoluble melanin. The great increase in dopachrome formation with added hydrogen peroxide and the similarity in configuration of curves with and without added hydrogen peroxide are consistent with a peroxidase dependency of the initial step of melanogenesis in this system.

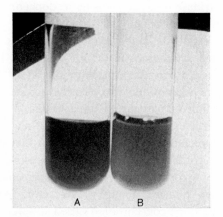

Fig. 6. The test tubes compare melanin suspension formed by the action of crude mouse melanoma supernatant on tyrosine with (tube a) and without (tube b) added hydrogen peroxide. Peroxidase-dependent melanogenesis is present. Our data indicate that the initial step of melanogenesis is entirely peroxidase-dependent. Oxidation of dopa represents the composite effect of catalase, peroxidase and aerobic dopa oxidase ('tyrosinase').

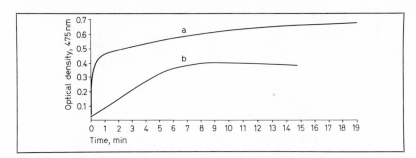

Fig. 7. Changes in the absorption at 475 nm (dopachrome) by the action of peroxidase on (a) tyrosine, dopa and hydrogen peroxide, and (b) dopa and hydrogen peroxide. The difference between the curves represents conversion of tyrosine to dopachrome by the enzyme.

pachrome curves with and without added hydrogen peroxide was similar (fig. 5) and aerobic dopa oxidase ('tyrosinase') isolated from this source had no ability to oxidize tyrosine.

Spectrophotometric Assay of Conversion of Tyrosine to Dopachrome by Isolated Peroxidase [12]

Without co-factor, plant peroxidase oxidized tyrosine to dopachrome at a relatively slow rate when hydrogen peroxide concentration was 10^{-2} M. This was believed to be based on autooxidation of tyrosine to small amounts of dopa, which then acted as co-factor for enzymatic hydroxylation of tyrosine. With hydrogen peroxide concentrations of 10^{-3} M or lower, peroxidase required initial dopa or dihydroxyfumaric acid as co-factor for the peroxidatic conversion of tyrosine to dopachrome. When dopa was used as co-factor, control experiments were carried out with dopa alone as substrate (fig. 7). Stoichiometric studies indicated that differential dopachrome formation recorded in the presence of tyrosine represented peroxidatic oxidation of tyrosine rather than enhancement of peroxidatic oxidation of dopa by tyrosine acting as co-factor. With tyrosine concentration constant and dopa concentration varied, differential dopachrome concentration was constant. With dopa concentration constant and tyrosine concentration varied, differential dopachrome concentration was approximately proportional to tyrosine concentration. Peroxidatic conversion of tyrosine to dopachrome in the presence of dopa cofactor was confirmed by Swan [13].

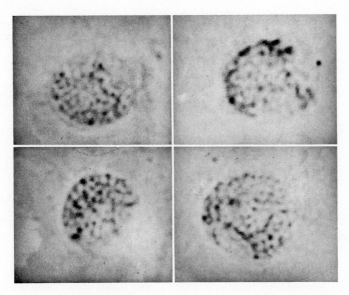

Fig. 8. Human eosinophils in unstained smear, viewed with brightfield illumination show granular pigmentation. × 2,000.

Demonstration that Preformed Melanin is a Normal Component of the Crystalloid Core of Human Eosinophil Granules [14]

Eosinophils in unstained blood smears from normal humans of Caucasoid, Mongoloid and Negroid race showed light grayish-brown granular pigment in their cytoplasm (fig. 8). The pigment had the histochemical characteristics of melanin: (a) it showed a positive Fontana-Masson silver reduction reaction; (b) it showed a positive Schmorl's reaction; (c) it showed a positive reaction with Lillie's ferrous iron uptake technique; (d) it showed basophilia with toluidine blue; (e) it was bleached with hydrogen peroxide; (f) it was non-acid fast; (g) it was not autofluorescent with ultraviolet illumination. With the electron microscopic Fontana-Masson silver reaction, the pigment was localized to the crystalloid core of eosinophil granules (fig. 9A). Specificity of this technique was increased by removal of sulfhydryl groups by preincubation with copper sulfate (fig. 9A). Melanosomes of Harding-Passey mouse melanoma, used as a control, showed a similar density of silver grains with this method (fig. 9B). It is likely that eosinophil melanin is synthesized by peroxidase in the matrix of eosinophil granules, acting alone (aerobic dopa oxidase ('tyrosinase') is

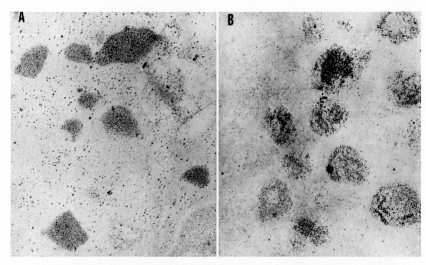

Fig. 9. A Electron micrograph of eosinophil subjected to the Fontana-Masson reducing silver reaction after pretreatment with copper sulfate shows dense aggregation of silver grains in the crystalloid core of eosinophil granules, indicating the presence of melanin. $\times$ 20,700; unstained. *B* Electron micrograph of Harding-Passey mouse melanoma cell subjected to the Fontana-Masson reducing silver reaction shows dense aggregation of silver grains in melanosomes similar to that observed in the crystalloid core of eosinophil granules. $\times$ 32,500; unstained.

not present in eosinophils). In a previous study [15], we showed that this peroxidase can convert tyrosine to melanin.

Since peroxidase is a widely distributed enzyme, its role must be suspected in the synthesis of other non-melanocytic melanins and melanin-containing pigments. We have published data supporting the role of peroxidase in neuromelanin and neuronal lipofuscin synthesis [16].

Summary

Biochemical studies with isolated mammalian 'tyrosinase' showed it to be an aerobic dopa oxidase with no ability to oxidize tyrosine.

Biochemical studies with crude melanoma preparations showed oxidation of tyrosine to be peroxidase-dependent. These studies also showed no evidence that mammalian 'tyrosinase' can oxidize tyrosine.

Spectrophotometric studies confirmed the ability of isolated peroxidase to convert tyrosine to dopachrome with dopa or dihydroxyfumarate as co-factor.

The presence of preformed melanin as a normal component of human eosinophils suggests that peroxidase, acting alone, can synthesize melanin in cells other than melanocytes.

References

1 PATEL, R.; OKUN, M.; YEE, W.; WILGRAM, G., and EDELSTEIN, L.: Inability of murine melanoma 'tyrosinase' (dopa oxidase) to oxidize tyrosine in the presence or absence of dopa or dihydroxyfumarate co-factor. J. invest. Derm. *61:* 55–59 (1973).

2 BROWN, F. and WARD, D.: Studies on mammalian tyrosinase. I. Chromatography on cellulose ion exchange agents. J. biol. Chem. *233:* 77–80 (1958).

3 RAPER, H.: The tyrosinase-tyrosine reaction. Biochem. J. *20:* 735–742 (1926).

4 POMERANTZ, S.: Separation, purification and properties of two tyrosinases from hamster melanoma. J. biol. Chem. *238:* 2351–2357 (1963).

5 EDELSTEIN, L.; CARIGLIA, N.; OKUN, M.; PATEL, R., and SMUCKER, D.: Inability of murine melanoma melanosomal 'tyrosinase' (L-dopa oxidase) to oxidize tyrosine to melanin in polyacrylamide gel systems. J. invest. Derm. *64:* 364–370 (1975).

6 PATEL, R.; OKUN, M.; EDELSTEIN, L., and CARIGLIA, N.: Peroxidatic oxidation of tyrosine to melanin in supernatant of crude mouse melanoma homogenates. Biochem. J. *142:* 441–443 (1974).

7 OKUN, M.; EDELSTEIN, L.; OR, N.; HAMADA, G., and DONNELLAN, B.: Histochemical studies of conversion of tyrosine and dopa to melanin mediated by mammalian peroxidase. Life Sci. *9:* 491–505 (1970).

8 OKUN, M.; EDELSTEIN, L.; OR, N.; HAMADA, G., and DONNELLAN, B.: The role of peroxidase vs the role of tyrosinase in enzymatic conversion of tyrosine to melanin in melanocytes, mast cells and eosinophils. An autoradiographic-histochemical study. J. invest. Derm. *55:* 1–12 (1970).

9 OKUN, M.; EDELSTEIN, L.; OR, N.; HAMADA, G.; DONNELLAN, B., and LEVER, L.: Histochemical differentiation of peroxidase-mediated from tyrosinase-mediated melanin formation in mammalian tissues. Histochemie *23:* 295–309 (1970).

10 FAHIMI, D.: Cytochemical localization of peroxidatic activity of catalase in rat hepatic microbodies (peroxisomes). J. Cell Biol. *43:* 275–288 (1969).

11 KNOX, W.: The action of peroxidases with enzymically generated peroxide in the presence of catalase. Biochim. biophys. Acta *14:* 117–126 (1954).

12 PATEL, R.; OKUN, M.; EDELSTEIN, L., and CARIGLIA, N.: Peroxidatic conversion of tyrosine to dopachrome. J. invest. Derm. *63:* 374–377 (1974).

13 SWAN, G.: Structure, chemistry and biosynthesis of the melanins. Fortschr. Chemie organ. Natur. *31:* 582 (1974).

14 OKUN, M.; DONNELLAN, B.; PEARSON, H., and EDELSTEIN, L.: Melanin: a normal component of human eosinophils. Lab. Invest. *30:* 681–685 (1974).

15 OKUN, M.; DONNELLAN, B., and PATEL, R.: Ultrastructural localization of melanin formed by peroxidatic oxidation of tyrosine in neutrophils and eosinophils. Lab. Invest. *37:* 151–155 (1972).

16 OKUN, M.; DONNELLAN, B.; LEVER, W.; EDELSTEIN, L., and OR, N.: Peroxidase-dependent oxidation of tyrosine or dopa to melanin in neurons. Histochemie *25:* 289–296 (1971).

Dr. MILTON R. OKUN, Department of Dermatology, Tufts University School of Medicine and Boston City Hospital, *Boston, MA 02111* (USA)

Pigment Cell, vol. 3, pp. 98–104 (Karger, Basel 1976)

Melanin Formation from
Adrenaline, Noradrenaline, Dopamine, and L-Dopa

McC. Goodall

Departments of Physiology and Pharmacology,
Duke University School of Medicine, Durham, N.C.

Introduction

It is generally believed that vertebrate melanin is a polyquinone and that the precursors of this quinone are specific phenols or catechols [1–10]. The most commonly cited precursors are tyrosine and L-dopa (3,4-dihydroxyphenylalanine), however, dopamine (3,4-dihydroxyphenylethylamine), noradrenaline (norepinephrine), and adrenaline (epinephrine) are also considered precursors [1–12]. The purpose of these studies is to determine the relative proportional importance of each of these precursors in the ultimate synthesis of vertebrate melanin in the human.

Methods

Four groups of subjects were selected and each group was infused with radioactive (^{14}C)-adrenaline, noradrenaline, dopamine or L-dopa. Urine was collected from each subject at various intervals up to 24 h for adrenaline and noradrenaline and continued for 120 h following the infusion of dopamine and L-dopa. Each urine sample was stored at –20 °C until assayed.

The various radioactive metabolic products in each urine sample were separated by column chromatography, identified and their radioactivity measured. The details of each infusion experiment and the separation and measurement of these radioactive metabolites has been previously described under the metabolism of adrenaline [13, 14], noradrenaline [15], dopamine [16], and L-dopa [17].

Results

DL-Adrenaline-2-¹⁴C infusion: From table I it appears that there are at least 14 metabolic products of adrenaline recovered in the urine. The principal metabolic products of adrenaline are the conjugates of the metadrenaline and 3-methoxy-4-hydroxymandelic acid (VMA, MOMA). Of the total amount of radioactivity infused $91.2 \pm 1.3\%$ was recovered within 24 h.

DL-Noradrenaline-2-¹⁴C infusion: Following an infusion of labeled noradrenaline, approximately 14 metabolic products of noradrenaline are recovered in the urine (table I). In addition, trace amounts of radioactivity are recovered as adrenaline or adrenaline metabolic products (fig. 1). The principal primary metabolic products of noradrenaline are 3,4-dihydroxymandelic acid (DOMA) and the conjugates of normetadrenaline and phenylglycol derivatives. The other metabolic products are listed in table I. $81.7 \pm 1.5\%$ of the total amount of radioactivity is recovered within a 24-hour postinfusion period and 100% within 192 h (table I) [18].

Dopamine-2-¹⁴C (3,4-dihydroxyphenylethylamine) infusion: There are 24 metabolic products of dopamine recovered in the urine (table I). Following an infusion, 75% of the circulating dopamine is converted directly into metabolic products of dopamine of which 3,4-dihydroxyphenylacetic acid (DOPAC) and its methylated product 3-methoxy-4-hydroxyphenylacetic acid (HVA) are the principal metabolites. The re-

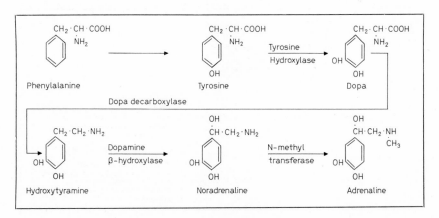

Fig. 1. Biosynthetic pathway to the formation of noradrenaline (norepinephrine) and adrenaline (epinephrine).

Table I. Excretion pattern of the metabolites and biosynthetic products of i.v. infused

Period	% of infused dose recovered	Adr.	Metadr.	Metadr. conj.	Nor.	Normet.	Normet and Nor. conj.	Dopamine	MT	Dopa	MOPEG and DOPEG
[13] Adrenaline 24 h	91.2±1.3	1.4	2.7	37.2	0	0	0	0	0	0	1.6
[15] Noradrenaline 24 h	81.7±1.5				4.3	2.5	14.7	0	0	0	tr.
[18] Noradrenaline 192 h	100.0										
[16] Dopamine 24 h	87.6±3.1	tr.			1.5	0.2	6.9	3.4	tr.		0.7
[16] Dopamine 120 h	97.2±3.5	tr.			1.5	0.3	9.3	3.4	tr.		0.8
[17] L-Dopa 24 h	71.6±3.1				tr.	tr.	tr.	16.5	2.4	1.4	
[17] L-Dopa 120 h	80.6±3.4				tr.	tr.	tr.	16.5	2.4	1.4	

Figures express the percent of the infused dose recovered. Adr., adrenaline; Metadr., metadrenaline; Metadr. conj., metadrenaline conjugate; Nor., noradrenaline; Normet., normetadrenaline; Normet. conj., normet conjugate; dopa, 3,4-dihydroxyphenylalanine; 3-M-Tyrosine, 3-methoxytyrosine; 3-MT, 3-methoxytyramine; 2-MT conj., 3-methoxytyramine conjugate; MOMA, 3-methoxy-4-hydroxymandelic acid; VA, vanillic acid; HVA, 3-methoxy-4-hydroxyphenylacetic acid; DOMA, 3,4-

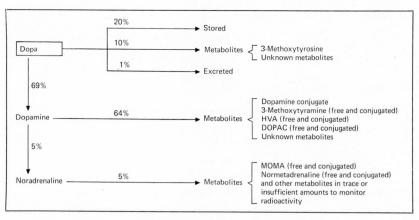

Fig. 2. Distribution of the intravenously infused L-dopa-3-^{14}C and its metabolites at 120 h postinfusion.

adrenaline-2-^{14}C, noradrenaline-2-^{14}C, dopamine-2-^{14}C, and L-dopa-3-^{14}C

3-M-Tyro.	MOMA	DOMA	3-MT	VA	MHPE and HHPE	Dopamine conj.	HVA	DOPAC	MHPE conj.	MOMA conj.	DOPAC conj.	HVA conj.	MT conj.	MOPEG and DOPEG conj.	Unk.	Number of Unk.
	22.5	1.6		1.2	2.3								0	3.2	13.8	(6)
	26.1	1.3		3.1	tr.								0	14.4	15.3	(6)
	7.7	0.6				0.7	1.5	27.5	2.0	4.2	2.1	5.9	4.8	6.3	11.6	(8)
	11.3	0.6				0.8	1.5	27.6	2.0	5.4	2.4	6.6	5.1	6.8	11.8	(8)
3.6	0.5	tr.					6.2	16.5	8.6	1.0	1.1	2.0	1.7	1.4	8.7	(16)
3.6	0.7	tr.					6.4	18.0	8.6	1.3	1.2	2.1	1.7	1.6	15.1	(16)

dihydroxymandelic acid; DOPAC, 3,4-dihydroxyphenylacetic acid; MOPEG and DOPEG, 3-methoxy-4-hydroxyphenylglycol and 3,4-dihydroxyphenylglycol; MHPE, 3-methoxy-4-hydroxyphenylethanol; HHPE, 3,4-dihydroxyphenylethanol; DOPAC conj., 3,4-dihydroxyphenylacetic acid conjugate; MOMA conj., 3-methoxy-4-hydroxymandelic acid conjugate; HVA conj., 3-methoxy-4-hydroxyphenylacetic acid conjugate; Unk., unknown metabolites.

maining 25% is synthesized into noradrenaline and appears in the urine as noradrenaline and metabolic products of noradrenaline. 87.6 ± 3.1% of the total amount of infused radioactivity is recovered in 24 h and 97.2 ± 3.5% in 120 h (table I).

L-dopa-3-^{14}C (3,4-dihydroxyphenylalanine) infusion: There are 35 metabolic products of L-dopa recovered in the urine (table I); 64% of the L-dopa is converted to dopamine, 5% to noradrenaline, 1% excreted as L-dopa and 10% as direct phenolic metabolic products of L-dopa (fig. 2). Approximately 20% of the infused radioactivity is unaccounted for and presumably stored in the sympathetic nerves and related structures, dopaminergic neurons and converted to melanin, etc. (fig. 3). 71.6 ± 3.1% of the radioactivity is recovered in 24 h and 80.6 ± 3.4% is recovered in 120 h (table I).

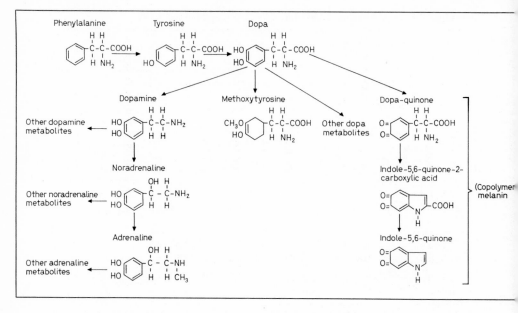

Fig. 3. Metabolic pattern of L-dopa following intravenously infused L-dopa-3-[14]C.

Discussion

Tyrosine and dopa are generally cited as the principal precursors of vertebrate melanin, albeit dopamine, noradrenaline and adrenaline are also referred to as melanin precursors [1–12]. When normal human subjects are infused with radioactive adrenaline, $91.2 \pm 1.3\%$ of the radioactivity is recovered in the urine within 24 h after the infusion as metabolic products of adrenaline (table I). Similar infusions with noradrenaline-2-^{14}C show a recovery of $81.7 \pm 1.5\%$ of the radioactivity in 24 h [15] and 100% in 192 h [18]. When studies are performed with radioactive dopamine, $87.6 \pm 3.1\%$ of the radioactivity is recovered in the urine within 24 h as dopamine biosynthetic or metabolic products, and in 120 h, $97.2 \pm 3.5\%$ of the radioactivity is recovered (table I) [16]. This, therefore, would lead one to conclude that adrenaline and noradrenaline in the human under normal conditions are not precursors of melanin and that dopamine, if at all, contributes little to the formation of melanin; only in those situations where dopamine might be converted back to L-dopa would it seem possible that any melanin might be derived from dopamine.

The situation with L-dopa as a precursor to vertebrate melanin is quite different. From figures 2 and 3 and table I, it can be seen that an undetermined amount of dopa is available for conversion to a quinone and ultimately to melanin. Following an infusion of L-dopa-3-^{14}C, even after 120 h, only 80.6 $\pm$ 3.4% of the total radioactivity was recovered in the urine as L-dopa related metabolic products (table I; fig. 2, 3) [17]. This means that approximately 20% of the radioactivity infused as L-dopa remains unaccounted for (fig. 2). Presumably some of this radioactivity is stored in the sympathetic nerves and dopaminergic neurons, but also it is quite reasonable to conclude that at least a portion is synthesized into melanin; certainly the work of SWAN [2, 6], DUCHON et al. [4, 8], HEMPEL [1], PIATELLI and NICOLAUS [3] and others [5, 7, 9] supports this conclusion.

Summary

Vertebrate melanin is a polyquinone, the precursors of which are specific phenols or catechols. Tyrosine and L-dopa are the most commonly cited precursors but dopamine, noradrenaline, and adrenaline are also considered precursors. The purpose of this study was to determine the relative proportional importance of these precursors in the human.

Normal subjects were individually infused with 100 μCi of adrenaline-2-^{14}C, noradrenaline-2-^{14}C, dopamine-2-^{14}C, and L-dopa-2-^{14}C. Urine was collected at different periods for five days. The various metabolic products found in the urine were separated by column chromatography, identified, and their radioactivity measured. Following infusion of adrenaline or noradrenaline or dopamine, approximately 90% of the radioactivity was recovered within 24 h in the urine as metabolic products; 120 h after infusion of dopamine-2-^{14}C, 97.2 $\pm$ 3.5% of the radioactivity was recovered. Since dopamine is the natural precursor of noradrenaline as well as adrenaline, the recovery of 97.2 $\pm$3.5% of the radioactivity in 120 h indicated that, under normal conditions, little or no adrenaline or noradrenaline or dopamine is incorporated in the synthesis of human melanin. In contrast, following an infusion of L-dopa-3-^{14}C, 71.6 $\pm$ 3.1% of the radioactivity is recovered in 24 h and only 80.6 $\pm$ 3.4% in 120 h. This means that approximately 20% is stored. Evidence indicates that at least part of this 20% is incorporated in the synthesis of melanin.

References

1 HAMPEL, K.: Investigation on the structure of melanin in malignant melanoma with H^3- and C^{14}-dopa labeled at different positions; in DELLA PORTA and MUHLBOCK Structure and control of the melanocyte, p. 162 (Springer, Berlin 1966).

2   SWAN, G. A.: Some studies on the formation and structure of melanins. Rend-
    ic. Accad. Sci. Fis. Mat. *31:* 1 (1964).
3   PIATTELLI, M. and NICOLAUS, R. A.: The structure of melanins and melanoge-
    nesis. I. The structure of melanin in sepia. Tetrahedron *15:* 66 (1961).
4   DUCHON, J. and MATOUS, B.: Identification of two new metabolites in mela-
    noma urine: 5-hydroxy-6-methoxyindole-2-carboxylic and 5-methoxy-6-
    hydroxyindole-2-carboxylic acids. Clin. chim. Acta *16:* 397 (1967).
5   RORSMAN, H.; ROSENGREN, A. M., and ROSENGREN, E.: Fluorimetry of a dopa
    peptide and dopa thioethers. 8th Int. Pigment Cell Conf., Sydney 1972.
6   SWAN, G. A.: Current knowledge of melanin structure. 8th Int. Pigment Cell
    Conf., Sydney 1972.
7   HINTERBERGER, H.; FREEDMAN, A., and BARTHOLOMEW, R. J.: Precursors of me-
    lanin in blood and urine of patients with malignant melanoma. 8th Int. Pig-
    ment Cell Conf., Sydney 1972.
8   DUCHON, J. and MATOUS, B.: Dopa and its metabolites in melanoma urine. 8th
    Int. Pigment Cell Conf., Sidney 1972.
9   GILBERT, F.; SKIBBA, J. L.; MCCORD, R. G.; CROFT, W. A., and FALLON, J. F.:
    Local recurrence and development of multiple primary melanomas following
    chronic oral administration of L-3,4-dihydroxyphenylalanine (L-dopa). 8th Int.
    Pigment Cell Conf., Sydney 1972.
10 DUCHON, J.; FITZPATRICK, T. B., and SEIJI, M.: Melanin. Yearbook of derma-
    tology (1968).
11 RILEY, V.: Pigmentation: its genesis and biologic control (Appleton Century
    Crofts, New York 1972).
12 KAWAMURA, T.; PITZPATRICK, T. B., and SEIJI, M.: Biology of normal and
    abnormal melanocytes (University of Tokyo Press, Tokyo 1971).
    Tokoy 1971).
13 ALTON, H. and GOODALL, McC.: Metabolic products of adrenaline (epineph-
    rine) during long-term constant rate intravenous infusion in the human. Bio-
    chem. Pharmacol. *17:* 2163 (1968).
14 SHARMAN, D. F.: The catabolism of catecholamines. Br. Med. Bull. *29:* 110
    (1973).
15 GOODALL, McC.; HARLAN, W. R., and ALTON, H.: Noradrenaline release and
    metabolism in orthostatic (postural) hypotension. Circulation *36:* 489 (1967).
16 GOODALL, McC. and ALTON, H.: Metabolism of 3-hydroxytyramine (dopamine)
    in human subjects. Biochem. Pharmacol. *17:* 905 (1968).
17 GOODALL, McC. and ALTON, H.: Metabolism of 3,4-dihydroxyphenylalanine
    (L-dopa) in human subjects. Biochem. Pharmacol. *21:* 2401 (1972).
18 GOLDSTEIN, M.; FRIEDHOFF, A. J.; SIMMONS, C., and PROCHOROFF, N. N.: Indi-
    rect evidence of synthesis of norepinephrine from 3-hydroxytyramine-1-C[14] *in
    vivo*. Proc. Soc. exp. Biol. Med. *103:* 137 (1960).

Dr. McC. GOODALL, Departments of Physiology and Pharmacology, Duke
University School of Medicine, *Durham, NC 27706* (USA)

Pigment Cell, vol. 3, pp. 105–112 (Karger, Basel 1976)

Hydroquinone Activation and Inhibition of Skin Tyrosinase[1]

Yu Min Chen and Walter Chavin

Department of Biology, Wayne State University, Detroit, Mich.

Introduction

The biochemical mechanism by which hydroquinone, a potent verte-brate melanocytolytic agent, produces depigmentation is not clear. Hy-droquinone has been considered a tyrosinase inhibitor [7] and a competi-tor with catechol as a substrate of tyrosinase [10]. The effects of hydro-quinone, quinone, and quinhydrone on skin tyrosinase were investigated to provide insight into the mechanisms responsible for tyrosinase activa-tion and inactivation.

Materials and Methods

28 black goldfish (*Carassius auratus* L) weighing 4.8 ± 0.25 g were utilized. Skin homogenate preparation and tyrosinase assay have been described previously [2]. The net enzymic activity (cpm) was the difference between the gross value (en-zyme preparation) and the control value (heat-inactivated enzyme; 100 °C, 5 min). ^{14}C-Hydroquinone replaced ^{14}C-L-tyrosine as substrate, and hydroquinone was used as the carrier, in place of L-tyrosine, in the hydroquinone utilization study. Thus, the calculated picomole conversion of substrate, either L-tyrosine or hydroquinone, from end product-^{14}C obtained is comparable to the tyrosinase unit [2]. The linear relationship between tyrosinase activity and time [2] is also present with hydroqui-none.

The tyrosinase activity of skin homogenate and fractions in the presence and ab-sence of hydroquinone, quinone and quinhydrone were determined. Further, the ef-fect of preincubation in the centrifuge tube of the homogenate sediment with and without hydroquinone upon tyrosinase activity was investigated (table III). The drug

1   Contribution Number 337, Department of Biology.

Table I. Tyrosinase activity of a pooled skin homogenate in the presence of hydroquinone, quinone and quinhydrone

Drug M		L-Tyrosine conversion pmol/5 mg skin	Activity % of normal
0 (Normal)		$1,142 \pm 10^a$	100.0
Hydroquinone	9×10^{-6}	$1,132 \pm 3$	99.2
	9×10^{-5}	$1,132 \pm 8$	90.1
	9×10^{-4}	113 ± 2	9.9
	4.5×10^{-3}	$1,774 \pm 3$	155.4
	9×10^{-3}	$3,406 \pm 13$	298.4
Quinone	9×10^{-6}	$1,708 \pm 6$	149.6
	9×10^{-5}	$2,029 \pm 11$	177.7
	9×10^{-4}	$6,274 \pm 16$	550.0
	4.5×10^{-3}	$11,794 \pm 42$	1,033.5
Quinhydrone	9×10^{-6}	$1,962 \pm 6$	171.8
	9×10^{-5}	$2,217 \pm 11$	194.5
	9×10^{-4}	$6,850 \pm 13$	600.0
	4.5×10^{-3}	$13,200 \pm 56$	1,156.2

[a] Mean $\pm$ SEM.

was directly dissolved in the enzyme preparation (sediment suspended in 0.1 M phosphate buffer, pH 6.8) and then centrifuged during preincubation. The resultant sediment was suspended in the above phosphate buffer without hydroquinone and centrifuged as above to obtain a washed sediment. The tyrosinase activities of all fractions were assayed.

The tyrosinase activity with and without hydroquinone was studied under different oxygen levels during incubation. The pO_2 was determined with a Beckman model 777 oxygen analyzer. Under standard assay conditions, the incubation tubes were loosely covered with a plastic film permitting free access of air (pO_2, 159 ± 1 mm). Oxygen supply was limited by sealing the tubes with rubber stoppers at the beginning of the incubation period (initial pO_2, 159 ± 1 mm; final pO_2, 144 ± 2 mm). Excess oxygen was supplied to other incubation tubes by flushing with oxygen for 5 min, then sealing and incubating (initial pO_2, 600 ± 3 mm; final pO_2, 560 ± 3 mm). Each of the pO_2 measurements utilized 10 assay tubes.

Results

The pH of the incubation mixture at the beginning and end of incubation remained constant (pH 6.8) despite the presence of hydroquinone,

Table II. Tyrosinase activity of enzyme preparations from a pooled skin homogenate in the presence of hydroquinone

Enzyme preparation[a]	L-Tyrosine conversion (picomoles per 5 mg skin)			
	normal	hydroquinone, M		
		9×10^{-4}	9×10^{-3}	4.5×10^{-2}
Homogenate	$1{,}373 \pm 11$[b]	123 ± 2	$1{,}776 \pm 25$	$6{,}227 \pm 30$
Sediment 1 (600 g)	663 ± 5	57 ± 2	$2{,}282 \pm 63$	$5{,}426 \pm 15$
Sediment 2 (144,000 g)	175 ± 6	156 ± 4	294 ± 10	$1{,}160 \pm 8$
Supernatant (144,000 g)	573 ± 5	0	$1{,}989 \pm 18$	$5{,}658 \pm 37$

[a] Sediment 1 was obtained by centrifugation of homogenate at 600 g (0–4 °C, 10 min). The supernatant thus obtained was centrifuged at 144,000 g (0–4 °C, 40 min) to obtain sediment 2 and the final supernatant.
[b] Mean ± SEM.

Table III. Tyrosinase activity of particulate tyrosinase (sediment of homogenate at 600 g, 0–4 °C, 10 min) preincubated with and without hydroquinone

Enzyme fractions[a]	L-Tyrosine conversion, pmol/5 mg skin			
	normal (preincubated in buffer)	preincubation with hydroquinone, M		
		9×10^{-4}	9×10^{-3}	4.5×10^{-2}
Sediment (800 g, 15 min) preincubated and washed	100 ± 2[b]	578 ± 11	710 ± 12	867 ± 14
Supernatant 1	62 ± 2	355 ± 8	$1{,}039 \pm 22$	$1{,}733 \pm 21$
Supernatant 2	0	0	19 ± 1	166 ± 3
Total activity	162	933	1,768	2,766
% Normal		580	1,091	1,713

[a] The particulate was suspended (0–4 °C, 40 min) in 0.1 M phosphate buffer, pH 6.8 with and without hydroquinone. The centrifugation (800 g, 15 min) was performed during incubation in the centrifuge tube. At the end of incubation-centrifugation, the original sediment was separated into sediment and supernatant 1. The sediment was suspended in phosphate buffer only and centrifuged (800 g, 0–4 °C, 15 min) again to obtain the washed sediment and supernatant 2 (washing).
[b] Mean ± SEM.

Table IV. Inhibition and activation of skin tyrosinase by hydroquinone as a function of oxygen availability

Hydroquinone concentration M	Standard assay condition		Oxygen restriction		Excess oxygen	
	L-tyrosine conversion pmol/5 mg skin	% normal	L-tyrosine conversion pmol/5 mg skin	% normal	L-tyrosine conversion pmol/5 mg skin	% normal
0 (normal)	1,142	100.0	1,085	100.0	689	100.0
4.5×10^{-7}	1,208	105.8	1,208	111.3	689	100.0
4.5×10^{-6}	1,227	107.4	1,208	111.3	481	69.9
4.5×10^{-5}	1,000	87.6	944	87.0	443	64.4
9.0×10^{-5}	1,028	90.1	821	75.7	311	45.2
1.8×10^{-4}	774	67.8	396	36.5	283	41.1
4.5×10^{-4}	198	17.4	160	14.8	887	128.8
9.0×10^{-4}	113	9.9	245	22.6	1,528	221.9
4.5×10^{-3}	1,774	155.4	1,066	98.3	7,416	1,076.7
9.0×10^{-3}	3,406	298.4	2,481	228.7	11,973	1,738.4

quinone or quinhydrone at any level used. Thus, possible changes in tyrosinase activity resulting from a pH shift were eliminated.

Skin tyrosinase activity was inhibited at low hydroquinone concentration, but activated at high hydroquinone concentration. For example, in one experiment, the normal tyrosinase activity (pM L-tyrosine converted/5 mg skin) was 2320 ± 256 (X $\pm$ SEM), but in the presence of 9×10^{-4} M hydroquinone, the activity was reduced to 405 ± 56 or 16.8% normal. However, in the presence of 9×10^{-3} M and 4.5×10^{-2} M hydroquinone, L-tyrosine conversion increased to $3,560 \pm 687$ (153.3%) and $5,590 \pm 766$ (240.9%), respectively. Similar results were obtained with a pooled skin homogenates and fractions (tables I, II).

Hydroquinone exerted inhibitory and activating effects on both particulate and soluble tyrosinase fractions. Preincubation of particulate tyrosinase with hydroquinone resulted in activation (table III).

In contrast to hydroquinone, quinone and quinhydrone produced only activation of tyrosinase at all concentrations tested (table I). This activation was greater than that of hydroquinone and increased with increase in drug concentration.

Table V. Utilization of labeled hydroquinone and labeled L-tyrosine by skin tyrosinase

Group	Substrate[a]	Concentration (M) of ^{14}C substrate	Net enzymic activity[b]
I	ULT	2.2×10^{-4}	$1,151 \pm 20$[c]
II	HQ	1.7 ± 10^{-4}	$20,130 \pm 450$
III	HQ	2.2×10^{-4}	$22,168 \pm 480$
IV	HQ	3.4×10^{-4}	$27,887 \pm 560$
V	HQ	5.1×10^{-4}	$27,710 \pm 270$
VI	HQ	6.8×10^{-4}	$27,762 \pm 510$
VII	HQ+T	1.7×10^{-4}	$8,538 \pm 60$
VIII	HQ+T	2.2×10^{-4}	$9,480 \pm 50$
IX	HQ+T	6.8×10^{-4}	$28,034 \pm 120$

[a] ULT = Uniformly labeled ^{14}C-L-tyrosine (spec. act. = 0.329 mCi/mmol); T = L-tyrosine (2.2×10^{-4} M); HQ = ^{14}C-hydroquinone-2, 3, 5, 6 (spec. act. = 0.159 mCi/mmol).
[b] Expressed as picomole conversion of ^{14}C substrate per 5 mg skin.
[c] Mean ± SEM.

The effects of hydroquinone on skin tyrosinase was modified by available oxygen (table IV). Under standard conditions, hydroquinone inhibition was maximal at 9×10^{-4} M and activation began at 4.5×10^{-3} M. Under conditions of restricted oxygen, maximum inhibition occurred at 4.5×10^{-4} M and activation now appeared at 9×10^{-3} M. With excess oxygen, maximal inhibition which was much less than that produced under normal or restricted oxygen conditions, occurred at a lower concentration (1.8×10^{-4} M). Despite lower normal values, the activation also appeared at a lower concentration and was greater than in the two former conditions. Tyrosinase activation was enhanced even further with higher concentrations of hydroquinone.

Skin tyrosinase utilized labeled hydroquinone (table V). Substrate saturation was reached at 3.4×10^{-4} M hydroquinone. Hydroquinone utilization was 19-fold greater than tyrosine (groups I and III) at the same molar concentration of ^{14}C-substrates. Tyrosine appeared to inhibit the utilization of hydroquinone at 1.7×10^{-4} M and 2.2×10^{-4} M, but not at 6.8×10^{-4} M. The small degree of tyrosine competition was probably reversed by the relatively high concentration of hydroquinone (6.8×10^{-4} M).

Discussion

The effects of hydroquinone in skin tyrosinase preparations are complex. Solutions of hydroquinone, quinone and quinhydrone are reversibly interconvertible through the semiquinone intermediate [12]. Quinhydrone formation from hydroquinone and quinone in phosphate buffer has been demonstrated [6]. Thus, the effects of hydroquinone on tyrosinase activity represent the total effects of three compounds in different proportions. Further, endogenous factors appear to be present in the skin enzyme preparations, inhibitors of tyrosinase which may react preferentially with quinone and accelerators of the oxidative melanogenic steps initiated by quinone. In addition, hydroquinone, quinone or quinhydrone, may liberate tyrosinase from the particulate state or convert the inactive enzyme into the active enzyme. Finally, hydroquinone, quinone and quinhydrone inhibit partially purified mushroom tyrosinase [6].

In skin enzyme preparations, hydroquinone inhibits tyrosinase activity at lower concentrations and activates the enzyme at higher concentrations. Quinone and quinhydrone greatly activate tyrosinase activity at all concentrations tested. Tyrosinase activation by high concentrations of hydroquinone may result from a high yield of quinone and quinhydrone. Since hydroquinone, quinone and quinhydrone inhibit comparatively purified mushroom tyrosinase, the skin enzyme preparations appear to contain endogenous factor(s), which may facilitate the quinone-initiated oxidative steps in melanogenesis.

The inhibitory effect of hydroquinone at lower concentrations may result from (a) reducing property of hydroquinone as reducing agents inhibit melanin formation [3, 7], (b) hydroquinone competition for oxygen with tyrosinase in the oxidative steps in the melanogenic pathway, as oxygen restriction reduces the hydroquinone concentration necessary for maximal inhibition and excess oxygen enhances the tyrosinase activity at lower hydroquinone concentration, and (c) hydroquinone competition with tyrosine as a substrate for tyrosinase.

Reduction of the maximal inhibitory effect and the enhancement of the activating effect of hydroquinone on skin tyrosinase is accomplished with increased oxygen tension. At low hydroquinone concentrations, a small degree of activation occurs only under the normal and the restricted oxygen conditions. This may result from the dopa-like catalytic action of hydroquinone on the tyrosine-dopa conversion at such concentrations.

The release of tyrosinase activity by preincubation of particulate ty-

rosinase with hydroquinone and by incubation of skin enzyme preparations in the presence of high levels of hydroquinone is interesting. The
washed sediment after preincubation with hydroquinone shows no inhibitory effect. Despite the presence of hydroquinone in supernatant 1 (table
III), tyrosinase activity was readily detectable and increased above the
control level. Such release of tyrosinase activity by hydroquinone may be
useful in the preparation of tyrosinase from tissue.

The presence of endogenous tyrosinase inhibitors in skin and melanomas have been reported. Various naturally occurring compounds ranging from reducing agents [3] to proteins [5] may be considered *in vivo* inhibitors of tyrosinase. Enhancement of tyrosinase activity may occur by
inactivation of the inhibitors [3, 4, 8, 11], labilization of melanosomal
membranes [1, 5, 9, 11], conversion of inactive protyrosinase into active
tyrosinase [8], and thermal agitation [1]. However, the activation of fish
skin tyrosinase by hydroquinone at high concentration is a type of activation previously unreported. Such activation may involve inhibitor-inhi-
bitor reactions, membrane-labilization and/or conversion of protyrosinase
into active tyrosinase. Resolution of the complex hydroquinone activation
and inhibition mechanisms may be achieved only by isolation and purification of the enzyme and endogenous factors concerned.

Summary

Studies of hydroquinone action *in vitro* have revealed that hydroquinone at
low concentrations inhibits, but at high concentrations activates, black goldfish skin
tyrosinase. The inhibitory effects of hydroquinone appear to be related to hydroquinone competition for oxygen with tyrosinase for oxidative steps in the melanogenic pathway and hydroquinone competition with tyrosine as a substrate for tyrosinase. The activation of fish skin tyrosinase may result from quinone formation during incubation, labilization of the particle membrane, and/or conversion of protyrosinase into active tyrosinase. Both ^{14}C-L-tyrosine and ^{14}C-hydroquinone were utilized
by fish skin tyrosinase.

References

1   CHEN, Y. M.: Thermal activation and inactivation of melanin formation in ver-
    tebrate skins and melanomas. J. invest. Derm. *64:* 77–79 (1975).
2   CHEN, Y. M. and CHAVIN, W.: Radiometric assay of tyrosinase and theoretical
    considerations of melanin formation. Analyt. Biochem. *13:* 234–258 (1965).

3   CHEN, Y. M. and CHAVIN, W.: Effects of depigmentary agents and related compounds upon *in vitro* tyrosinase activity; in RILEY Pigmentation: its genesis and control, pp. 593–606 (Appleton Century Crofts, New York 1972).

4   CHEN, Y. M. and CHAVIN, W.: Tyrosinase activity in a highly pigmented human melanoma and a negro skin. Proc. Soc. exp. Biol. Med. *145:* 695–697 (1974).

5   CHEN, Y. M. and CHAVIN, W.: Melanogenesis in human melanomas. Cancer Res. *35:* 606–612 (1975).

6   CHEN, Y. M. and CHAVIN, W.: Unpublished data.

7   LERNER, A. B. and FITZPATRICK, T. B.: The control of melanogenesis in human pigment; in GORDON Pigment cell growth, pp. 319–333 (Academic Press, New York 1953).

8   McGUIRE, J. S.: Activation of epidermal tyrosinase. Biochem. biophys. Res. Commun. *40:* 1084–1089 (1970).

9   MENON, I. A. and HABERMAN, H. F.: Activation of tyrosinase in microsomes and melanosomes from B-16 and Harding-Passey melanomas. Archs Biochem. Biophys. *137:* 231–242 (1970).

10 MILLER, W. H.; MALLETTE, M. F.; ROTH, L. J., and DAWSON, C. R.: A new method for the measurement of tyrosinase catecholase activity. II. Catecholase activity based on the initial reaction velocity. J. Am. Chem. Soc. *66:* 514–519 (1944).

11 SEIJI, M.: Enzymatic digestion of smooth surfaced membrane of mouse melanoma. J. Biochem. *63:* 670–674 (1968).

12 WEBB, J. L.: Quinones; in WEBB Enzyme and metabolic inhibitors, vol. 3, pp. 421–594 (Academic Press, New York 1966).

Dr. WALTER CHAVIN, Department of Biology, 5104 Second, Wayne State University, *Detroit, MI 48202* (USA)

Pigment Cell, vol. 3, pp. 113–120 (Karger, Basel 1976)

Tyrosinase as Glycoprotein

Kazuhiro Miyazaki and Noriko Ohtaki

Department of Dermatology, Tokyo Medical and Dental University, Tokyo

Introduction

One of the most reliable and useful methods to elucidate the mechanism of melanization is an immunochemical method. Many attempts have been made to isolate and purify tyrosinase from melanoma and other sources, and multiple forms of the enzymes have been demonstrated [1, 3, 11].

Recently, Burnett [3] has reported the presence in mouse melanoma of two soluble tyrosinases (T1 and T2). They show definite differences in molecular weight, amino acid composition, and electrophoretic mobility. We have reported a highly purified tyrosinase preparation from mouse melanoma melanosome [8], which showed only one active component consistent with that of T1. Antiserum against this enzyme was obtained [9]. In our previous paper, both T1 and T2 tyrosinases were partially purified from 11,000 g supernatant fraction, mainly to obtain a T2 tyrosinase preparation [10]. We described with emphasis that despite a definitive difference of isoelectric points and difference of molecular weights between tyrosinase T1 and T2, they have quite similar immunologic and enzymic properties. It is indispensable, therefore, for further immunochemical studies to clarify the relation of both T1 and T2 tyrosinases and characterize their properties precisely.

The present paper deals with our attempts to clarify the possible factors responsible for such a definitive difference of isoelectric points.

Materials and Methods

Harding-Passey mouse melanoma was serially transplanted into a strain of Swiss mice. The entire actively growing melanoma was excised when it had developed to about 2.0 cm in diameter and the tumor was either used immediately or frozen.

Tyrosinase T1 was purified from melanosomes by the method of MIYAZAKI and SEIJI [8]. Tyrosinase T2 was partially purified from the microsomal and soluble fraction of melanoma according to the method of our previous paper [9]. Tyrosinase was solubilized with trypsin (twice crystallized type III) purchased from the Sigma Chemical Co., St Louis, Missouri. The enzyme preparation was concentrated with Diaflo Ultrafiltration membrane PM 30 (Amicon Corporation) which was operated under nitrogen at 80 psi.

Tyrosinase activity was determined colorimetrically [12] with L-dopa (1 μmol/ml) as substrate in 0.1 M potassium buffer, pH 6.8, in a total volume of 1.0 ml in cuvette with a 1-cm light path. The optical density was determined with Beckman spectrophotometer, model 24. The rate of change in absorbancy at 475 nm was scanned with a recorder; the molar absorbancy coefficient of dopachrome is 3,600 [7]. A unit of enzyme was expressed according to the international unit. Protein was determined according to LOWRY et al. [6].

Neuraminidase from *Clostridium perfringens* was obtained from Boehringer Mannheim Corporation (Germany).

Acrylamide gel electrophoresis was carried out according to the method of DAVIS [4]. Electrophoresis equipment was manufactured by Mitsumi Kagaku Co., Tokyo. Electrophoresis was carried out at 3 mA per gel. The distribution of enzymes was stained with Amido Black [4]. The carbohydrate component in gel was stained according to ZACHARIUS et al. [13] with periodic acid-Shiff's reagent (PAS).

Results

Treatment of T1 Tyrosinase with Neuraminidase

Purified tyrosinase T1 was incubated with neuraminidase either with or without Ca++, because there is a report that neuraminidases from different sources are activated, inhibited, or not influenced by Ca++ ions. This effect is also reported to be substrate-dependent [5]. The experiment was, therefore, carried out as described in table I. The results showed that no significant incubation effect was caused by 5×10^{-3} M Ca++.

After incubation at 37 °C for 5 h, the samples were immediately transferred to ice-cold boxes or frozen until required. Repeated freezing and thawing of the samples were not recommended, because of decomposition of the enzyme. Samples of No. 1 (incubated with Ca++ and neuraminidase) and No. 3 (incubated with neuraminidase) were subjected to gel filtration, G-100 super fine, 1.5×30 cm, in order to exclude neuraminidase fraction from tyrosinase. Fractions of 1.0 ml were collected. Protein was measured at 280 nm. Tyrosinase was determined colorimetrically. Both blue dextran 2000 and phenol red were eluted as marker substances, which were measured at 620 and 470 nm, respectively. As shown in figure 1, neuraminidase was clearly separated from the tyrosinase fraction.

Table I

No.	Tyrosinase[1] ml	Buffer[2], ml		Neurami- nidase[3], ml	Water	Total tyrosinase activity, mU
		Ca(+)	Ca(−)			
1	0.1	0.1		0.2		9.6
2	0.1	0.1			0.2	9.0
3	0.1		0.1	0.2		9.5
4	0.1		0.1		0.2	9.5
5	0.1				0.3	9.8

1 Tyrosinase in 20 mM phosphate buffer; 100 mU/ml.
2 0.1 M phosphate-citrate buffer, pH 6.0. Ca(+) means that the buffer contained 20 mM CaCl₂.
3 Neuraminidase was dissolved (1 mg/2 ml) in the same buffer.

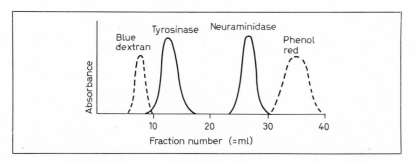

Fig. 1. G-100 gel filtration to exclude neuraminidase from incubation mixture. The column, 1.5×30 cm, was equilibrated with 20 mM phosphate-citrate buffer, pH 6.0. Each sample was applied on top of the column. Fractions of 1.0 ml were collected Protein was measured at 280 nm. Tyrosinase activity was determined colorimetrically. Blue dextran and phenol red were measured at 620 and 470 mn, respectively.

Decrease in Anodic Mobility of T1 Tyrosinase by Treatment with Neuraminidase

Each sample described above was subjected to disc electrophoresis. After electrophoresis, detection of the separated substances were carried out by staining with L-dopa (for tyrosinase activity), Amido Black (for protein) and PAS (for carbohydrate), respectively. Both samples No. 1 and No. 3 showed essentially the same distribution patterns following electrophoresis. Three samples, No. 2, 4, and 5, showed identical patterns. Accordingly, gel of No. 1 (neuraminidase-digested samples) and No. 5 (incubated controls) were demonstrated in figure 2. As shown here, if purified T1 tyrosinase was incubated with neuraminidase, the T1 tyrosinase band (dopa-stained) was transformed into a new electrophoretically slower-moving form without its original enzymic activity (A to a). The staining band of protein was also converted into one less acidic, retaining its color intensity (C to c), which was completely consistent with the dopa-stained band.

The most fascinating results are demonstrated in PAS staining of gels. The staining bands of original purified tyrosinase T1 was split off into the three slower-moving bands. The other two were much slower-moving bands, and completely free of peptide and enzymic activity. These two simple sugar components were not separated from complexed glycoprotein moiety during the gel filtration procedure, but clearly separated

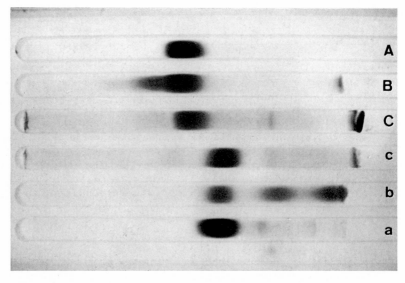

Fig. 2. Acrylamide gels of both purified native tyrosinase T1 (A, B, C) and neuraminidase-treated T1 tyrosinase (a, b, c). A and a = Tyrosinase patterns stained with L-dopa (dark brown); 2 mU of tyrosinase were applied on both gels. B and b = PAS-stained (violet); 100 mU of tyrosinase were applied on both gels. C and c = Protein-stained with Amido Black (dark blue); 50 mU of tyrosinase were applied on both gels. Right = Cathode; left = anode.

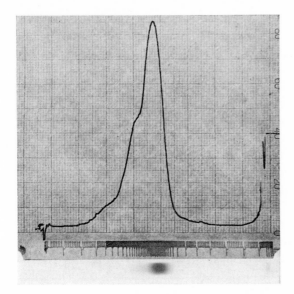

A

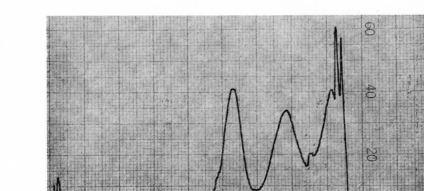

B

Fig. 3. Densitometer traces of carbohydrated components in both purified native T1 tyrosinase (A) and neuraminidase-treated T1 tyrosinase (B). The preparations having identical tyrosinase activity (both A and B = 100 mU), were applied to gels and electrophoresis was carried out, followed by staining with PAS. Densitometric scans were carried out at 570 nm.

on disc electrophoresis. This result suggested that neuraminidase-split sugar components were presumably electrostatically attached to the tertiary structure of the glycoprotein molecule with tyrosinase activity.

Quantitative Scans of the PAS-Positive Bands

Quantitative scans of PAS-stained bands on the gels were carried out with Fujiox densitometer FD-A IV at 570 nm. As shown in figure 3, the integrated densitometric value of native T1 tyrosinase was 400, and those of neuraminidase-treated sample separated into three bands were 103, 117, and 175, respectively, and the total of those three was 395, which was almost equal to that of the single PAS-stained band of native tyrosinase T1.

This result means that the carbohydrate moiety of T1 tyrosinase has been split quantitatively into three, one of which is a glycoprotein with tyrosinase activity. This glycoprotein contains carbohydrate residues bound to amino acid residues of polypeptide, for example, serine and aspargine, etc., forming relatively stable carbohydrate-peptide linkages. The other two sugar groups contained sialic acids presumably free of peptide chain.

Discussion

Multiple forms of tyrosinase have been reported in mammalian melanomas since 1950s [1, 3, 11]. BURNETT [2, 3] isolated two forms of tyrosinase, which she designated T1 and T2. T1 and T2 were reported to have similar molecular weights, but to be different in amino acid composition, and not to undergo interconversion.

Recently, we reported that only one form of soluble tyrosinase could be purified from the melanosomes of Harding-Passey mouse melanoma which corresponded to T1 tyrosinase described by BURNETT [3], and reported also that in contrast to the melanosomal fraction, 11,000 g supernatant fraction contained both T1 and T2 tyrosinases. In the same paper, we stated that T1 and T2 tyrosinases had similar enzyme characteristics and completely identical antigenic properties [10], which suggested fairly common amino acid sequences, especially at their antigenic sites. We stressed that, despite these similarities, there was a definitive difference in the isoelectric points of the 2 forms of tyrosinase.

A recent paper by JUTISZ and DE LA LLOSA [5] stated that fundamental differences between some isoenzymes, previously believed due to different electrophoretic mobility, may lie in their different contents of sialic acid groups. The acidic forms were thus shown to have decreased their electrophoretic mobilities after treatment with neuraminidase and conversion into the basic forms giving similar patterns on electrophoresis. They stated also that the catalytic and antigenic properties were essentially retained after removal of sialic acid.

In the present paper, purified T1 tyrosinase was shown, by the treatment with neuraminidase, to have decreased its mobility but retained its original tyrosinase activity. These facts strongly suggest that T1 tyrosinase is an acidic glycoprotein containing sialic acid groups that can be removed by neuraminidase, and that it also contains, as shown in figure 3, presumably neutral sugars which were not attacked by neuraminidase.

It seems a reasonable interpretation that the large difference in isoelectric points and the small difference in molecular weights of T1 and T2 tyrosinases are mainly ascribable to their different contents of carbohydrate residues, especially sialic acids, though we would have appreciated some contribution of protein moieties to such a difference. It is true that neuraminidase-treated T1 tyrosinase and native T2 have very similar electrophoretic mobilities and enzymic characteristics, but the detailed molecular configuration of both tyrosinases still remain to be clarified.

Further sugar and peptide analysis of T1 and T2 tyrosinases, using sufficient amounts of highly purified tyrosinase, must be carried out for the elucidation of this problem.

Summary

Purified tyrosinase T1 was incubated with neuraminidase. The catalytic activity of tyrosinase was essentially retained, after this treatment. The tyrosinase band (dopa-stained) was transformed into a new less anodic form, similar to tyrosinase T2, on disc electrophoresis. The band of protein was also converted to the same position as the dopa-stained.

On the other hand, the single PAS-stained band of native tyrosinase T1 was split into three slower-moving bands. One was consistent with the dopa- and protein-stained band. The other two were much slower and completely free of peptide and enzymic activity. The PAS-densitometric value of native tyrosinase T1 was almost equal to the sum of the three separated bands.

These results suggest that the large difference in isoelectric points and the small difference in molecular weights of both T1 and T2 tyrosinase are mainly ascribable to their different contents of carbohydrate residues, especially sialic acid groups.

References

1 BROWN, F. C. and WARD, D. N.: Studies on mammalian tyrosinase. I. Chromatography on cellulose ion exchange agents. J. biol. Chem. *233:* 77–80 (1958).

2 BURNETT, J. B.; SEILER, H., and BROWN, I. V.: Separation and characterization
of multiple forms of tyrosinase from mouse melanoma. Cancer Res. *27:*
880–889 (1967).

3 BURNETT, J. B.: The tyrosinase of mouse melanoma. J. biol. Chem. *246:*
3079–3091 (1971).

4 DAVIS, B. J.: Electrophoresis. II. Method and application to human serum protein. Ann. N.Y. Acad. Sci. *121:* 404–427 (1964).

5 JUTISZ, M. and LLOSA, P. DE LA: Glycoproteins as hormones and as enzymes; in Glycoproteins: their composition, structure and function (Elsevier,
Amsterdam 1972).

6 LOWRY, O. H.; ROSENBROUGH, N. J.; FARR, A. I., and RANDALL, R. J.: Protein
measurement with Folin phenol reagent. J. biol. Chem. *66:* 265–275 (1951).

7 MASON, H. S.: The chemistry of melanin. III. Mechanism of oxidation of dihydroxyphenylalanine by tyrosinase. J. biol. Chem. *172:* 83–99 (1948).

8 MIYAZAKI, K. and SEIJI, M.: Tyrosinase isolated from mouse melanoma melanosome. J. invest. Derm. *57:* 81–86 (1971).

9 OHTAKI, N. and MIYAZAKI, K.: Antiserum against tyrosinase from mouse melanoma. J. invest. Derm. *58:* 238–241 (1972).

10 OHTAKI, N. and MIYAZAKI, K.: Immunologic homogeneity and electrophoretic
heterogeneity of mouse melanoma tyrosinases. J. invest. Derm. *61:* 339–343
(1973).

11 POMERANTS, S. H.: Separation and properties of two tyrosinases from hamster
melanoma. J. biol. Chem. *238:* 2351–2357 (1963).

12 POMERANTS, S. H. and PEH-CHEN, LI, J.: Tyrosinases (hamster melanoma); in
Methods in enzymology, vol. 17A (Academic Press, New York 1970).

13 ZACHARIUS, R. M.; ZELL, T. E.; MORRISON, J. H., and WOODLOCK, J. J.: Glycoprotein staining following electrophoresis on acrylamide gels. Analyt. Biochem.
30: 148–152 (1969).

KAZUHIRO MIYAZAKI, MD, Department of Dermatology, School of Medicine,
Tokyo Medical and Dental University, 1-5-45, Yushima, Bunkyo-ku, *Tokyo* (Japan)

Pigment Cell, vol. 3, pp. 121–126 (Karger, Basel 1976)

Particulate and Soluble Tyrosinases of Human Malignant Melanoma[1]

KENJI NISHIOKA and MARVIN M. ROMSDAHL[2]

Departments of Surgery, Surgical Research Laboratory and Biochemistry, The University of Texas System Cancer Center M. D. Anderson Hospital and Tumor Institute, Houston, Tex.

Introduction

The enzyme tyrosinase (o-diphenol:O_2 oxidoreductase, EC 1.10.3.1) is considered to be a key enzyme in melanogenesis, controlling the initiation of a sequence of reactions converting tyrosine to the complex insoluble pigment polymer, melanin. Pigment control mechanisms appear to escape control in malignant melanoma and, while alternative factors may be wholly or partially responsible, attention has focused principally on tyrosinase due to its prominent role. A majority of biochemical investigations concerning tyrosinase have utilized enzyme derived from bacterium, plant and animal sources [1, 2, 4, 8, 10, 11]. Unlike plants and bacteria which contain only soluble tyrosinase, mammalian tissue contains active tyrosinase in both naturally soluble and insoluble particulate forms. Studies of mammalian tyrosinases have been generally conducted on the soluble form of the enzyme, which usually accounts for 20% or less of total enzyme activity. 80% or more of enzyme obtained after melanoma tissue homogenization is of a particulate nature [4] and has not been easily released in soluble form. Investigations of human tyrosinase are very scarce, due in part to the lesser availability of human melanoma tumor material for re-

1 This investigation was supported by the Robert A. Welch Foundation Grant No. G-548 and USPHS Grant CA 05831.
2 The authors appreciate the excellent technical assistance of P. K. TROSTLE and E. FAUSTO.

search purposes. However, BURNETT and SEILER [3], using an extract of human melanoma homogenate, showed that there were two kinds of soluble tyrosinase (T^1 and T^2) as well as insoluble tyrosinase (T^3) with polyacrylamide gel electrophoresis. Following treatment of the particulate fraction of disrupted human melanoma cells with lipase, CHEN [5] reported that tyrosinase thus solubilized was very similar to the naturally soluble enzyme in regard to activity and gel electrophoresis patterns. We have attempted to solubilize the particulate enzyme by detergents without using enzymatic digestion, to obtain the intact form of tyrosinase. This report concerns the nature of the particulate form of tyrosinase obtained from human malignant melanoma by detergents and sonication and its potential relationship to the soluble form of the enzyme.

Materials and Methods

Human melanoma tissue is acquired by surgical excision from patients with widespread metastasis or at autopsy. For these particular experiments, melanotic melanoma tissue was obtained postmortem from metastatic deposits in the liver. Tumor material was sliced and stored at –20 °C prior to the thawing and purification of enzyme.

Particulate fraction containing small and large granules was obtained according to SEIJI et al. [12]. 16 g of human malignant melanoma tumor was homogenized in isotonic sucrose solution, pH 7.1. The homogenate was centrifuged at 700 g. The supernatant thus obtained was further centrifuged at 143,000 g for 1 h to obtain the particulate fraction, contained in the resulting pellet. The ratio between soluble and particulate tyrosinases is usually 1:4 or less.

Tyrosinase activity was measured by two methods. The first method, a modification of the procedure described by POMERANTZ and LI [9], measures 3,4-dihydroxphenylalanine (dopa) oxidation spectrophotometrically at 475 nm. A sample of the enzyme is incubated at room temperature in 0.1 M sodium phosphate buffer, pH 6.8, with 0.005% gelatine (USP, Curtin) and 1 mM dopa (Schwarz/Mann) in a cuvette with a total volume of 1 ml and a 1-cm light path. The rate of change in absorbancy at 475 nm is recorded for the first 2 min. The second method employed concerns a measurement of tyrosine hydroxylation as described by POMERANTZ and LI [9] with slight modifications. The reaction mixture contains the following for each 1.5 ml:3,5-^{3}H-L-tyrosine (1.6 μCi), L-tyrosine (1 μmol), 17.5 μg gelatine and enzyme. The mixture is incubated with occasional shaking at 37 °C; the reaction is stopped by adding 1.15 ml of 50% TCA. To measure ^{3}HOH, the reaction mixture was mixed with 150 mg charcoal (Norit A, MC & B). After standing for 15 min at room temperature, the mixture was filtered through EH Millipore filter. The filter was washed with water. Washings were combined with the filtrate and the volume adjusted to 10 ml. 1 ml was taken, mixed with 10 ml Aquasol (New England Nuclear) and counted in a Packard Tri-carb Scintillation Spectrometer.

Acrylamide gel electrophoresis was run according to DAVIS [6], using a standard Tris-glycine system. For this study, 3.5% spacer gels and 7% running gels were utilized. 3 mA for each column was applied for the gel electrophoresis. For activity, gels were stained with 0.3% dopa in 0.1 M sodium phosphate buffer, pH 6.8. The dopa-stained gels were traced at 475 nm with a gel scanner (Vicon Industries, Inc.) and a linear logarithmic intergrating recorder (Brinkman, W+W) attached to Zeiss spectrophotometer.

Results

Solubilization of particulate tyrosinase was attempted by freezethawing, sonication and lastly by the detergents Triton X-100 and deoxycholate. The particulate fraction obtained from human malignant melanoma tissue was treated by the above methods. Freeze-thawing and sonication were totally ineffective as determined by tyrosinase activity in the 143,000 g supernatant. However, treatment of the particulate fraction with the detergents, Triton X-100 and deoxycholate-combined with sonication, released 100% of activity into 143,000 g supernatant. This solubilized tyrosinase, following ammonium sulfate fractionation and Sephadex G-200 chromatography, yielded a single active peak which was active with both substrates, dopa and ^{3}H-tyrosine. The active fraction was examined by 7% acrylamide gel electrophoresis (fig. 1). Solubilized tyrosinase moved through the 3.5% spacer gel but did not migrate into the 7% gel, suggesting a very high molecular weight for this active component. However, we were also able to observe a smaller fast-migrating tyrosinase band which migrated into the 7% gel and showed a Rf value of 0.5. Since a molecule of this size should have been eliminated by the previous Sephadex G-200 column chromatography, it suggested that this smaller fast-migrating tyrosinase was formed by the action of some contaminating proteases. Therefore, in order to examine the susceptibility of this solubilized tyrosinase to a protease, we incubated two aliquots of this fraction, one with trypsin and the other without trypsin at 4 °C overnight. Both samples were then examined by 7% gel electrophoresis. The results are shown in figure 1. The sample on the right, incubated with trypsin, showed augmentation of the fast-migrating tyrosinase after reacting with dopa. These gels, when traced using a densitometer at 475 nm (fig. 2), clearly indicated that trypsin released the smaller tyrosinase from the larger detergent-solubilized tyrosinase.

The naturally soluble tyrosinase fraction was also compared with this

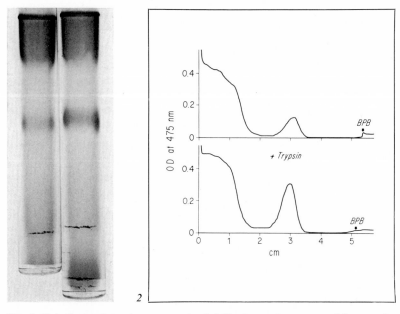

Fig. 1. Gel electrophoresis pattern of solubilized tyrosinase treated by trypsin. Particulate tyrosinase was solubilized by detergents and partially purified by ammonium sulfate fractionation and Sephadex G-200 column chromatography. 0.2 ml of the enzyme solution, containing 20 μg of protein, was incubated in 0.01 M Tris-HCl buffer pH 7.4 with 0.5% Triton X-100 overnight at 4 °C with and without 1 μg of trypsin. These samples were examined by 7% polyacrylamide gel and stained by dopa to locate enzyme activities as described in Methods. The right gel depicts the gel pattern of solubilized tyrosinase treated with trypsin. The left sample was a control, indicating solubilized tyrosinase which was not treated by trypsin. The gels were run from the top (cathode) to the bottom (anode).

Fig. 2. Gel scanning pattern of trypsin-treated solubilized tyrosinase. The gels shown in figure 1 were traced at 475 nm. The above pattern was obtained from the left gel (control) in figure 1, the lower profile was derived from trypsin-treated solubilized tyrosinase.

smaller trypsin-released enzyme. Results indicated that the small tyrosinase thus obtained corresponds to T^1 tyrosinase as described by BURNETT and SEILER [3] from its Rf value of 0.5. This enzyme form is one of the most dominant tyrosinases in the soluble tyrosinase fraction. Our findings suggest that soluble tyrosinase (T^1) in the homogenate of human malignant melanoma may result from proteolysis of the particulate form of tyrosinase.

Discussion

Particulate tyrosinase, solubilized by detergents and sonication, has been found to yield a smaller fast-migrating tyrosinase which appears to correspond to one of the naturally soluble forms of this enzyme (T^1). In addition, treatment of the larger particulate enzyme form with trypsin augmented the development of the faster migrating tyrosinase. Treatment of human malignant melanoma homogenate with a serine protease inhibitor, phenylmethylsulfonyl fluoride, appears to block the release of the smaller tyrosinase.

Evidence that cathepsins are not responsible for the breakdown of particulate tyrosinase is afforded by the following considerations. Most cathepsins are not sensitive to phenylmethylsulfonyl fluoride. Since the pH during our purification procedures was kept at neutral, where cathepsins are not active, contaminating proteases would not appear to be typical lysosomal proteases.

Mechanisms which relate the relationship between particulate intracellular tyrosinase with the soluble enzyme are not known at this time. Purification of naturally soluble tyrosinase from human malignant melanoma will permit one to compare such a form with the one released by trypsin. Our findings are compatible with the results obtained by CHEN [5] who found that lipase-solubilized, particulate tyrosinase was very similar to the naturally soluble enzyme in regard to activity and gel electrophoresis pattern. Both investigations support our interpretation of the dynamic transition of the particulate form of tyrosinase to the soluble form.

HABERMAN and MENON [7], using the B-16 mouse melanoma system, showed that melanoma-bearing mice have circulating tyrosinase in their sera and that the circulating enzyme was of the soluble form. It may be found that tyrosinase in serum may represent soluble tyrosinase released from particulate tyrosinase by proteolytic action during melanoma cell destruction.

Summary

Particulate tyrosinase was solubilized by Triton X-100 and deoxycholate combined with sonication and then partially purified. Evidence is presented which indicates that particulate tyrosinase, which is bound to melanosomes, will yield soluble enzyme by treatment with trypsin. This soluble enzyme appears to correspond to one of the most dominant of the naturally soluble forms previously characterized.

Since soluble tyrosinase is a minor part of total tyrosinase activity in most mammalian systems, our findings suggest that soluble tyrosinase might be a proteolytic product of particulate tyrosinase.

References

1 BALASINGAM, K. and FERDINAND, W.: The purification and properties of a ribonucleoenzyme, *o*-diphenol oxidase, from potatoes. Biochem. J. *118:* 15–23 (1970).
2 BARISAS, B. G. and McGUIRE, J. S.: A proteolytically activated tyrosinase from frog epidermis. J. biol. Chem. *249:* 3151–3156 (1974).
3 BURNETT, J. B. and SEILER, H.: Multiple forms of tyrosinase from human melanoma. J. invest. Derm. *52:* 199–203 (1969).
4 BURNETT, J. B.: The tyrosinases of mouse melanoma. J. biol. Chem. *246:* 3079–3091 (1971).
5 CHEN, Y. M.: Solubilization and activation of mammalian melanoma particulate tyrosinase by lipase digestion. Cancer Res. *34:* 3192–3196 (1974).
6 DAVIS, B. J.: Disc electrophoresis. II. Method and application to human serum proteins. Ann. N. Y. Acad. Sci. *121:* 404–427 (1964).
7 HABERMAN, H. F. and MENON, I. A.: Presence and properties of tyrosinase in sera of melanoma-bearing animals. Acta derm.-vener., Stockh. *51:* 407–412 (1971).
8 MAKINO, N.; McMAHILL, P.; MASON, H. S., and MOSS, T. H.: The oxidation state of copper in resting tyrosinase. J. biol. Chem. *249:* 6062–6066 (1974).
9 POMERANTZ, S. H. and LI, J. P.-C.: Tyrosinase (hamster melanoma); in TABOR and TABOR Methods in enzymology, vol. 17, pp. 620–626 (Academic Press, New York 1970).
10 POMERANTZ, S. H. and LI, J. P.-C.: Purification and properties of tyrosinase isozymes from hamster melanoma. Yale J. Biol. Med. *46:* 541–552 (1973).
11 POMERANTZ, S. H. and MURTHY, V. V.: Purification and properties of tyrosinases from *Vibrio tyrosinaticus*. Archs Biochem. Biophys. *160:* 73–82 (1974).
12 SEIJI, M.; SHIMAO, K.; BIRBECK, M. S. C., and FITZPATRICK, T. B.: Subcellular localization of melanin biosynthesis. Ann. N. Y. Acad. Sci. *100:* 497–533 (1963).

Dr. KENJI NISHIOKA, Surgical Research Laboratory - RI 409, The University of Texas System Cancer Center, M. D. Anderson Hospital and Tumor Institute, 6723 Bertner Avenue, *Houston, TX 77030* (USA)

Pigment Cell, vol. 3, pp. 127–137 (Karger, Basel 1976)

Effect of Irradiation on Tyrosinase Isozymes Activity in Mammalian Pigment Cells

K. TODA, T. KOBORI, F. MORIKAWA, K. OKAZAKI, M. UZUKA and F. FUKUDA

Department of Dermatology, Tokyo Teishin Hospital, Tokyo, and Shiseido Laboratories, Yokohama

Introduction

Certain furocumarins, commonly called psoralens, are used in the treatment of pigmentary disorders, such as vitiligo, and to increase the tolerance of skin to solar radiation. In the presence of long-wave UV radiation (320–400 nm), these substances induce a reversible cutaneous photosensitivity manifested by augmented sunburn reaction and subsequent hyperpigmentation [6]. It has been clearly demonstrated that exposure of Caucasoid skin to long-wave UV light after administration of psoralens resulted in an increase in pigmentation of skin and in the average size of the melanosomes. Also, the distribution pattern of melanosomes within keratinocytes was changed from aggregated form to single, discrete, non-aggregated form, because the size of the melanosome is the determining factor of the distribution pattern of melanosomes within keratinocytes [7].

Recently, NAKAYAMA et al. [5] suggested that melanin pigmentation of mammalian skin can be stimulated by long-wave UV light after administration of 4,5′,8-trimethylpsoralen (TMP) without inducing any recognizable phototoxic reactions, such as erythema, edema, vesiculation and bulla-formation.

The purpose of this study is to investigate the photobiologic effects of long-wave UV light in the presence of TMP on the mammalian pigmentary system both *in vivo* and *in vitro*, using melanocytes in guinea pig epidermis and melanocytes in a mono-layer cell culture system.

Materials and Methods

1. In vivo *Study*

Adult brown guinea pigs were used. After epilation the animals received 35.0 mg/kg body weight of TMP. 2 h after administration of TMP, animals were exposed to the black light (energy dose; 8.0×10^7 erg sec/cm²). Seven days after irradiation, specimens were taken from the exposed area. Specimens were fixed with 2.5% glutaraldehyde in 0.1 M cacodylate buffer for 2 h, washed with 0.1 M cacodylate buffer, fixed again with 1% osmium tetroxide in 0.1 M cacodylate buffer, then embedded in Epon 812, and observed with a Hitachi HU 12 electron microscope.

2. In vitro *Study*

Small skin specimens were obtained from adult brown guinea pig ears. The specimens were incubated in 1% trypsin solution for 30 min at 37 °C. The epidermis was separated from the dermis and then squeezed, shaken and pulled about with fine forceps. The resulting cell suspension was centrifuged at 1,000 rpm for 5 min. The sediment was resuspended in Eagle's MEM supplemented with 20% fetal bovine serum. The cells were grown in 35 mm in diameter Falcon tissue culture dishes, of which inside surface had been precoated with Epon 812. Seven days later, when the culture had been established, 0.05 μg/ml TMP was added to the culture medium and then cells were exposed to long-wave UV light (energy dose; 8.0×10^6 erg sec/cm²). Soon after the exposure, the culture medium was changed to regular Eagle's MEM.

a) Electron Microscopy

The cells were fixed, as they were, in Petri dishes with 2.5% glutaraldehyde and 2% osmium tetroxide in 0.06 M veronal acetate buffer pH 7.2 containing 4.5% sucrose for 20 min at 4 °C, and 3, 12, 24, 72 h after the exposure. They were then washed with 50% ethanol, and counterstained with uranylacetate solution for 10 min, then dehydrated with graded series of ethanol. The resulting cells were infiltrated in 50% Epon 812 in ethanol for 30 min before final embedding. The thin sections were examined with a Hitachi HU-12 electron microscope.

b) Acrylamide-Gel Electrophoresis

At 12, 24 and 72 h after exposure, cells were homogenized with a Potter-Elvehjem glass homogenizer in 4–5 ml of 0.25 M sucrose, respectively. Each homogenate was centrifuged for 30 min at 20,000 *g* and 0 °C. Aliquots of the supernatant were then subjected to acrylamide-gel electrophoresis according to the methods of Davis [3] with the exceptions that the upper and lower bath buffers were not diluted and the sample gel was omitted; the enzyme preparation was layered directly on top of the spacer gel. After electrophoresis, gels were neutralized with 1 M phosphate buffer, pH 6.7, 30 min and the multiple forms of tyrosinase visualized by incubation in a solution of 0.1 M phosphate buffer, pH 6.8, containing 0.15% L-dopa, for several hours.

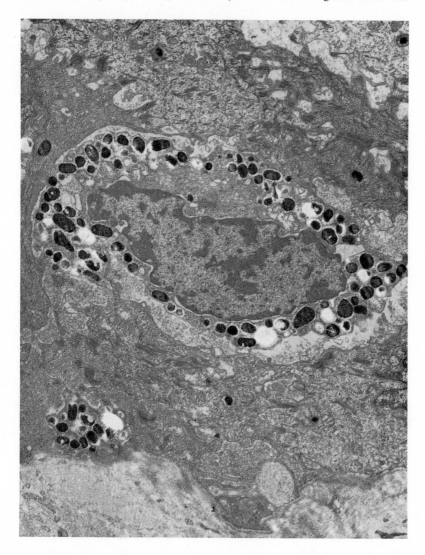

Fig. 1. A melanocyte in the treated site showing fully melanized melanosomes and well-developed membranous system.

Results

1. In vivo *Study*

An electron micrograph of a melanocyte taken from the pigmented area and without any evidence of erythema reaction after TMP administration and long-wave UV light exposure, showed remarkable changes, such as many fully melanized melanosomes, melanosomes in different stages of development and well-developed membranous system in the cytoplasm (fig. 1). An electron micrograph taken from the untreated control area showed a melanocyte which had very few barely recognizable melanosomes, many thick microfilaments around the nucleus and poorly developed membranous systems; in the adjacent keratinocytes, a few melanosomes could be observed (fig. 2).

2. In vitro *Study*

a) Electron Microscopy

72 h after exposure, melanocytes as well as keratinocytes from the culture exposed to long-wave UV light following addition of TMP to the culture medium, were apparently darker than those from control cultures (fig. 3, 4). It was clearly demonstrated by electron microscopy that melanosomes in different stages of development and well-developed membranous systems could be observed in the melanocytes from the treated culture, but not in those from the control culture (fig. 5, 6). This suggests that long-wave UV light exposure following addition of TMP to the culture medium can induce melanogenesis in melanocytes in monolayer cell culture.

b) Acrylamide-Gel Electrophoresis

Tyrosinase extracted from the culture cells at 24 h after UV exposure following the addition of TMP to culture medium was found to exist in as many as 2 distinct molecular forms (T_1, T_2), separable by acrylamide-gel electrophoresis. The location of the diverse tyrosinases in acrylamide-gel was demonstrated by deposition of dark melanin pigment at restricted sites on incubation in dopa reagent. Tyrosinase extracted from the control culture cells was found to exist in only one fast-moving separable band (T_1). Figure 7 shows activity patterns of tyrosinase from cultured cells. Marked (a) is acrylamide-gel electrophoresis of tyrosinase from the control culture cells, showing only one broad band. Marked (b) is acrylamide-gel electrophoresis of tyrosinases from cultured cells after exposure

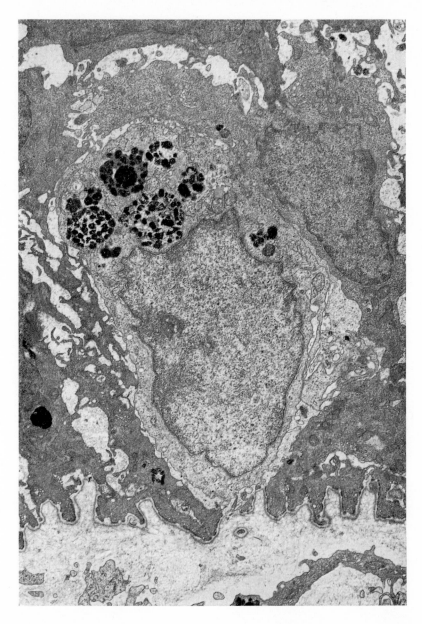

Fig. 2. A melanocyte in the untreated control site showing bearly recognizable melanosomes which appear to be autophagosomes, thick aggregation and microfilaments around a nucleus and poorly developed membranous system.

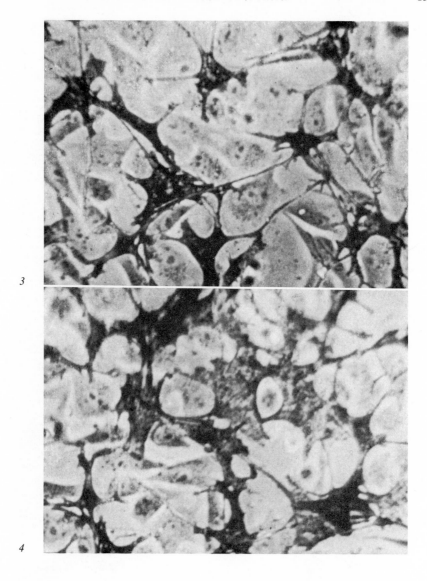

Fig. 3, 4. In the culture 72 h after exposure to long-wave UV light following the addition of TMP to the culture medium, melanocytes as well as keratinocytes (fig. 3) were apparently darker than those (fig. 4) in the control culture.

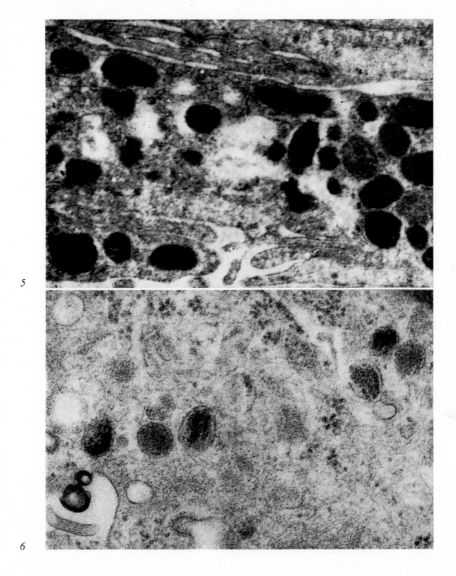

Fig. 5. A melanocyte from the treated culture showing many melanosomes in different stages of development. 72 h after the exposure of long-wave UV light following addition of TMP to the culture medium.

Fig. 6. A melanocyte from the control culture showing a few melanosomes in a poorly developed stage.

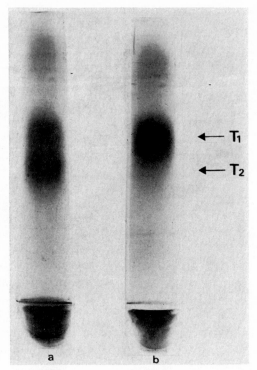

Fig. 7. Acrylamide-gel electrophoresis patterns: left, tyrosinase extracted from the control culture, T_1 can be found; right, tyrosinase extracted from the treated culture, T_1 and T_2 can be found.

to long-wave UV light following addition of TMP to the medium, showing two distinct broad bands.

It appears that exposure to long-wave UV light after the addition of TMP to the culture medium results in new synthesis of tyrosinase in the melanocytes in the cell culture system, because tyrosinase extracted from all active melanocytes, which are synthesizing melanosomes, is found to exist in as many as 3 distinct molecular forms (T_1, T_2, T_3), separable by acrylamide-gel electrophoresis.

Discussion

It has been believed that the epidermal melanocyte-keratinocyte pool, known as the epidermal melanin unit, serves as a structural and functional unit for the understanding of variation in skin color and hyper-pigmentation stimulated by psoralen [6]. In our study, however, not only the epidermal melanin unit but also melanocytes in monolayer cell culture system can be stimulated by psoralen and long-wave UV light irradiation.

The augmentation of melanin pigmentation in the normal epidermis, *in vivo*, by topical or oral administration of psoralens like TMP and exposure to long-wave UV light involves the close interaction of melanocytes and keratinocytes. During this process, increases are observed in: (1) tyrosinase activity in melanocytes; (2) number of functional melanocytes as the result of proliferation; (3) number of melanosomes in melanocytes as well as in keratinocytes; (4) number of melanosomes transferred from melanocytes to keratinocytes as the result of more rapid synthesis of melanosomes in melanocytes, and (5) the size of melanosomes which determine the distribution pattern of melanosomes within keratinocytes; large melanosomes distributed as single, discrete, and non-aggregated form as in Negroid epidermal keratinocytes, and small melanosomes distributed as an aggregated group form like melanosomes in Caucasoid epidermal keratinocytes. In the epidermis of brown guinea pig skin, we observed changes of the epidermal melanin unit similar to that of Caucasoid skin after administration of TMP and long-wave UV light irradiation.

In the mono-layer cell culture system, however, we could only observe increases in tyrosinase activity, the number of melanosomes synthesized in melanocytes, and the number of melanosomes transferred from melanocytes to keratinocytes.

These different results between conditions *in vivo* and *in vitro* seem to depend on the different interrelationship between melanocytes and keratinocytes, i.e. organized cell structure in the epidermis, and unorganized cell structure in the mono-layer cell culture. It may be necessary for control of the size of melanosomes to exist in both melanocytes and keratinocytes in the organized structure of the epidermis.

It is well-known that multiple forms of tyrosinase are present in crude extracts of mammalian pigment cells and that these tyrosinases are separated into 3 typical forms by acrylamide-gel electrophoresis [2, 4]. There are two soluble tyrosinases called T_1 and T_2 and an insoluble membrane-bound tyrosinase called T_3.

T_2 appears first in the newborn skin or during hair cycle of the black C-57 mouse; T_3 and T_1 appear next; T_2 disappears earlier than T_3; T_1 is demonstrable for a long period. Incorporation of ^{3}H-amino acids into T_1, T_2 and T_3, using Cain's method for the radioactivity of ^{3}H-protein in acrylamide-gel, shows that T_2 is the first labeled, T_3 is second, and T_1 is last. The peak of radioactivity among the three fractions moves from T_2 to T_3 and to T_1. Finally, radioactivity can be found in T_1 but not in T_2 and T_3. It is suggested that T_2 is the precursor of T_3 and T_1, and T_3 is the precursor of T_1; T_2 is tyrosinase in the process of being synthesized; T_3 is a membrane-bound form which is active in catalyzing melanin synthesis *in vivo*, and T_1 is an inhibited form *in vivo* because it is covered by layered melanoprotein in the melanosome, but it is easily extracted or inactivated [8].

The presence of T_2 band in acrylamide-gel electrophoresis of tyrosinase extracted from the cells after addition of TMP and the exposure of the cell culture system to long-wave UV light, suggests that the exposure to long-wave UV light and addition of TMP can stimulate melanin synthesis in the melanocyte in mono-layer cell culture. These data also suggest that pigment synthesis can be stimulated by UV light exposure and psoralen administration without any recognizable phototoxic reaction, and that skin pigmentation can be induced by UV light exposure and psoralen administration without any erythema reaction.

Under both *in vitro* and *in vivo* conditions, psoralens photoreact with native DNA, forming C_4-cycloaddacts with pyrimidine bases. Besides this monofunctional photoaddition reaction, psoralen can photoreact as bifunctional reagents and give interstrand cross-linkage in the native DNA of epidermal cells. Repair synthesis of UV-damaged DNA following psoralen administration and UV irradiation can be demonstrated in normal epidermal cells in about 12–20 h, but not in those from xeroderma pigmentosum [1]. Additional investigations revealed that bleomycin and other drugs also inhibit the repair synthesis of photo-damaged DNA and increase pigmentation after UV irradiation [9]. It may be speculated that photo-damage of DNA is closely related to the pigmentation of the skin but this relationship has not yet been clearly demonstrated.

Summary

Cells from brown guinea pig ears were grown in mono-layer cell culture system with 0.05 μg of TMP and exposure to the long-wave ultraviolet light. In the control culture, T_3 and T_1 were present and T_2 was weakly demonstrable. In the treated culture, however, T_2 was strongly demonstrable, and an increase in numbers of melanosomes could be observed with electron microscopy. These results suggest that tyrosinase and melanin synthesis in the melanocyte can be stimulated by psoralen and ultraviolet light irradiation in the mono-layer cell culture system.

References

1 BADEN, H. P.; PARRINGTON, J. M., and DELHANTY, J. D. A.: DNA synthesis in normal and xeroderma pigmentosum fibroblasts following treatment with 8-methoxypsoralen and longwave ultraviolet light. Biochim. biophys. Acta 262: 247–255 (1972).

2 BURNETT, J. B.; HOLSTEIN, T. J., and QUEVEDO, W. C., jr.: Electrophoretic variations of tyrosinase in follicular melanocytes during the hair growth cycle in mice. J. exp. Zool. 171: 369–373 (1969).

3 DAVIS, B. J.: Disc electrophoresis. II. Methods and application to human serum protein. Ann. N. Y. Acad. Sci. 121: 404–427 (1964).

4 HOLSTEIN, T. J.; BURNETT, J. B., and QUEVEDO, W. C., jr.: Genetic regulation of multiple forms of tyrosinase in mice. Action of a and b loci. Proc. Soc. exp. Biol. Med. 126: 415–418 (1967).

5 NAKAYAMA, Y.; MORIKAWA, F.; FUKUDA, M.; HAMAO, M.; TODA, K., and PATHAK, M. A.: Monochromatic radiation and its application laboratory studies on the mechanism of erythema and pigmentation induced by psoralen; in PATHAK et al. Sunlight and man, p. 591 (University of Tokyo Press, Tokyo 1974).

6 PATHAK, M. A.; KRÄMER, D. M., and FITZPATRICK, T. B.: Photobiologic and photochemistry of furocoumarins; in PATHAK et al. Sunlight and man, p. 335 (University of Tokyo Press, Tokyo 1974).

7 TODA, K.; PATHAK, M. A.; PARRISH, J. A.; FITZPATRICK, T. B., and QUEVEDO, W. C., jr.: Alteration of racial differences in melanosome distribution in human epidermis after exposure to ultraviolet light. Nature new Biol. 236: 143–145 (1972).

8 TODA, K.; BURNETT, J. B., and FITZPATRICK, T. B.: Biologic function of isoenzymes of tyrosinase in mammalian pigment cells. J. invest. Derm. 58: 260 (1972).

9 TODA, K.; IKEMURA, I.; MORIKAWA, F.; NAKAYAMA, Y., and PATHAK, M. A.: The size of the melanosome and photo-damage of DNA. Yale J. Biol. Med. 46: 428 (1973).

K. TODA, MD, PhD, Department of Dermatology, Tokyo Teishin Hospital, 2-14-23, Fujimi, Chiyoda-Ku, Tokyo (Japan)

Pigment Cell, vol. 3, pp. 138–151 (Karger, Basel 1976)

Acid Phosphatase Activity during Pigment Transfer in Three Genotypes of the Fowl [1]

ROGER R. BOWERS and GARY T. TANOUYE [2]

Department of Biology, California State University, Los Angeles, Calif.

Introduction

In the regenerating breast feather of the fowl, two developmental processes are evident: feather growth or keratinization, and melanization. During feather growth, the basal keratinocytes form a collar from which the rachis (shaft) and barb ridges differentiate. The feather melanocytes, initially located in the dermal papillae below the collar, divide and migrate towards the barb ridge apex. From this position, the melanocytes produce and transfer pigment to the differentiating barb ridge cells which will form the barbs and barbules of the definitive feather [29].

The process of pigment transfer in the fowl has previously been described [30] and closely resembles the same process found in mammalian epidermis *in vivo* [21, 22, 24, 26, 28, 31, 34] and *in vitro* [4, 9, 18, 19, 27]. Generally, the transfer process consists of the following four steps: (1) invagination of the tip of the melanocyte process into the epithelial cell; (2) incorporation of the tip of the melanocyte process into the epithelial cell; (3) transformation of the incorporated process into a melanosomal complex [11], and (4) dissolution of the melanosomal complex and dispersion of melanosomes within the cytoplasm of the epithelial cell [19, 30].

By definition, the melanosome complexes are analogous to the phagosomes of phagocytic cells and have been shown to contain acid hydro-

1   This work was supported in part by CSULA Institutional Grant A4028914.
2   The authors are extremely grateful to Dr. JOHN A. BRUMBAUGH who supplied the three Fowl genotypes and to Mr. JOSE APODACA for his excellent technical assistance.

lases in mammals [12, 14, 18, 23, 24, 32, 34, 37] and in the fowl [5]. Based on this, WOLFF and HÖNIGSMAN [34] concluded that melanosome complexes and single melanosomes within keratinocytes represent secondary lysosomes.

If the transferred pigment granules stimulate phagolysosome formation, would the lysosomal response vary if the chemical composition of the melanin granule differed? The present investigation was performed in an attempt to answer this question.

Materials and Methods

A. Materials

Pigment transfer in regenerating breast feathers of adult wild-type, pink-eye, and albino-like males was examined. Wild-type males ($+E/+E$, $+Pk/+Pk$, $+C/+C$) have black breast feathers, pink-eye males (E/E, pk/pk, $+C/+C$) have gray feathers, and albino-like males (ey/ey, $+Pk/+Pk$, c/c) have white feathers. These genotypes are distinguished ultrastructurally in that the wild-type melanocyte produces a fully melanized melanosome (stage IV), the pink-eye melanocyte produces a partially melanized melanosome (stages II, III), and the albino-like melanocyte produces premelanosomes that contain no apparent melanin (stage I). Stocks are maintained by Dr. JOHN A. BRUMBAUGH in the School of Life Sciences, University of Nebraska-Lincoln. The wild-type stock is of the junglefowl origin [8]. The pink-eye stock was previously described [6] and the albino-like effect is due to the presence of the recessive white (c) mutation [15]. All feathers used in this investigation were from homozygotes. Henceforth, the three tissue genotypes will be designated as wild-type, pink-eye, and albino-like.

B. Methods

14 day-old regenerating breast feathers of the three genotypes, wild-type, pink-eye, and albino-like, were carefully plucked and immediately placed in a solution of 3% glutaraldehyde in 0.1 M cacodylate buffer, pH 7.3. Dissection was immediately begun in the fixative solution. Each feather was split longitudinally along the forming rachis or primordial shaft. The central feather pulp was then removed and each piece was placed outer sheath down and the barb ridges removed from the sheath by carefully sliding a probe between the two structures. Thus, 2 tissue pieces, approximately 7 mm long, were obtained from each feather and consisted primarily of barb ridges.

After the 2-hour fixation period, the barb ridge tissues were rinsed 5 times (10 min each) in a cold 10% sucrose solution in 0.1 M cacodylate buffer. After routine rinsing in sucrose, the tissues were incubated for 2 h at 37 °C in the Gomori medium as modified by BARKA and ANDERSON [3], but with the omission of the ammonium sulfide step. Control feather pieces were treated exactly the same except the substrate (sodium glycerophosphate) for the enzyme, acid phosphatase, was omitted in the incubation medium. Distilled water was then used to bring the medium to the correct volume.

After incubation, postfixation was accomplished by placing the tissues in buffered 2% osmium tetroxide for 1 h (pH 7.3). After washing in buffer, the pieces were stained 10 min in a 2% uranyl acetate solution and then carefully dehydrated in a graded series of ethyl alcohol solutions. After the alcohol was replaced by propylene oxide, the tissues were embedded in an Epon-812 mixture. The blocks were cast in flat silicone embedding molds so that the pieces could be oriented for convenient sectioning.

1-μm, 'thick' sections were made in the pre-barb ridge area of the tissue until the barb ridges first appeared. These 'thick' sections were mounted on glass slides and stained with 1% toluidine blue in 1% borax solution. They provided information regarding the earliest level or site in each genotype where pigment transfer occurred in substantial amounts. Sections were made using a Porter-Blum MT-2 ultramicrotome equipped with diamond knives. The previously stained sections were viewed and photographed with a RCA-EMU3-G electron microscope at 50 kV.

To perform the determination of the area of acid phosphatase activity in the intact cell, a calibrated transparency overlay was made with each square equal to 0.1 μm^2. The negatives, which were all taken at a magnification of 7,500×, were photographically enlarged 4× for a total of 30,000×. Thus, the overlay was calibrated for this particular magnification and carefully placed over the printed electron micrograph. The data was determined from 20 cells of each of the 3 genotypes studied. Acid phosphatase activity is given as the ratio between the area of enzymatic activity either associated with the granules or cytoplasmic to the total area of cytoplasm of the host keratinocyte.

Results

Pigment transfer in the wild-type regenerating feather occurred in substantial amounts approximately 100 μm distal to the area where the barb ridges first formed. The ultrastructure of a typical wild-type feather melanocyte at this level is shown in figure 1. Three stages of melanosome formation are evident: the fully melanized stage IV melanosome (m, fig. 1); the partially melanized stage III premelanosome (pm, fig. 1); and the protein backbone stage II [33] premelanosome (arrow, fig. 1). In ma-

Fig. 1. Wild-type melanocyte incubated in Gomori medium for acid phosphatase. × 47,500.

Fig. 2. Wild-type keratinocyte containing transferred melanosomes incubated in Gomori medium for acid phosphatase. × 19,100.

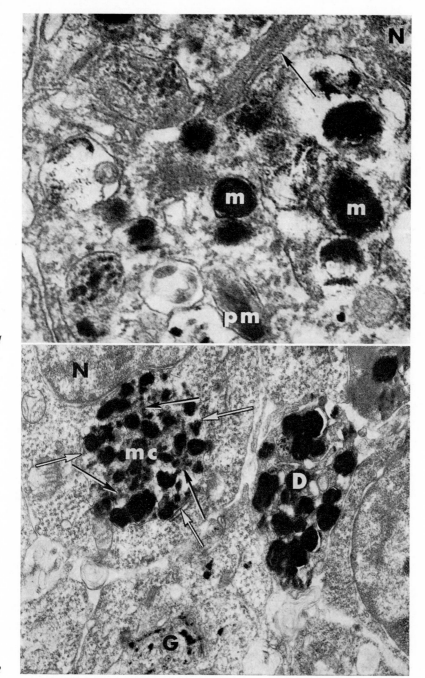

ture melanocytes of this genotype, stage IV melanosomes were the dominant type present. Acid phosphatase activity was found in the Golgi complex and scattered lysosomes, but little or no reaction product was observed associated with the developing melanosomes.

Figure 2 illustrates the presence of acid phosphatase in wild-type keratinocytes at the same level as figure 1. Acid phosphatase was located in several areas within the cytoplasm of these cells. As might be expected, it is present in the Golgi complex (G, fig. 2) of the cells. In an adjacent cell, however, it is associated with a melanosome complex (mc, fig. 2) which had been phagocytized by the keratinocyte from a melanocyte. Enzyme activity is located around these pigment granules (black arrows, fig. 2). The membranes of the individual melanosomes and the outer one around the melanosome complex appear to be broken or missing (white arrows, fig. 2). The melanosomes themselves are irregular in shape with acid phosphatase reaction product located at their edges.

Melanosomes in a melanocyte dendrite (D, fig. 2), located next to the keratinocyte just described, do not show this enzyme activity and serve as a control. The pigment granules are more regular in shape and do not show obvious acid phosphatase produced precipitate. Control sections did not visibly illustrate the enzyme and the melanosomes appeared normal as in the dendrite of figure 2.

Pigment transfer in the pink-eye regenerating feather occurred in substantial amounts approximately 175 μm distal to the area where the barb ridges first formed. Stage III premelanosomes (pm, fig. 3) are the dominant type present in the pink-eye melanocyte at this level as shown in figure 3. Surrounding the partially melanized premelanosomes are numerous vesicles and dilated rough endoplasmic reticulum. Slight amounts of acid phosphatase activity were seen in the rare Golgi complexes, but no enzymatic activity was seen associated with the melanosomes.

Figure 4 illustrates the presence of transferred melanosomes in the pink-eye keratinocyte at the same level as figure 3. Acid phosphatase activity was observed both in the cytoplasm (Golgi complex and lysosomes) and associated with the melanosomes (m, fig. 4). The enzymatic activity

Fig. 3. Pink-eye melanocyte incubated in Gomori medium for acid phosphatase. × 40,000.

Fig. 4. Pink-eye keratinocyte containing transferred melanosomes incubated in Gomori medium for acid phosphatase. × 33,750.

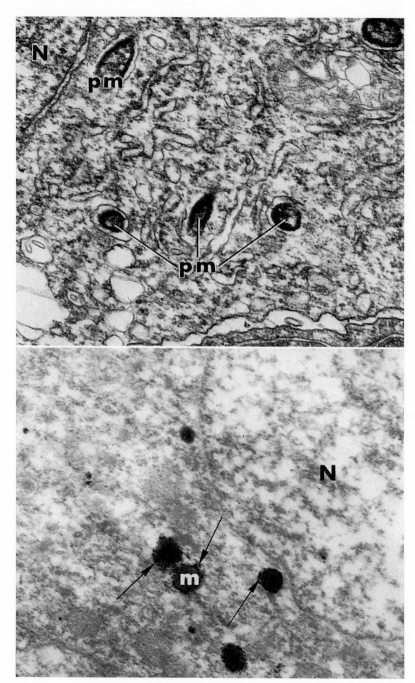

3

4

(arrows, fig. 4) is scattered around the melanosomes which in cross-section appear more dense than they really are. In longitudinal sections, they resembled the premelanosomes shown in figure 3. Control sections did not show enzymatic activity and the melanosomes appeared as in figure 3.

Pigment transfer in the albino-like regenerating feather occurred in substantial amounts approximately 225 μm distal to the area where the barb ridges first formed. The ultrastructure of a typical albino-like melanocyte at this level is shown in figure 5. The cell has an abundance of Golgi complexes in which acid phosphatase activity is found (arrows, fig. 5). The premelanosomes (pm, fig. 5) are of the stage I [33] variety in that they consist of membrane-bound spherical vesicles. No acid phosphatase activity was observed associated with these premelanosomes.

Figure 6 shows an albino-like keratinocyte from the same level as in figure 5. No acid phosphatase activity is observed associated with the premelanosome complex (pmc, fig. 6), and the double membrane (arrow, fig. 6) created by phagocytosis is still intact around the premelanosome complex. Cytoplasmic acid phosphatase activity is present, however, in the Golgi complex (G, fig. 6). Control sections appeared identical to the experimental with the exception of no demonstrated cytoplasmic acid phosphatase activity.

Before analyzing the quantitative results of acid phosphatase activity, it was necessary to compare the amount of melanosome transfer in each of the three genotypes studied. There was little or no difference between the number of transferred melanosomes observed between the wild-type and the pink-eye keratinocytes. However, the number of transferred premelanosomes observed in the albino-like keratinocyte was reduced significantly to approximately one half of that in the other two genotypes.

The data for the number of transferred melanosomes is summarized in table I.

The results of the calibrated levels of acid phosphatase activity for each genotype is summarized in table II. Interactions between granule-associated enzymatic activity and cytoplasmic (nongranule) enzymatic activity were significant for all 3 genotypes studied. Thus, the presence (as shown in the wild-type and pink-eye keratinocyte) or absence (as shown

Fig. 5. Albino-like melanocyte incubated in Gomori medium for acid phosphatase. $\times 25,000$.

Fig. 6. Albino-like keratinocyte containing transferred melanosomes incubated in Gomori medium for acid phosphatase. $\times 25,000$.

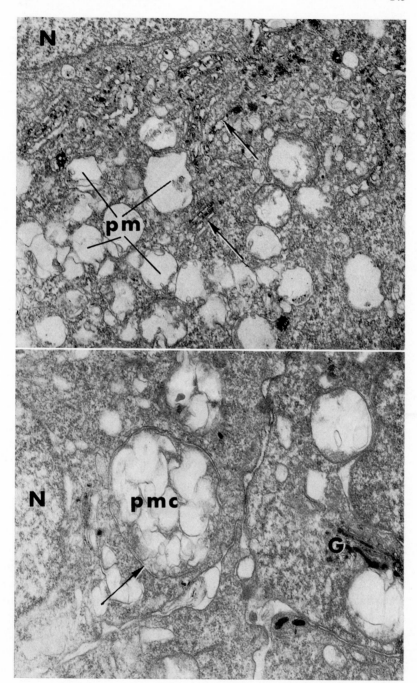

5

6

Table I. Number of transferred pigment granules

Genotype	Total number of transferred granules	Number of identical area samples	Standard mean ± SD
Pink-eye	237	20	11.85 ± 5.78[+]
Albino-like	123	20	6.15 ± 3.06[+],[*]
Wild-type	232	20	11.60 ± 6.49[*]

The differences within the pairs of values marked [+],[*] are significant (p<0.01).

Table II. Levels of acid phosphatase activity in the three genotypes

Genotype	Location of activity	Total enzyme activity[1]	Number of identical area samples	Standard mean ± SD
Wild-type	granule	0.937	20	0.047 ± 0.025[*]
	nongranule			
	cytoplasm	0.057	20	0.003 ± 0.005[*]
Pink-eye	granule	0.106	20	0.005 ± 0.004[**]
	nongranule			
	cytoplasm	0.022	20	0.001 ± 0.002[**]
Albino-like	granule	0.000	20	0.000 ± 0.000[***]
	nongranule			
	cytoplasm	0.159	20	0.008 ± 0.006[***]

1 Total enzymatic activity is the ratio between the area of enzymatic activity to the area of cytoplasm of the host keratinocyte. The differences within the pairs of values marked [*], [**], [***] are significant (p<0.001).

in the albino-like keratinocyte) of granule-associated acid phosphatase activity appeared to be directed.

In comparing the three genotypes studied as to the degree of granule-associated acid phosphatase activity and the degree of cytoplasmic acid phosphatase activity, there appeared to be certain trends. The data from table II has been retabulated in tables III and IV to facilitate the demonstration of these trends. As shown in table III, the wild-type keratinocyte had the highest level of granule-associated acid phosphatase activity while the albino-like keratinocyte had no enzymatic activity, and the pink-eye

Table III. Granule-associated acid phosphatase activity levels in the host keratinocyte

Genotype	Total granule-associated acid phosphatase activity[1]	Number of samples	Standard mean ± SD
Wild-type	0.937	20	0.047 ± 0.025*,+
Pink-eye	0.106	20	0.005 ± 0.004*,**
Albino-like	0.000	20	0.000 ± 0.000**,+

1 Total granule-associated acid phosphatase activity is the ratio between the area of granule enzymatic activity to the area of the cytoplasm of the host keratinocyte. The differences within the pairs of values marked*, **, + are significant.

Table IV. Cytoplasmic acid phosphatase levels in the host keratinocyte

Genotype	Total cytoplasmic acid phosphatase activity[1]	Number of samples	Standard mean ± SD
Wild-type	0.057	20	0.003 ± 0.005*
Pink-eye	0.032	20	0.001 ± 0.002+
Albino-like	0.159	20	0.008 ± 0.006*,+

1 Total cytoplasmic acid phosphatase activity is the ratio between the area of non-granule enzymatic activity to the area of cytoplasm of the host keratinocyte. The differences within the pairs of values marked *, + are significant ($p < 0.01$).

keratinocyte had an intermediate level of enzymatic activity. Interactions of the three genotypes shown in table III were significant.

The cytoplasmic acid phosphatase activities in the host keratinocyte of the three genotypes are shown in table IV. The albino-like keratinocyte had a significantly higher level of cytoplasmic acid phosphatase activity than either of the other two genotypes studied. No significant difference of cytoplasmic enzymatic activity between wild-type and pink-eye keratinocytes was found.

Discussion

By definition, a lysosome is any membrane-bound vacuole which contains acid phosphatase. Within this group, there may be those which

digest exogenous material termed heterophagic lysosomes [10]. Keratinocytes receive exogenous material in the form of transferred melanosomes.
The results of this study, based on acid phosphatase activity, suggest that
there is a differential lysosomal response to the transfer of the three melanosome types (table III).

The albino-like mutation is probably due to an altered tyrosinase
molecule while the pink-eye melanocytes possibly have altered premelanosome components [7]. In either case, the production of melanin is affected in the premelanosome. It would be justified to suggest that the presence of melanin in varying quantities is influencing lysosomal activity.

Although lysosomal recognition of phagosomes has been attributed
to the chemical composition of the membranes [10, 20] there is evidence
that the contents of the phagosome may influence phagolysosome formation.

AXLINE and COHN [2] reported increased levels of *total* cellular acid
phosphatase after phagocytosis of digestible material and no increase with
undigestible material. However, in both cases, no inhibition of phagosomes fusion with secondary lysosomes was observed and acid phosphatase was seen cytochemically in the phagosome vacuoles of each type.
ARMSTRONG and D'ARCY HART [1] suggested that intracellular fusion of
lysosomes with *M. tuberculosis*-containing phagosomes was inhibited in
cultured mouse macrophages until the bacteria were no longer viable.
Similar situations were demonstrated in mouse macrophages infested with
Toxoplasma gondii [16] and in *Paramecium bursaria* symbiotically har-
boring *Chlorella* [17]. If the presence of melanin is influencing acid phosphatase activity, it is still not known whether this occurs before or after
phagolysosome formation.

Statistical results of table I show that the total number of granules
transferred did not differ significantly between the wild-type and the pink-
eye mutant. Even though the total number of transferred granules is
markedly reduced in the albino-like mutant, the results between the wild-
type tissue and the pink-eye mutant indicate that any difference in lysosomal response to the transferred granules is due to some intrinsic characteristic of the melanosome complex and not to any difference in the number of granules transferred.

Interactions of the results of table II indicate that there is distinct dichotomy between cytoplasmic and transferred-granule acid phosphatase
activity. As shown in table IV, there is a significantly greater amount of
cytoplasmic acid phosphatase activity in the albino-like keratinocyte. This

quantity of enzymatic activity could be due to the lack of an apparent shift to the phagosomes. Certain levels of cytoplasmic acid phosphatase would normally be present in feather keratinocytes to aid in the degradative phase of keratinization [5], and would be stimulated by the process of phagocytosis alone [2].

No acid phosphatase activity was seen associated with the various stages of melanosomes in the three types of melanocytes. In contrast, acid phosphatase activity has been reported associated with melanosomes in mammalian melanocytes [24, 35, 36]. Cytoplasmic acid phosphatase was evident particularly in the Golgi complexes of the three types of feather melanocytes.

This is the first report of albino-like melanosome transfer in the fowl. It corresponds with the work of PARAKKAL [25] and HASHIMOTO [13], who reported mammalian keratinocytes phagocytizing nonmelanized premelanosomes.

Summary

The lysosomal (acid phosphatase) responses to transferred melanosomes in the regenerating breast feather from three genotypes of the male jungle-fowl were studied utilizing cytochemical and electron microscope techniques. The particular genotypes were utilized because their melanosomes differ in degree of melanization: the wild-type melanosomes are fully melanized; the pink-eye mutant melanosomes are partially melanized protein backbones, and the albino-like mutant melanosomes are nonmelanized vacuoles.

The greatest lysosomal response was to the wild-type transferred melanosomes, while the pink-eye mutant-transferred melanosomes showed an intermediate amount of lysosomal activity, and the albino-like mutant-transferred melanosomes had no observable lysosomal activity. This varied lysosomal response was apparently independent of the number of transferred melanosomes for each genotype. Since the lysosomal response was directly proportional to the degree of melanosome melanization, it was suggested that the amount of melanin polymer present may stimulate variable lysosomal responses.

References

1   ARMSTRONG, J. A. and D'ARCY HART, P.: Response of cultured macrophages to *Mycobacterium tuberculosis*, with observations on fusion of lysosomes with phagosomes. J. exp. Med. *134:* 713–740 (1972).

2 AXLINE, S. G. and COHN, Z. A.: *In vitro* induction of lysosomal enzymes by phagocytosis. J. exp. Med. *131:* 1239–1260 (1970).

3 BARKA, T. and ANDERSON, P. J.: Histochemistry (Harper & Row, New York 1963).

4 BLOIS, M. S.: Phagocytosis of melanin particles by human epidermal cells *in vitro.* J. invest. Derm. *50:* 336–337 (1968).

5 BOWERS, R. R.: An ultrastructural study of keratinization in the regenerating fowl feather and the concomitant stimulation of lysosomal activity; PhD thesis, Lincoln (1971).

6 BRUMBAUGH, J. A.: Ultrastructural differences between forming eumelanin and pheomelanin as revealed by the pink-eye mutation in the fowl. Devl Biol. *18:* 375–390 (1968).

7 BRUMBAUGH, J. A.; BOWERS, R. R., and CHATTERJEE, G. E.: Genotype substrate interactions altering Golgi development during melanogenesis. Pigment Cell, vol. 1, pp. 47–54 (Karger, Basel 1973).

8 BRUMBAUGH, J. A. and HOLLANDER, W.: A further study of the *E* pattern *locus* in the fowl. Iowa State J. Sci. *40:* 51–64 (1965).

9 COHEN, J. and SZABÓ, G.: Study of pigment donation *in vitro.* Expl Cell Res. *50:* 418–434 (1968).

10 DUVE, C. DE and WATTIAUX, R.: Functions of lysosomes. A. Rev. Physiol. *28:* 435–492 (1966).

11 FITZPATRICK, T. B.; QUEVEDO, W. C.; LEVENE, A. L.; McGOVERN, V. J.; MISHIMA, Y., and OETTLE, G. A.: Terminology of vertebrate melanin containing cells. Science *152:* 88–89 (1965).

12 GAZZOLO, L. and PRUNIERAS, M.: Melanin granules in keratinocytes *in vitro.* J. invest. Derm. *51:* 186–189 (1968).

13 HASHIMOTO, K.: An electron microscopic study of balloon cell nevus. Cancer *30:* 530–540 (1972).

14 HORI, Y.; TODA, K.; PATHAK, M. A.; CLARK, W. H., jr., and FITZPATRICK, T. B.: A fine structure study of the human epidermal melanosome complex and its acid phosphatase activity. J. Ultrastruct. Res. *25:* 109–120 (1968).

15 HUTT, F. B.: Genetics of the fowl (McGraw Hill, New York 1949).

16 JONES, T. C. and HIRSCH, J. G.: The interaction of *Toxoplasma gondii* and mammalian cells. II. The absence of lysosomal fusion with phagocytic vacuoles containing living parasites. J. exp. Med. *136:* 1173–1194 (1972).

17 KARAKASHIAN, M. W. and KARAKASHIAN, S. J.: Intercellular digestion and symbiosis in *Paramecium bursaria.* Expl Cell Res. *81:* 111–119 (1973).

18 KLAUS, S. N.: Post-transfer digestion of melanosome complexes and saltatory movement of melanin granules within mammalian epidermal cells. J. invest. Derm. *53:* 440–444 (1969).

19 KLAUS, S. N.: Pigment transfer in mammalian epidermis. Archs Derm. *100:* 756–762 (1969).

20 LUCY, J. A.: Lysosomal membranes; in DINGLE and FELL Lysosomes in biology and pathology, vol. 2, pp. 313–341 (North-Holland, Amsterdam 1969).

21 MOTTAZ, J. H. and ZELICKSON, A. S.: Melanin transfer: a possible phagocytic process. J. invest. Derm. *49:* 605–610 (1967).

22 MOTTAZ, J. H. and ZELICKSON, A. S.: The phagocytic nature of the keratinocyte in human epidermis after tape stripping. J. invest. Derm. *54:* 272–278
(1970).
23 NORDQUIST, R. E.; OLSON, R. L., and EVERETT, M. A.: The transport, uptake,
and storage of ferritin in human epidermis. Archs Derm. *94:* 482–490 (1966).
24 OLSON, R. L.; NORDQUIST, J., and EVERETT, M. A.: The role of epidermal lysosomes in melanin physiology. Br. J. Derm. *83:* 189–199 (1970).
25 PARAKKAL, P. F.: Transfer of premelanosomes into the keratinizing cells of albino hair follicle. J. Cell Biol. *35:* 473–477 (1967).
26 POTTER, B. and MEDENICA, M.: Ultramicroscopic phagocytosis of synthetic melanin by epidermal cells *in vivo.* J. invest. Derm. *51:* 300–303 (1968).
27 PRUNIERAS, M.: Interactions between keratinocytes and dendritic cells. J. invest. Derm. *52:* 1–17 (1969).
28 QUEVEDO, W. C.: Epidermal melanin units: melanocyte-keratinocyte interactions. Am. Zoologist *12:* 35–41 (1972).
29 RAWLES, M. E.: The integumentary system; in MARSHALL The biology and
comparative physiology of birds, vol. 1, pp. 190–240 (Academic Press, New
York 1960).
30 RUPRECHT, K. W.: Pigmentierung der Dunenfeder von *Gallus domesticus* L.
Licht- und elektronenmikroskopische Untersuchungen zur Melanosomen-
übertragung. Z. Zellforsch. *112:* 396–413 (1971).
31 SATO, S. and KUKITA, A.: Electron microscopic study of melanin phagocytosis
by cutaneous vessels in cellular blue nevus. J. invest. Derm. *52:* 528–532
(1969).
32 SEIJI, M. and KUKUCHI, A.: Acid phosphatase activity in melanosomes. J. invest. Derm. *52:* 212–216 (1969).
33 TODA, K. and FITZPATRICK, T. B.: Ultrastructural and biochemical studies of
the formation of melanosomes in the embryonic chick retinal pigment epithelium; in RILEY Pigmentation: its genesis and biological control (Appleton Century Crofts, New York 1972).
34 WOLFF, K. and HÖNIGSMANN, H.: Are melanosome complexes lysosomes? J. invest. Derm. *59:* 170–176 (1972).
35 WOLFF, K. and SCHREINER, E.: Melanosomal acid phosphatase. Arch. Derm.
Forsch. *241:* 255–272 (1971).
36 ZELICKSON, A. S.; MOTTAZ, J. H., and HUNTER, J. A.: An electron microscopic
study on the effect of ultraviolet irradiation on human skin. I. Autophagy and
melanosome degradation in melanocytes; in RILEY Pigmentation: its genesis
and biologic control (Appleton Century Crofts, New York 1969).
37 ZELICKSON, A. S.; WENDHORST, D. B.; WHITE, J. G., and GOOD, R. A.: The
Chediak-Higashi syndrome: formation of giant melanosomes and the basis of
hypopigmentation. J. invest. Derm. *49:* 575–581 (1967).

ROGER R. BOWERS, Department of Biology, California State University, *Los
Angeles, CA 90032* (USA)

Pigment Cell, vol. 3, pp. 152–164 (Karger, Basel 1976)

Hypopigmentation of Skin Lesions in Leprosy and Occurrence of o-Diphenoloxidase in Mycobacterium leprae[1]

K. Prabhakaran, E. B. Harris and W. F. Kirchheimer

US Public Health Service Hospital, Carville, La.

Introduction

Leprosy is an ancient disease of mankind; the causative agent, *Mycobacterium leprae*, specifically invades the skin and the peripheral nerve tissues in the human body. The discovery of *M. leprae* was reported in 1874. However, several problems regarding the infection still remain unresolved. No established procedure is as yet available for cultivation of the organisms *in vitro*. Why do the bacilli evince such an affinity for tissues of ectodermal origin? What causes the hypopigmentation of skin lesions characteristic of leprosy?

Because of recurring failures of attempts at cultivation of the organisms in chemically defined media and in tissue cultures, no basic studies have been conducted on the metabolic properties of the bacilli until recently. In the course of our investigations using concentrates of *M. leprae* separated from infected human tissues, we accidentally found that these organisms possess an active *o*-diphenoloxidase (EC 1.10.3.1) [6, 11]. The present report deals with: (a) certain distinguishing features of the *o*-diphenoloxidase in *M. leprae*, and (b) experimental evidence suggesting a possible mechanism of the pigment loss in skin lesions of leprosy.

1   This investigation was supported in part by the US-Japan Cooperative Medical Science Program of the National Institute of Allergy and Infectious Diseases, Department of Health, Education and Welfare (AI-07890). We thank I. Aravindakshan Menon, University of Toronto, Ontario, Canada, for the molecular model of diethyldithiocarbamate.

Materials and Methods

Bacilli and Cell Cultures

Concentrates of the bacilli were separated from lepromatous tissues. In advanced cases of leprosy, the organisms become blood-borne and large numbers of *M. leprae* occur in internal organs like the spleen. The tissues were homogenized and the bacilli were separated by differential and density-gradient centrifugations in solutions of sucrose and KCl. The preparation of *M. leprae* was washed with saline and water, and sometimes treated with trypsin, acetone, ether and dilute NaOH to remove any material adsorbed from the host tissue. The bacilli were used in the intact state or were disrupted by ultrasonic oscillation. After disintegration, the bacterial particles were collected by centrifugation at 126,000 g for 60 min. The *o*-diphenoloxidase activity was almost exclusively localized in the particulate fraction [10].

Melanocyte cultures derived from Cloudman S-91 melanoma were purchased from the American Type Culture Collection. The cells were grown at 37 °C in Ham's F-10 medium containing 10% fetal calf serum.

Chemicals

L-Tyrosine [3,5-³H] (aqueous solution containing 2% ethanol, 1 Ci/mmol) and DL-dopa [³H(G)] (labeling distributed generally, 250 mCi/mmol) were purchased from Amersham-Searle Corporation, Arlington Heights, Ill. The scintillation solution (Aquasol) was a product of New England Nuclear Corporation, Boston, Mass. Glass counting vials were obtained from Beckman Instruments, Inc., Fullerton, Calif. D-Dopa was purchased from Sigma Chemical Company, St. Louis, Mo., or from ICN Life Sciences Group, Cleveland, Ohio. Other commercially available chemicals of the highest purity were used.

Enzymes

Lyophilized mushroom tyrosinase was purchased from Sigma Chemical Co. or from ICN Life Sciences Group. Cultured melanoma cells or a particulate fraction prepared from Harding-Passey mouse melanoma served as sources of mammalian *o*-diphenoloxidase. A 10% homogenate of the melanoma was centrifuged at 10,000 g for 10 min to remove the coarse particles and the 'mitochondrial' fraction. The 'microsomal' fraction collected by centrifugation of the supernatant at 126,000 g for 60 min was used in the study.

Enzyme Assay

The *o*-diphenoloxidase of the preparations was assayed by measuring the quinone or the water produced in the reaction, or by determining the amount of oxygen taken up.

In the spectrophotometric procedure [9] where the absorbance maximum of the quinone formed was measured, the reaction system consisted of the following constituents in the final concentrations indicated: Na_2HPO_4-KH_2PO_4 buffer (pH 6.8), 0.1 M; *M. leprae*, 1.5–2 mg protein; melanoma extract, 3–5 mg protein; mushroom tyrosinase, 10–20 μg; substrates, 0.002 M; inhibitors, 0.004 M; volume, 3 ml; temperature, 37 °C; time, 30 min.

Oxygen uptake by the bacilli in presence of dopa was measured by convention-al Warburg manometric technique or polarographically using a Gilson Oxygraph, Model K-1C, equipped with a Clark electrode (Gilson Medical Electronics, Inc., Middleton, Wisc.). The reaction system used for the manometric method was essen-tially the same as for the spectrophotometric procedure, except that the bacterial concentration had to be 10–15 times higher. The Oxygraph method also contained the same reaction components as in the spectrophotometric technique, except that the volume was 2 ml. The duration of the experiments for measuring oxygen uptake was 2–3 h.

In the liquid scintillation counting procedure where the activity of the tritiated water formed was determined [5, 10], the reaction system consisted of: Na_2HPO_4-KH_2PO_4 buffer (pH 6.8), 40 μmol; ^{3}H-dopa or ^{3}H-tyrosine, 1 μCi; unlabeled dopa or tyrosine, 1 μmol; bacilli, 1.2 mg protein; melanoma extract, 2.9 mg protein; mush-room tyrosinase, 20 μg; volume, 2 ml; temperature, 37 °C; time, 60 min. Radioactiv-ity of the labeled water produced was determined in a Beckman LS-250 liquid scin-tillation counter. The counting efficiency was in the range of 41–44%, as deter-mined by the combined external standard channel ratio method.

Detergent Treatment

In attempts at releasing the *o*-diphenoloxidase activity from the bacterial and melanoma particles, several detergents were tried. Sodium dodecyl sulfate 1% (w/v) was the most effective for *M. leprae* and sodium deoxycholate 0.5% (w/v) was the most effective for the melanoma preparation [10]. After detergent treatment at 0 °C for 30 min, the suspensions were centrifuged at 126,000 g for 60 min. The enzyme activities of both the sediment and the supernatant fractions were assayed spectro-photometrically.

Protein was determined by the method of Lowry *et al.* [2], with crystalline bovine serum albumin as standard. Each experiment was carried out at least 3 times; the results reported are for typical experiments.

Results and Discussion

M. leprae *Purified from Tissue*

Table I shows the fractionation scheme employed in the preparation of concentrates of bacilli from infected tissues. The final preparations were examined by routine staining procedures and contained no visible tissue debris.

Oxidation of Substrates

The uptake of oxygen in the oxidation of dopa by *M. leprae*, as mea-sured by the manometric and the polarographic techniques, is presented in table II. In the presence of substrate, the organisms show considerable increase in utilization of oxygen over auto-oxidation of dopa or endogen-

Table I. Fractionation scheme for separation of *M. leprae* from lepromatous tissue

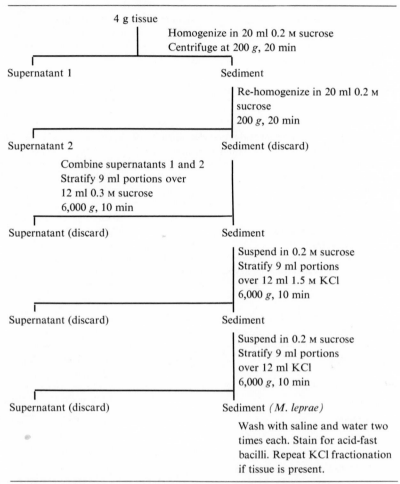

ous respiration of the bacilli. Table III illustrates the results on the oxidation of dopa by *M. leprae* and by plant and mammalian tyrosinases, as measured by the radioisotope tracer technique. It may be noted that heating the preparations at 100 °C for 30 min leads to considerable loss of enzyme activity.

Results of the oxidation of a variety of phenolic compounds by *M. leprae* and by plant and mammalian tyrosinases, as measured by the spectrophotometric method, are presented in table IV. Mammalian tyrosinase

Table II. Oxidation of dopa by *M. leprae:* O_2 uptake

Reaction system	Manometry $\mu l\ O_2$	Polarography nmol O_2
M. leprae + L-dopa	72	355.8
M. leprae	9	66.3
L-Dopa	12	122.7

Table III. Oxidation of tritium-labeled dopa by *M. leprae* and by plant and mammalian tyrosinases: pmol ^{3}H-dopa oxidized

Enzyme source	Unheated enzyme	Heated enzyme
M. leprae	122.0	33.6
Mushroom tyrosinase	298.9	22.2
Melanocytes	139.4	0

Values corrected for nonenzymic oxidation of substrate.

Table IV. Oxidation of phenolic compounds by *M. leprae* and by plant and mammalian tyrosinases: increase in absorbance

Substrate	*M. leprae*	Mushroom tyrosinase	Melanoma extract
L-Dopa	0.170 (540)	0.120 (480)	0.250 (480)
D-Dopa	0.187 (540)	0.120 (480)	0.020 (480)
3,4-Dihydroxybenzoic acid (protocatechuic acid)	0.125 (560)	0.202 (350)	0
3,4,5-Trihydroxybenzoic acid (gallic acid)	0.104 (560)	0.155 (380)	0
3,4-Dihydroxycinnamic acid (caffeic acid)	0.135 (600)	0.160 (480)	0
3-(3,4-Dihydoxycinnamoyl) quinic acid (chlorogenic acid)	0.143 (500)	0.110 (775)	0
Epinephrine	0.205 (480)	0.130 (480)	0
Norepinephrine	0.330 (480)	0.150 (480)	0
Isoproterenol	0.100 (490)	0.155 (490)	0

Values in parentheses indicate absorbance maxima in nm.

Table V. Oxidation of tyrosine-3,5-³H by mushroom tyrosinase and *M. leprae:* pmol ³H-tyrosine oxidized

Enzyme source	Unheated enzyme	Heated enzyme
Mushroom tyrosinase	50.8	0.6
M. leprae	0.9	0.9
M. leprae + ³H-dopa	122.1	18.6

Values corrected for nonenzymic oxidation of substrate.

Table VI. Release of *o*-diphenoloxidase from *M. leprae* particles and from 'microsomal' fraction of melanoma by detergents: increase in absorbance

Detergent	*M. leprae* (540 nm)		Melanoma (480 nm)	
	residue +L-dopa	supernatant +L-dopa	residue +L-dopa	supernatant +L-dopa
Sodium dodecyl sulfate	0.075	0.230	0.110	0.290
Deoxycholate	0.100	0.010	0.084	0.254

is highly restricted in its substrate requirement, whereas the enzyme in *M. leprae* resembles plant tyrosinase in the wide range of substances oxidized. These data are in conformity with the generalization that substrate-specificity of tyrosinase becomes restricted with rise in the phylogenetic scale [3]. The absorption maximum of the quinone formed from dopa by *M. leprae* is characteristic of indole-5,6-quinone, which is a decarboxylation product [1, 3]. With plant or mammalian tyrosinase, the quinone produced is dopachrome. However, when compounds with no carboxyl groups were oxidized, the absorption maxima of the quinones were identical for *M. leprae* as well as plant tyrosinase. The results suggest that probably the *o*-diphenoloxidase in the bacillus is associated with an active decarboxylase [9].

To see whether the enzyme in *M. leprae* possesses monophenolase activity, tritium-labeled tyrosine was used as substrate. Table V shows that the bacilli do not oxidize tyrosine, whereas mushroom tyrosine readily oxidizes the substrate. The bacterial preparation was active, as is evidenced by the oxidation of ³H-dopa. Apparently, *M. leprae* separated from tissues is devoid of monophenolase activity.

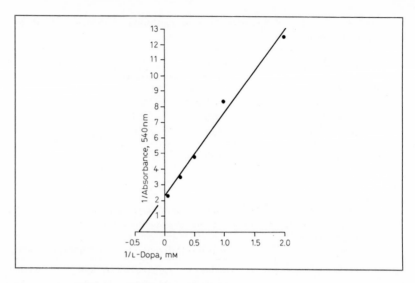

Fig. 1. Lineweaver-Burk plot (●) of 1/v against 1/(S) for the oxidation of dopa by *M. leprae.* —— = Line of best fit by regression analysis.

Release of o-Diphenoloxidase from Particles

Approximately two thirds of the activity of the bacterial particles could be released by treatment with sodium dodecyl sulfate (SDS). Other detergents tested were ineffective. Both SDS and deoxycholate (DOC) released the activity of the melanoma particles, the latter being more effective (table VI). Liberation of melanoma tyrosinase by DOC has been reported earlier [12].

Effect of Substrate Concentration

When the concentration of dopa in the reaction system was increased, the results with *M. leprae* gave a hyperbolic curve, whereas with the melanoma extract, high substrate levels produced an inhibitory effect. Because the preparations used are crude, no definitive conclusions could be drawn from these data. One obvious explanation would be that the mammalian tyrosinase binds the substrate at two sites, while in the bacilli, the enzyme binds dopa at only one site [10]. Lineweaver-Burk plot of the data obtained with *M. leprae* is given in figure 1. The K_m value for the bacterial enzyme was 2.35×10^{-3} M. Under identical experimental contitions, K_m for the mushroom tyrosinase was 2.55×10^{-3} M and for mela-

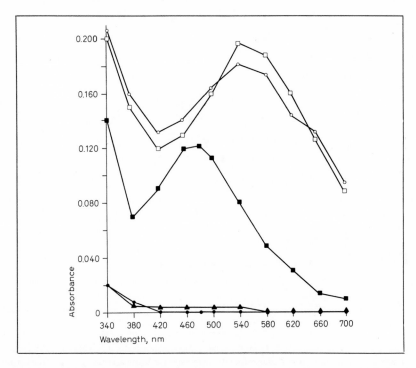

Fig. 2. Oxidation of dopa by *M. leprae* in presence of ascorbic acid and effect of GSH and ascorbic acid on mammalian tyrosinase. ○ = *M. leprae* + L-dopa; □ = *M. leprae* + L-dopa + ascorbate; ■ = melanoma extract + L-dopa; ● = melanoma + L-dopa + ascorbate; ▲ = melanoma + L-dopa + GSH.

noma tyrosinase was 4.5×10^{-4} M. It may not be valid to compare these values with those obtained with purified enzyme preparations.

Reducing Agents and Metal Chelators

The effect of reduced glutathione (GSH), ascorbic acid or cysteine was tested on the oxidation of dopa to quinone by *M. leprae*. Surprisingly, the reducing agents showed no influence on the conversion of the substrate to quinone by the bacilli. On the other hand, with plant and mammalian tyrosinases, no quinone formation from dopa was detected in presence of the reducing agents [7]. Figure 2 shows the effect of ascorbic acid and GSH on oxidation of dopa by melanoma extract, and the conversion of dopa to quinone by the bacilli in presence of ascorbic acid. Figure 3 shows the oxidation of dopa by *M. leprae* in the presence of GSH and the

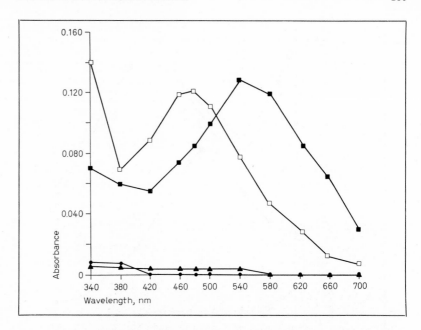

Fig. 3. Oxidation of dopa by *M. leprae* in presence of GSH and effect of ascorbic acid and GSH on mushroom tyrosinase. ■ = *M. leprae*+L-dopa+GSH; □ = mushroom tyrosinase+L-dopa; ● = mushroom tyrosinase+L-dopa+ascorbate; ▲ = mushroom tyrosinase+L-dopa+GSH.

effect of GSH and ascorbic acid on mushroom tyrosinase. The results obtained with *M. leprae* are not due to permeability barrier of the bacterial cell membrane, since the preparations used were disrupted by ultrasonic oscillation. It is likely that the active site of the enzyme in *M. leprae* is not easily accessible to the reducing agents and that it has a higher affinity for dopa than in plant or mammalian tyrosinase. Cyanide, a potent inhibitor of metalloenzymes, completely suppressed oxidation of dopa by mushroom tyrosinase and melanoma extract; however, it showed little effect on the enzyme in the bacilli, under similar experimental conditions. Penicillamine, a copper chelator, produced total inhibition of plant and mammalian tyrosinases; but it did not inhibit the bacterial *o*-diphenoloxidase. On the other hand, another copper chelator, diethyldithiocarbamate (DDC), inhibited the enzyme from all the three sources (table VII). In fact, DDC could penetrate even intact *M. leprae* and completely suppress its enzyme activity. A molecular model of DDC shows that it has two ethyl

Table VII. Effect of metal chelators on oxidation of dopa by *M. leprae* and by plant and mammalian tyrosinases: increase in absorbance

Inhibitor	M. leprae		Mushroom tyrosinase		Melanoma	
	−inhibitor	+inhibitor	−inhibitor	+inhibitor	−inhibitor	+inhibitor
Sodium cyanide	0.115	0.105	0.270	0	0.225	0
Penicillamine	0.130	0.160	0.290	0	0.240	0
Diethyldithiocarbamate	0.105	0	0.225	0	0.230	0

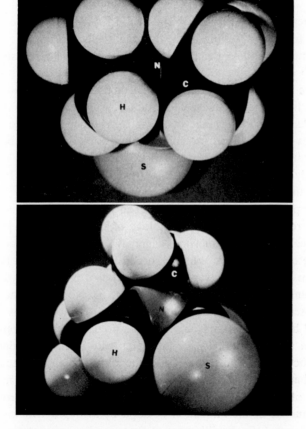

a

b

Fig. 4. Molecular model of diethyldithiocarbamate. C = Carbon; H = hydrogen; O = oxygen; N = nitrogen; S = sulfur. *a* Frontal view; *b* lateral view.

groups (nonpolar masses) which more or less shadow the sulfurs (the polar region) (fig. 4). The presence of the lipid-soluble ethyl groups would enable the compound to easily pass through lipid-predominant pores.

Significance of o-diphenoloxidase in M. leprae

The data reported above demonstrate that the leprosy bacilli possess a characteristic o-diphenoloxidase enzyme. In the range of substrates utilized, in the nature of the quinones formed and in the effects of reducing agents and metal chelators, the o-diphenoloxidase of M. leprae was distinct from similar enzymes of plant and mammalian origin. The exact physiological role of the enzyme in the bacillus has not yet been established. In experimental mice, M. leprae failed to multiply when the animals were treated with tyrosinase inhibitors, indicating that o-diphenoloxidase may be of metabolic significance in the bacilli [9]. The leprosy organisms have been found to multiply in the Schwann cells, the dorsal root ganglia of spinal nerves and in the adrenal medulla, besides other sites like the skin which contain melanocytes. It may be significant that M. leprae proliferates in tissues of neural crest origin or tissues which contain cells derived from the neural crest, where metabolism of dopa and its derivatives is important. The occurrence of an active o-diphenoloxidase in the bacilli indicates that the organisms might utilize dopa or its metabolites at the sites where they multiply. In advanced cases of leprosy, the iris and the ciliary body of the eye are invaded by M. leprae. Presence of free dopa at these sites in the mammalian eye has been reported [4].

An in vitro experimental system was designed to see whether M. leprae would interfere with the normal physiology of the melanocytes [8]. When melanoma cells are grown in vitro, aggregates of melanin pigment can be seen in the culture (fig. 5). When a suspension of live leprosy bacilli prepared from skin biopsies was added to cultures of melanocytes, formation of melanin pigment was suppressed (fig. 6). Normal pigment formation was observed in untreated cultures, as well as the cultures to which were added heat-killed bacilli or organisms prepared from autopsy material. The data show that M. leprae interferes with pigment production by the melanocytes. The presence of o-diphenoloxidase in the bacilli suggests that the bacilli in vivo utilize dopa, which is a precursor of melanin. The failure of normal pigment formation in skin lesions of leprosy might be a consequence of the utilization of dopa by M. leprae. In well-defined lesions of leprosy, the bacilli occur at the spreading outer margins which become hypopigmented, while the healing middle regions often re-

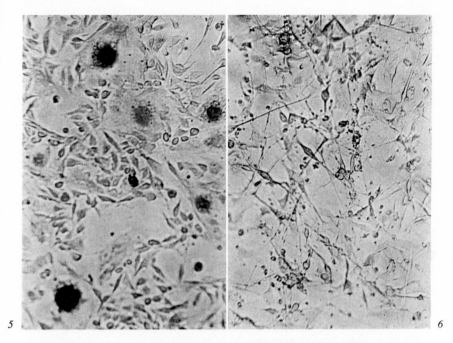

Fig. 5. Culture of melanocytes. From PRABHAKARAN *et al.* [8]. × 58.56.

Fig. 6. Melanocyte culture to which live *M. leprae* was added. From PRABHAKARAN *et al.* [8]. × 58.56.

gain the pigment. In the advanced cutaneous form of leprosy, the skin contains numerous mast cells loaded with catecholamines. In these areas, the bacilli are distributed diffusely. We have shown that *M. leprae* readily oxidizes catecholamines. This unusual metabolic requirement of the leprosy bacilli also might explain why innumerable attempts over the past one hundred years to culture the organisms have not yet met with success.

Summary

Mycobacterium leprae contains a characteristic *o*-diphenoloxidase. The enzyme converts a wide range of phenolic compounds to quinones *in vitro*. The *M. leprae* preparations show no monophenolase activity. In the human body, the bacilli multiply at sites such as the skin and the peripheral nerves where metabolism of dopa or its derivatives is important. Hypopigmentation of skin lesions is a characteristic feature of leprosy. When suspensions of *M. leprae* are added to cultures of melanoma cells, formation of melanin pigment by the cells is suppressed. The utilization of dopa, a precursor of melanin, by *M. leprae* could result in loss of normal pigmentation in skin lesions of leprosy. This unusual metabolic requirement of the organisms, not possessed by any other mycobacteria, might also explain the failure of repeated attempts at culture of *M. leprae in vitro*.

References

1 LERNER, A. B. and FITZPATRICK, T. B.: Biochemistry of melanin formation. Physiol. Rev. *30:* 91–126 (1950).
2 LOWRY, O. H.; ROSENBROUGH, N. J.; FARR, A. L., and RANDALL, R. J.: Protein measurement with the folin phenol reagent. J. biol. Chem. *193:* 265–275 (1951).
3 MASON, H. S.: Comparative biochemistry of the phenolase complex. Adv. Enzymol. *16:* 105–184 (1955).
4 PIRIE, A.: Reaction of tyrosine oxidation products with proteins of the lens. Biochem. J. *109:* 301–305 (1968).
5 POMERANTZ, S. H.: The tyrosine hydroxylase activity of mammalian tyrosinase. J. biol. Chem. *241:* 161–168 (1966).
6 PRABHAKARAN, K.: Phenoloxidase of *Mycobacterium leprae*. Nature, Lond. *215:* 436–437 (1967).
7 PRABHAKARAN, K.: Unusual effects of reducing agents on *o*-diphenoloxidase of *Mycobacterium leprae*. J. Bact. *107:* 787–789 (1971).
8 PRABHAKARAN, K.; HARRIS, E. B., and KIRCHHEIMER, W. F.: Interaction of *Mycobacterium leprae* and melanocytes *in vitro*. Cytobios *4:* 93–95 (1971).
9 PRABHAKARAN, K.; HARRIS, E. B., and KIRCHHEIMER, W. F.: The nature of the phenolase enzyme in *Mycobacterium leprae*. Microbios *5:* 273–281 (1972).
10 PRABHAKARAN, K.; HARRIS, E. B., and KIRCHHEIMER, W. F.: Particulate nature of *o*-diphenoloxidase in *Mycobacterium leprae* and assay of the enzyme by the radioisotope technique. Microbios *8:* 151–157 (1973).
11 PRABHAKARAN, K. and KIRCHHEIMER, W. F.: Use of 3,4-dihydroxyphenylalanine oxidation in the identification of *Mycobacterium leprae*. J. Bact. *92:* 1267–1268 (1966).
12 SEIJI, M.: Subcellular particles and melanin formation in melanocytes; in MONTAGNA and HU Adv. Biol. Skin, vol. 8, pp. 189–222 (Pergamon Press, Oxford 1967).

Dr. K. PRABHAKARAN, Biochemistry Research Department, Laboratory Research Branch, US Public Health Service Hospital, *Carville, LA 70721* (USA)

Pigment Cell, vol. 3, pp. 165–176 (Karger, Basel 1976)

Types of Genetic Mechanisms Controlling Melanogenesis in the Fowl[1]

J. A. BRUMBAUGH and K. W. LEE

School of Life Sciences, University of Nebraska, Lincoln, Nebr.

For several years, we have been analyzing 4 pigment mutants of the fowl. This report will survey the results of ultrastructural analyses of each mutant locus, suggest the melanogenic steps involved, and postulate the types of genetic mechanisms which are operating.

Materials and Methods

Melanocytes from regenerating feathers, embryos, and cell cultures were used for analyses of the *pk, I, c,* and *Bl* loci. Each mutant was compared to its respective heterozygote and standard. Genetic stocks were produced in the School of Life Sciences of the University of Nebraska-Lincoln.

Four basic aspects of gene action at each locus were determined as follows: (1) the basic phenotype and genetic dominance were noted; (2) the presence or absence of dopa oxidase was ascertained using the ultrastructural dopa reaction of BRUMBAUGH and ZIEG [4]; (3) the ultrastructure of retinal and neural crest melanocytes from embryos were compared, and (4) high resolution autoradiographic determinations of ^{3}H-leucine and ^{3}H-dopa incorporation in melanocyte cell cultures were calculated.

Glutaraldehyde was used for fixation except after radioactive labeling when paraformaldehyde was used to reduce nonspecific binding of label to tissues [11]. Ultrastructural observations were made with an RCA EMU 3-B (modified) electron microscope.

Autoradiographic analyses were of neural crest melanocytes cultured according to the method of ZIMMERMAN *et al.* [17]. Since the labeling experiments were done over a 3-year period, there have been variations as methods have evolved. In every case, however, a particular mutant, its heterozygote and respective standard have

1 This work was supported by PHS Research Grant GM18969 and by PHS Research Career Development Award GM42355 to J. A. B.

been examined simultaneously so that comparisons within a locus grouping are valid. It should be noted that radioactive analysis of the *c* locus is only preliminary until the mutant is transferred to a genetic background more conducive to melanin synthesis in culture.

Melanocyte cultures of 6, 7, or 8 days were labeled with ³H-leucine (50 Ci/mmol) at either 0.500 or 0.250 mCi/ml for 1 h in leucineless medium. This was followed by 3×10 min changes of medium at 4.6 mM 'cold' leucine. Replicate cultures were labeled with ³H-dopa (35 Ci/mmol) at either 0.500 or 0.375 mCi/ml for 4 h. This was followed by 3×10 min changes of regular medium.

After labeling, the cultures were fixed *in situ*, dehydrated and embedded in epon. Ultrathin sections were coated with Ilford L4 emulsion, according to the method of BRUMBAUGH and FROILAND [3] or YOUNG [16]. ³H-leucine-labeled cells were exposed for 8 days and ³H-dopa-labeled cells for 35 days before being developed in Microdol-X (2 min).

From 12 to 49 cells of each genotype and treatment were randomly selected and photographed. Each grain was assigned to a melanosome or other cytoplasmic organelle by viewing each negative with a dissecting microscope. The area occupied by melanosomes was also determined, using the method of BRUMBAUGH and FROILAND [3]. Background was less than 0.027 grains/μm², so no correction for background was made.

The mean percent of cytoplasmic ³H-leucine grains over melanosomes was determined for each genotype. In the case of the *c* locus grouping, the percent of cytoplasmic area was substituted for the percent ³H-leucine. The mean number of grains per μm² of melanosome for each genotype and treatment was also determined. Confidence intervals (95%) and tests for significance between means were calculated using Student's *t* distribution. The mean number of ³H-dopa grains/μm² was divided by the mean number of ³H-leucine grains/μm² to determine the dopa/leucine ratio. For comparative purposes, the data for heterozygotes and homozygous mutants are reported as a proportion of their respective standard genotypes which were arbitrarily set at 1.000.

Results

Pinkeye (*pk*) is a recessive mutation first described by WARREN [15] which reduces feather pigmentation to gray and which severely restricts retinal pigmentation. At the gross phenotypic level the heterozygote is indistinguishable from standard (upper left grouping, fig. 1). The dominant white *(I)* mutation whitens primarily eumelanic feathers, but does not affect retinal pigmentation. It is a dominant mutation, but heterozygotes are revealed by black flecks in the feathers which indicate instability (lower left grouping, fig. 1; note arrows). The recessive white *(c)* mutation whitens all body regions and also reduces retinal pigmentation. Its heterozygote is indistinguishable from standard (upper right grouping, fig. 1). Blue

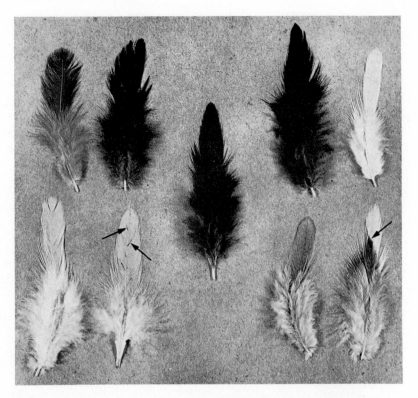

Fig. 1. Male breast feathers of each genotype. Upper left = *pk/pk*; *pk/+*; upper right = *c/+*; *c/c*; center = *+/+*(standard); lower left = *l/l*; *l/+* with reverted flecks (arrows); lower right = *Bl/+*; *Bl/Bl* with reverted area (arrow).

(Bl) is a semi-dominant mutation which reduces pigmentation primarily in eumelanic feathers. It does not affect retinal pigmentation. The heterozygote is clearly distinguishable from both the standard and the homozygote. Heterozygous feathers are 'blue' (gray) and contain flecks of standard black. The homozygote *(Bl/Bl)* is characterized by much instability which is aptly described by the fanciers as 'blue-splashed white'. Flecks of heterozygote-like blue are frequent and often large. These blue areas may contain 'doubly reverted' black flecks (lower right grouping, fig. 1; note arrow). (See HUTT [9] for a more complete description of each of these mutants.)

Cytochemically, all genotypes, except recessive white *(c/c)* and homozygous blue *(Bl/Bl)*, were dopa oxidase positive. This was true for both

BRUMBAUGH/LEE168

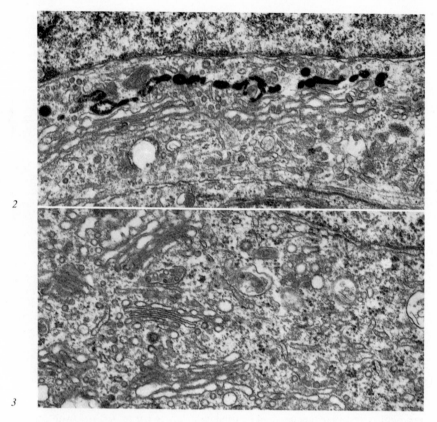

Fig. 2. pk/pk melanocyte showing dopa oxidase-positive reaction products in Golgi-related vesicles and cisternae. × 25,000.

Fig. 3. c/c melanocyte showing absence of dopa oxidase reaction products in Golgi-related vesicles and cisternae. × 25,000.

regenerating feather melanocytes and melanocytes in cell culture. All possessed deposits of electron-opaque, dopa-melanin reaction product in their Golgi-related cisternae and vesicles, like the pinkeye *(pk/pk)* cell shown in figure 2; *c/c* (fig. 3) and *Bl/Bl* melanocytes, however, formed no reaction product in their Golgi systems.

Melanocytes are derived from two embryonic sources, the optic cup and the neural crest. Figure 4 shows typical melanosomes from embryonic retinal melanocytes (column one) and neural-crest derived choroidal (column two) and feather (column three) melanocytes. Samples were tak-

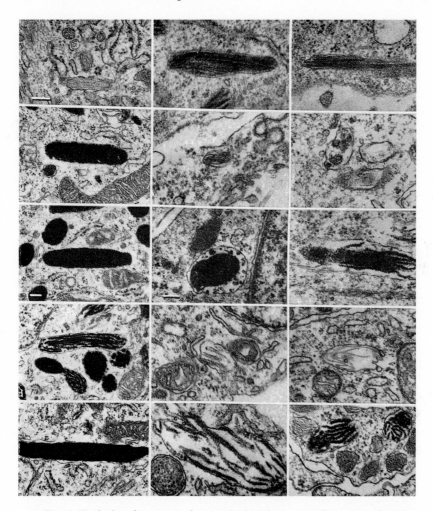

Fig. 4. Typical melanosomes from retinal melanocytes (first column) and neural crest derived choroidal (second column) and feather (third column) melanocytes. Row 1 = *pk/pk*; row 2 = *I/I*; row 3 = standard; row 4 = *c/c*; row 5 = *Bl/Bl*. Retinal melanosomes at × 12,500 except *pk/pk* and all neural crest melanosomes which are at × 20,000.

en from homozygous 9-day embryos except for *c/c* embryos which were 14 days old. *pk/pk* and *c/c* embryos have aberrant melanosomes in all tissues regardless of embryonic origin (compare rows 1 and 4 with 3, fig. 4). *I/I* and *Bl/Bl* embryos, however, have abnormal melanosomes only in

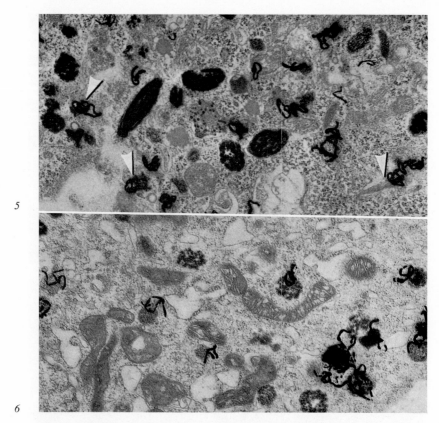

Fig. 5. ³H-Leucine-labeled *pk/+* melanocyte. Arrows point to 3 of the labeled melanosomes. × 18,000.

Fig. 6. ³H-Dopa-labeled +/+ melanocyte. All grains are associated with melanosomes. × 18,000.

their neural-crest derived melanocytes (compare rows 2 and 5 with 3, fig. 4).

It should be noted that the melanosomes pictured from *Bl/Bl* choroidal and feather melanocytes are probably from heterozygote-like 'reverted' cells since *Bl/Bl* cells are almost completely devoid of melanosomes.

³H-Leucine is not a melanogenically specific molecule and was incorporated into all compartments of the cytoplasm and nucleus (fig. 5). The percentage of cytoplasmic ³H-leucine incorporated into melanosomes, however, indicated the proportion of newly synthesized protein molecules which were melanosomic (arrows, fig. 5).

The *pk* and *c* loci did not seem to extensively alter the proportionate quantity of melanosomic molecules. This is particularly evident in the heterozygotes which have values similar to standard (first data column, table I). Although *pk/pk* cells have a significantly lower mean than standard, it is not nearly as low as the *I/I* and *Bl/Bl* values. In the *c* series the percent area occupied by melanosomes and/or melanosomic vesicles was used as a substitute for radioactive data which were not available. Percent ^{3}H-leucine grains compared to percent area determinations for other genotypes have shown them to be reasonable substitutes [unpublished data].

The *I* and *Bl* loci definitely reduce melanosomic quantity as shown by the homozygotes. At both loci, the heterozygotes also have reduced melanosomic quantities in spite of the fact that 'revertants' are frequently encountered (first data column, table I). Heterozygote-like 'revertant' melanocytes in *Bl/Bl* cultures were not used in determining *Bl/Bl* values. Revertants in *I/I* cultures were not easily discerned and therefore were included.

The melanogenic specificity of ^{3}H-dopa is shown by the fact that nearly all of the grains in figure 6 are associated with melanosomes. The number of ^{3}H-dopa grains/μm^2 of melanosome shows the effect each locus had upon dopa incorporation.

The *pk* mutation significantly reduced ^{3}H-dopa incorporation both in the homozygote and heterozygote (second data column, table I. The *c* locus also seemed to reduce ^{3}H-dopa incorporation. The heterozygote and homozygote values are similar, however. These *c* locus data are preliminary and are based on a small sample from a melanogenically undesirable genetic background (second data column, table I).

Based on heterozygote expression, the *I* and *Bl* loci do not seem to affect ^{3}H-dopa incorporation since their means are not significantly different from standard (second data column, table I). Both homozygotes, however, do have significantly reduced ^{3}H-dopa incorporation. It should be noted, however, that *I/I* melanocytes have a higher ^{3}H-dopa incorporation than *pk/+* cells.

The number of ^{3}H-leucine grains/μm^2 of melanosome indicates the synthetic activity of the cells, with regard to melanogenesis, and is important in calculating the dopa/leucine ratio. Cultures within a locus grouping incorporated the same amount of ^{3}H-leucine with the exception of *pk/pk* melanocytes which incorporated significantly more, and *I/+* cells which incorporated significantly less (third data column, table I).

Since replicate cultures of each genotype were labeled in ^{3}H-dopa

Table I. Comparative[a] autoradiographic analysis of the four loci

Genotype	Melanosomic ³H-leucine, %	³H-Dopa: grains/μm² of melanosome	³H-Leucine: grains/μm² of melanosome	Ratio: ³H-dopa/μm² / ³H-leucine/μm²
Pinkeye (*pk/pk*)	0.518±0.110 (p<0.001)	0.061±0.020 (p<0.001)	1.667±0.267 (0.01>p>0.005)	0.038
Heterozygote (*pk/+*)	1.066±0.171	0.469±0.082 (p<0.001)	1.000±0.105	0.462
Standard (+/+)	1.000±0.149	1.000±0.122	1.000±0.158	1.000
Dominant white (*I/I*)	0.310±0.107 (p<0.001)	0.475±0.200 (0.005>p>0.001)	1.000±0.269	0.467
Heterozygote (*I/+*)	0.797±0.137 (0.10>p>0.05)	0.850±0.200	0.692±0.115 (0.01>p>0.005)	1.267
Standard (+/+)	1.000±0.137	1.000±0.275	1.000±0.192	1.000
Recessive white (*c/c*)[b]	0.803±0.162[c]	0.723±0.253	–	–
Heterozygote (*c/+*)[b]	1.170±0.203[c]	0.724±0.260	–	–
Standard (+/+)[b]	1.000±0.133[c]	1.000±0.249	–	–
Blue-splashed white (*Bl/Bl*)[d]	0.197±0.113 (p<0.001)	0.066±0.079 (p<0.001)	0.827±0.323	0.080
Heterozygote (*Bl/+*)	0.814±0.205	0.880±0.137	1.063±0.173	0.832
Standard (+/+)	1.000±0.137	1.000±0.333	1.000±0.156	1.000

Expressed intervals are at the 95% confidence level. Probabilities of means significantly different from their respective standards are expressed in parentheses. Data in this table involve 34,922 grains from 388 cells.
a All values are proportional to the respective standard value for each locus of 1.000.
b Only preliminary data available.
c Based on the percent of cytoplasmic area which was melanosomic.
d Heterozygote-like revertants excluded.

and ^{3}H-leucine at the same time, the dopa/leucine ratio estimates the amount of ^{3}H-dopa incorporated at that stage of differentiation per unit of melanogenic protein (shown by ^{3}H-leucine incorporation) that was concurrently synthesized. The ratio tends to 'level out' differences in cellular maturity that might exist between cultures. The dopa/leucine ratios in the last column of table I corroborate the information derived from the ^{3}H-dopa/μm^2 values.

Discussion

Because of the survey nature of this paper the Discussion will deal primarily with hypotheses concerned with the function of each locus and its genetic mechanism. The authors are aware that other interpretations are possible, but have limited themselves to what seem to them to be the most obvious.

The 4 loci suggest that melanogenesis involves two major components. One component, dopa oxidase, is affected by the c and Bl loci. The other component, premelanosomal matrix protein, is affected by the pk and I loci. The existence of a single, major premelanosomal protein is substantiated by the fact that HEARING and EPPIG [8] found only a single major protein in chick eye melanosomes.

The c mutation severely reduces dopa oxidase activity, but apparently possesses altered enzyme since c/c melanocytes have hypertrophied Golgi systems and can become functional in the presence of excess tyrosine [5]. The Bl mutation apparently reduces the amount of enzyme produced without affecting the Golgi network.

The pk mutation affects the ability of premelanosomes to incorporate dopa, even in the heterozygote. Since eumelanin is bound to the premelanosome, possibly through thioether linkages [3], it is possible to suggest that the pk mutation alters this ability to bind dopa and/or its melanin intermediates. The I mutation reduces the number and area occupied by melanosomes in both the heterozygote [2] (also present data) and homozygote. Since dopa oxidase is present, even in the homozygote, it seems likely that the I mutation reduces premelanosomal synthesis.

STANBURY et al. [12] suggest that two broad functional classes of mutations exist: structural mutations and control gene mutations. Even though control gene mutations are not clearly defined they must exist [12]. In this study, structural mutations would be expected to affect the *quality* of melanogenic molecules while control gene mutations would affect only their *quantity* or *distribution*. The embryological, autoradiographic and genetic data, when considered together, suggest that *pk* and *c* are structural loci and that *I* and *Bl* are control gene loci.

Nucleic acid hybridization studies show that multiple copies of 'unique' DNA sequences are rarely encountered in eukaryotes [1, 6, 7, 13, 14]. Thus, it is very likely that the same set of structural genes is utilized by both retinal and neural crest melanocytes. If this is the case, then the *I* and *Bl* mutations would be control gene mutations since only neural crest melanocytes are affected. On the other hand, the *pk* and *c* mutations would appear to be structural since *both* retinal and neural crest melanocytes are affected. These two melanocyte lineages are apparently controlled by different genetic mechanisms.

The quantity of melanogenic molecules was estimated by the % ^{3}H-leucine values (% melanosomic area for the *c* locus). Observed reductions in quantity were caused by the *I* and *Bl* mutations in heterozygotes as well as homozygotes. The *pk* and *c* mutations did not affect quantity in heterozygotes. The reduced values for homozygotes could be attributed to the poor assembly of premelanosomes or their degradation. Based on the definitions given previously, the *I* and *Bl* loci again seem likely control gene loci by virtue of their quantitative effect.

The quality of melanogenic molecules was estimated by the ^{3}H-dopa/μm^2 and dopa/leucine values. Observed reductions in ^{3}H-dopa incorporation were caused by the *pk* and *c* mutations in heterozygotes as well as homozygotes. The *I* and *Bl* mutations did not appreciably affect this quality in heterozygotes. The reduced values for homozygotes could be attributed to the resolving limitations of ultrastructural autoradiography. It should also be noted that *Bl/Bl* melanocytes are devoid of dopa oxidase. If dopa must be oxidized before it is attached to the premelanosome [3], then *Bl/Bl* cells would not incorporate dopa and would possess only 'naked' premelanosomes. Such was the case (data columns 2, 4, table I). Based on the definitions given previously, the *pk* and *c* mutations again seem likely structural mutations by virtue of their effect on melanosome quality.

PATTERSON *et al.* [10] have suggested that control genes can be expected to have dominant rather than recessive expressions. It is interesting to note that *I* and *Bl* are both dominant mutations which have unstable expressions. Although the frequency of reverted clones in feathers of *I*/+, *Bl*/+, and *Bl/Bl* individuals have not been determined, it appears to be high enough to support explanations other than back mutation. The 'reverted' cells of these genotypes may represent melanocytes that have 'escaped' from the melanogenic suppression controlled by these two mutations.

Based on the evidence presented, a working hypothesis of melanogenesis in the fowl follows: Both retinal and neural crest melanocytes require the product of the *pk* locus, premelanosomal protein, and the product of the *c* locus, tyrosinase (dopa oxidase). Neural crest melanocytes, unlike retinal melanocytes, utilize the *I* and *Bl* loci during differentiation. A normal *I* locus responds to differentiative 'cues' by causing premelanosome synthesis. A normal *Bl* locus responds by causing tyrosinase synthesis. Thus, the *I* locus seems to be the quantitative controller or 'regulator' of the *pk* locus, while the *Bl* locus seems to be the quantitative controller or 'regulator' of the *c* locus.

Summary

The *pk, I, c,* and *Bl* loci of the fowl were analyzed using six criteria: genetic expression, the cytochemical dopa test, ultrastructural comparisons of retinal and neural crest melanocytes, percent cytoplasmic ^{3}H-leucine grains melanosomic, the number of ^{3}H-dopa grains/μm^2 of melanosome, and the dopa/leucine ratio. The results indicate that the *c* and *Bl* mutants affect tyrosinase (dopa oxidase) while the *pk* and *I* mutants affect premelanosomes. The results also indicate that *pk* and *c* are structural mutations, while *I* and *Bl* are control genes or 'regulatory' mutations. The structural mutations affected both retinal and neural crest melanocytes and were qualitative having autoradiographically detectable heterozygotes with suppressed ^{3}H-dopa/μm^2 and dopa/leucine ratios. 'Regulatory' mutations affected only neural crest melanocytes and were quantitative, having reduced percentages of ^{3}H-leucine grains melanosomic. They also were mosaic, possessing 'reverted' melanocyte clones.

It is hypothesized that the *I* locus regulates the premelanosomal synthesizing *pk* locus while the *Bl* locus regulates the tyrosinase synthesizing *c* locus.

References

1   BISHOP, J.; PEMBERTON, R., and BAGLIONI, C.: Reiteration frequency of haemoglobin genes in the duck. Nature new Biol. *235:* 231–234 (1972).

2   BRUMBAUGH, J.: The ultrastructural effects of the *I* and *S* loci upon black-red melanin differentiation in the fowl. Devl Biol. *24:* 392–412 (1971).

3   BRUMBAUGH, J. and FROILAND, T.: Dopa and cysteine incorporation into premelanosomes. Effects of cycloheximide and gene substitution. J. invest. Derm. *60:* 172–178 (1973).

4   BRUMBAUGH, J. and ZIEG, R.: The ultrastructural effects of the dopa reaction upon developing retinal and epidermal melanocytes in the fowl; in RILEY Pigmentation: its genesis and biologic control, pp. 107–123 (Appleton Century Crofts, New York 1972).

5   BRUMBAUGH, J.; BOWERS, R., and CHATTERJEE, G.: Genotype-substrate interactions altering Golgi development during melanogenesis. Pigment Cell, vol. 1, pp. 47–54 (Karger, Basel 1973).

6   DAVIDSON, E. and BRITTEN, R.: Organization, transcription and regulation in the animal genome. Q. Rev. Biol. 48: 565–613 (1973).

7   HARRISON, P.; HELL, A.; BIRNIE, G., and PAUL, J.: Evidence for single copies of globin genes in the mouse genome. Nature, Lond. 239: 219–221 (1972).

8   HEARING, V. and EPPPIG, J., jr.: Electrophoretic characterization of melanosomal proteins extracted from normal and malignant tissues. Experientia 17: 1011–1013 (1974).

9   HUTT, F.: Genetics of the fowl (McGraw-Hill, New York 1949).

10 PATTERSON, D.; KAO, F., and PUCK, T.: Genetics of somatic mammalian cells. Biochemical genetics of Chinese hamster cell mutants with deviant purine metabolism. Proc. natn. Acad. Sci. USA 71: 2057–2061 (1974).

11 PETERS, T., jr. and ASHLEY, C.: Binding of amino acids to tissues by fixatives; in ROTH and STUMPF Autoradiography of diffusible substances, pp. 267–278 (Academic Press, New York 1969).

12 STANBURY, J.; WYNGAARDEN, J., and FREDRICKSON, D.: Inherited variation and metabolic abnormality; in STANBURY, WYNGAARDEN and FREDRICKSON The metabolic basis of inherited disease, pp. 3–28 (McGraw-Hill, New York 1972).

13 SULLIVAN, D.; PALACIOS, R.; STAUNEZER, J.; TAYLOR, J.; FARAS, A.; KIELY, M.; SUMMERS, N.; BISHOP, J., and SCHIMKE, R.: Synthesis of deoxyribonucleic acid sequence complementary to ovalbumin messenger ribonucleic acid and quantitation of ovalbumin genes. J. biol. Chem. 248: 7530–7539 (1973).

14 SUZUKI, Y.; GAGE, L., and BROWN, D.: The genes for silk fibroin in Bombyx mori. J. molec. Biol. 70: 637–649 (1972).

15 WARREN, D.: Inheritance of pinkeye in the fowl. J. Hered. 31: 291–292 (1940).

16 YOUNG, R.: The role of the Golgi complex in sulfate metabolism. J. Cell Biol. 57: 175–189 (1973).

17 ZIMMERMAN, J.; BRUMBAUGH, J.; BIEHL, J., and HOLTZER, H.: The effect of 5-bromodeoxyuridine on the differentiation of chick embryo pigment cells. Expl Cell Res. 83: 159–165 (1974).

Dr. J. A. BRUMBAUGH, School of Life Sciences, University of Nebraska, Lincoln, NB 68508 (USA)

Pigment Cell, vol. 3, pp. 177–183 (Karger, Basel 1976)

Studies on the Expression of Genes for Melanogenesis *in vivo* and *in vitro*

TAKUJI TAKEUCHI, TAKASHI IKEJIMA and YUJI SUGITA

Biological Institute, Tohoku University, Aoba-yama, Sendai

Introduction

Melanogenesis is a metabolic event in which the functions of genes at several loci are involved. In the mouse, a locus designated c is known to control the synthesis of tyrosinase, which is the key enzyme in melanogenesis. Some loci are considered to control the formation of melanosomes, the site of melanogenesis. Another type of gene conditions the environment in which the expression of the major genes for melanogenesis takes place. It has been demonstrated that the genes at a locus express in the cells adjacent to the melanocytes of hair bulbs indirectly influencing the melanogenesis in the melanocytes [6, 7, 9]. Thus, the presence of A^y gene, a dominant allele at a locus, leads to the formation of yellow melanin (phaeomelanin) in the melanocytes of hair bulbs, while a mouse homozygous for a allele produces black melanin (eumelanin) in the melanocytes.

An attempt was made in this study to induce black melanin formation in genotypically yellow skin and to induce the formation of yellow melanin in genotypically black skin of mice, in order to understand the mode of action of genes at a locus. We also studied the expression of genes for melanogenesis *in vitro*, utilizing a cell line derived from B16 mouse melanoma. It has been reported that the 5-bromodeoxyuridine (BrdU) completely diminished melanogenesis in cultured melanoma cells [10, 12]. We investigated the alteration in the synthesis of messenger RNA in BrdU-treated melanoma cells.

Materials and Methods

Young adult mice *(Mus musculus)* with genotypes A^y/A and A^y/a of strains, C3H/HeNSa and C57BL/6, were used in this experiment. Their dorsal hair was removed either by plucking or clipping, and the dorsal skin exposed to UV (254 nm) of 1.0×10^6 erg/cm² per day for ten consecutive days, using a Nippo UV lamp (GL-6W) at the distance of 3.5 cm. Organ culture of the skin explants was performed as previously reported [11]. The materials were fixed with buffered formalin solution, pH 7.2, for 24 h. They were then lyophilized and mounted with balsam on slide glasses. The electrophoresis of the skin homogenate was carried out as reported elsewhere [3].

The cells used in this experiment were line G4 cloned in our laboratory from the line 440B established by KITANO and HU [4] from B16 mouse melanoma. The cells were grown in monolayer culture in Eagle's medium supplemented with 10% calf serum.

For the enzyme assay, the cells were homogenized in 30 mM phosphate buffer, pH 7.4, and the homogenate was centrifuged at 600 g for 5 min. The resulting supernatant was used for the assay of enzyme activity. Tyrosinase activity was estimated spectrophotometrically by the initial rate of increase in optical density at 475 nm with 1 mg/ml of L-dopa in M/10 phosphate buffer, pH 6.8. Cytochrome oxidase activity was assayed spectrophotometrically by following the disappearance of ferrocytochrome C.

Polysomal RNA was isolated from the melanoma cells at the late exponentially growing period using the method described by ADESNIK and DARNELL [1]. Prior to the preparation, the cells were incubated with 2.5 µCi/ml of ³H-labeled uridine (specific activity, 18.7 Ci/mmol) for 100 min. The polysomal RNA was fractionated by affinity chromatography on poly(U)-Sepharose [2]. The RNA fractionated on poly(U)-Sepharose was analyzed by polyacrylamide gel electrophoresis by the method reported by LOENING [5], except that the gel was allowed to polymerize overnight.

Results and Discussion

A. Induction of Black Pigment Formation in the Genotypically Yellow Skin by UV Irradiation

Small black foci were found in the dorsal skin of the genotypically yellow mice 7 days after the beginning of the irradiation in most cases. The foci gradually expanded in area and finally became black or smear patches. The darkening of the irradiated skin was detected in 6 out of 11 mice with the genotype A^y/A and in 4 out of 7 mice with genotype A^y/a. The microscopic observation showed that the darkening occurred in both hair shafts and hair bulbs indicating that eumelanin, instead of phaeomelanin, is produced in the melanocytes. This result is in accord with QUEVEDO and MCTAGUE [8].

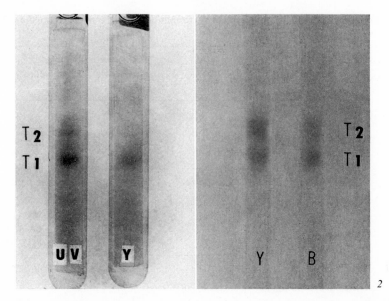

Fig. 1. Multiple forms of tyrosinase from the UV-irradiated yellow skin (left) and from the nonirradiated yellow skin (right) as visualized by polyacrylamide gel electrophoresis.

Fig. 2. Electrophoretic bands of tyrosinase in the skin explants cultured in actinomycin D-containing medium (left) and in the normal medium (right).

In the genotypically yellow mice, only one tyrosinase band, T_1, was detected by polyacrylamide gel electrophoresis. After the UV irradiation, however, the darkened part of the skin from the yellow mouse was demonstrated to possess T_2-form of tyrosinase beside the T_1 band (fig. 1). Electron microscopic observation also showed that melanosomes of eumelanin type were present in the hair-bulb melanocytes of the irradiated mice.

B. Induction of Yellow Pigment Formation in the Genotypically Black Skin

The explants from the dorsal skin of 1.5-day-old black mice (C57BL/10, *a/a*) were cultured in the medium containing actinomycin D (10 μg/ml, Merck) for 3 days. Yellow pigments were found in the hair follicles of the explants while no change was detected in the color of the hair follicles in the control culture (table I). The yellow pigment was soluble to ethanol and disappeared during the regular histological preparation.

Table I. Induction of yellow pigment formation by actinomycin D in the genotypically black mouse skin

Experiments	Number of explants	Number of hair follicles observed	Number of yellow bulbs
Control			
I	5	451	0 (0)
II	8	689	0 (0)
III	5	535	0 (0)
Total	18	1,675	0 (0)
Actinomycin D, 10 μg/ml			
I	9	940	940 (100)
II	7	676	676 (100)
III	9	841	841 (100)
Total	25	2,457	2,457 (100)
Cycloheximide, 500 μg/ml			
I	7	576	0 (0)
II	6	525	0 (0)
III	5	308	0 (0)
Total	18	1,409	0 (0)

Percentages are given in parentheses.

Therefore, the explants were lyophilized to preserve the pigments. It is demonstrated, however, by polyacrylamide gel electrophoresis, that both T_1 and T_2 bands of tyrosinase were present in the explants cultured with actinomycin D as well as in the control cultures (fig. 2). Melanosomes observed in the hair bulbs in the explants were rod-shaped, one of the characteristics of eumelanin, instead of being round-shaped, one of the characteristics of yellow melanosomes. On the other hand, in the explants cultured with cycloheximide (500 μg/ml, Wako), no yellow pigment was detected (table I). In order to demonstrate the requirement for tyrosinase in the induction of the yellow pigment found in the genotypically black skin, explants from albino skin (BALB/c) were cultured in the actinomycin D-containing medium. Contrary to our expectation, yellow pigments appeared in the albino explants. The yellow pigments found in this study do not seem to be phaenomelanin in the general sense, and the nature of the pigment is the subject for a future study.

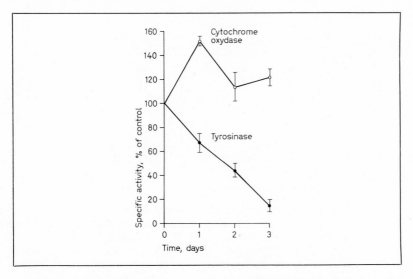

Fig. 3. Enzyme activities of melanoma cells cultured in BrdU-containing medium.

C. m-RNA Synthesis in BrdU-Treated Melanoma Cells

The cells, when inoculated with the density of 1.5×10^4/ml, grew in the medium containing BrdU (3 μg/ml, Sigma) at a rate similar to the control cells during the first 6 days after the inoculation, but reached the stationary phase earlier (6×10^4/ml) than the control cells (5×10^5/ml). They seemed to divide twice in the BrdU-containing medium. The pattern of growth was essentially the same when cells were inoculated with the density of 6×10^4/ml. The cells grown in the medium containing BrdU showed a distinct morphological change. They were epithelial-like with transparent cytoplasm, whereas the control cells were fibroblast-like and contained numerous melanosomes in the cytoplasm. A gradual decrease in tyrosinase activity was seen in the BrdU-treated melanoma cells, while some increase was detected in the activity of cytochrome oxidase in the same culture (fig. 3).

The polysomal RNA prepared by poly(U)-Sepharose chromatography, which has been considered to be cytoplasmic messenger RNA [2] from BrdU-treated melanoma cells, was analyzed by polyacrylamide gel electrophoresis. The electrophoretic pattern of the RNA prepared from the control cells showed a broad distribution in radioactivity, indicating the presence of RNAs with heterogeneous molecular weights. In the

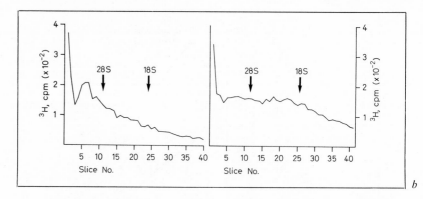

Fig. 4. Electrophoretic pattern of polysomal RNA prepared by poly(U)-Sepharose chromatography from the BrdU-treated melanoma cells (a) and the control (b).

BrdU-treated cells, the radioactivity in the region smaller than 28S was much lower than that of the control (fig. 4). This result indicates that BrdU affects the synthesis of a wide variety of messenger RNAs, including those for melanogenesis.

Summary

The formation of eumelanin was induced in the skin of genotypically yellow mice by UV irradiation. The T_2 band was demonstrated by gel electrophoresis in the irradiated skin. A kind of yellow pigment was found in the explants from the genotypically black and albino skin when cultured with actinomycin D. Polysomal RNA prepared from the BrdU-treated melanoma cells was analyzed by gel electrophoresis. Reduction in the synthesis of a wide variety of messenger RNAs was demonstrated.

Acknowledgments

We are indebted to Dr. F. Hu for providing us with the cell line, to Mr. S. Ohtomo and Miss A. Momoki for their technical assistance. This work was partly supported by a grant (944008) from the Ministry of Education.

References

1   ADESNIK, M. and DARNELL, J. E.: Biogenesis and characterization of histone messenger RNA in HeLa cells. J. molec. Biol. *67:* 397–406 (1972).

2   ADESNIK, M.; SALDITT, M.; THOMAS, W., and DARNELL, J. E.: Evidence that all messenger RNA molecules (except histone messenger RNA) contain poly(A) sequences and that the poly(A) has a nuclear function. J. molec. Biol. *71:* 21–30 (1972).

3   IKEJIMA, T. and TAKEUCHI, T.: Genetic modification of the molecular forms of tyrosinase in the house mouse. Jap. J. Genet. *49:* 37–43 (1974).

4   KITANO, Y. and HU, F.: Melanin versus protein synthesis in melanocytes *in vitro*. Expl Cell Res. *64:* 83–88 (1971).

5   LOENING, U. E.: The fractionation of high-molecular-weight ribonucleic acid by polyacrylamide-gel electrophoresis. Biochem. J. *102:* 251–257 (1967).

6   MAYER, T. C. and FISHBANE, J. L.: Mesoderm-ectoderm interaction in the production of the agouti pigmentation pattern in mice. Genetics *71:* 297–303 (1972).

7   POOLE, T. W.: Dermal-epidermal interactions and the site of action of the yellow (*A^y*) and nonagouti (*a*) coat color genes in the mouse. Devl Biol. *36:* 208–211 (1974).

8   QUEVEDO, W. C., jr. and MCTAGUE, C. F.: Genetic influences on the response of mouse melanocytes to ultraviolet light. The melanocyte system of hair-covered skin. J. exp. Zool. *152:* 159–168 (1963).

9   SILVERS, W. K. and RUSSELL, E. S.: An experimental approach to action of genes at the agouti locus in the mouse. J. exp. Zool. *130:* 199–220 (1955).

10 SILAGI, S. and BRUCE, S. A.: Suppression of malignancy and differentiation in melanotic melanoma cells. Proc. Nat. Acad. Sci. USA *72:* 47–50 (1970).

11 TAKEUCHI, T.: Regulating function of agouti gene in the mouse; in KAWAMURA, FITZPATRICK and SEIJI Biology of normal and abnormal melanocytes, pp. 117–124 (University of Tokyo Press, Tokyo 1971).

12 WRATHALL, J. R.; OLIVER, C.; SILAGI, S., and ESSNER, E.: Suppression of pigmentation in mouse melanoma cells by 5-bromodeoxyuridine. Effects on tyrosinase activity and melanosome formation. J. Cell Biol. *57:* 406–423 (1973).

Dr. TAKUJI TAKEUCHI, Biological Institute, Tohoku University, Aoba-yama, *Sendai 980* (Japan)

Pigment Cell, vol. 3, pp. 184–190 (Karger, Basel 1976)

Studies on the Mechanism of the Inherited Red Skin Color Found among New Guineans

P. F. NIXON

Department of Biochemistry, John Curtin School of Medical Research, Australian National University, Canberra, and the Papua New Guinea Institute of Medical Research, Goroka

Inbreeding of clan groups in the New Guinea highlands has resulted in frequent expression of genetic variants inherited in an autosomal recessive manner. Several skin color variants are found among the highland people, who are normally dark brown. The most interesting and perhaps unique variant is characterized by red skin, pale brown (not red) hair and sometimes by nystagmus [2]. The red skin color is moderately dark; certainly darker than some other New Guinea highlanders whose skin color is that of milk coffee and who are termed pale brown in this paper. Previous light microscopic studies [1] have shown that the melanocytes of red skin can be distinguished under the light microscope by their numerous, thick, multipolar dendrites.

To determine if the red color of red skin could be attributed to a red melanin, the visible spectra of melanin granules were recorded by a Zeiss Universal Microspectrophotometer I. Unstained sections of 5 μm thickness were used with suitable controls. Spectra of melanin granules recorded over the wavelength range 360–700 nm were converted to the form $\log_{10}A$ (absorbance) to remove the effects of concentration and thickness and confine attention to the shape of the absorbance spectrum. In common with other melanins, neither spectra exhibited any characteristic narrow absorbance peaks. However, the broad absorbance curves were such that pigment granules of red skin absorbed comparatively less strongly in the red region 600–750 nm and more strongly in the complementary region 490–500 nm than did granules from control pale or dark brown skin. To quantitate redness, the difference between $\log_{10}A_{500\,nm}$ and $\log_{10}A_{675\,nm}$ was measured and was found to be significantly greater for red than for control skins (p = 0.003). Such spectra are consistent with the proposition that the red quality of red skin is due to redness of the melanin granules.

The studies described below were therefore carried out with the objective of understanding the ultrastructural and chemical characteristics of this red melanin found in human skin apparently as a unique variant (i.e. mutant) phenotype. Our long-term objective is to describe the pathway of its biosynthesis. Since this red melanin is found in the skin, but not the hair of these subjects, only non-follicular melanocytes were examined.

In a search for known melanin precursors in melanocytes, freeze-dried specimens were exposed to formaldehyde vapor, embedded, sectioned at 7 and 10 μm and examined for melanocyte fluorescence characteristic of dopa or cysteinyldopa (excitation at ≤ 420 nm and emission at ≥ 460 nm). Fluorescence was detected in melanocytes from half the control skin samples but from no red skin samples suggesting that fluorogenic melanin precursors might not accumulate in the melanocytes of red skin. This negative result does not allow of any conclusion regarding the nature of the immediate precursors of the melanin of red skin, but it does suggest that there is no block in its biosynthetic pathway.

To determine their ultrastructural features, skin samples were fixed in glutaraldehyde-formaldehyde, embedded in Durcopan and examined in the electron microscope. Some skin was incubated with dopa after fixation and before embedding. The first ultrastructural difference to be noticed between red and control skin was in the distribution of melanin granules. In red skin (fig. 1A, B), the melanosomes were more frequently found in melanocyte dendrites than in keratinocytes. The dendrites of red skin were consequently large and obvious. In contrast, the melanocyte dendrites of dark brown skin were hard to find and contained few melanosomes. These differences do not appear to depend only on the amount or intensity of total melanin granules, since the distribution of melanosomes between dendrites and keratinocytes of pale brown skin was intermediate between that of dark brown and red skin (table I), but the pigmentation of pale skin was more dilute than that of red skin.

The melanocytes of red skin, like those of controls, preferentially absorbed and oxidized dopa to melanin which was deposited in vesicles associated with the Golgi apparatus and endoplasmic reticulum (fig. 1C). In fact, the melanocytes of red skin were stained more deeply than were those of control skin by the melanization which followed incubation in dopa. This histochemical finding also suggests that there are no total blocks in the pathway of melanin biosynthesis in the melanocytes of red skin.

Melanosomes found in keratinocytes of red skin were more frequently in complexes (fig. 1D, E) than were those of control skin. However, some melanosome complexes were regularly found even in dark skin and as many as half of the melanosomes of pale brown skin were found in complexes. Both single and complex melanosomes of red skin were frequently incompletely melanized, but premelanosomes were found even more frequently in pale brown skin and were occasionally found even in dark brown skin.

The external dimensions of melanosomes were measured and, where possible, the internal structure of premelanosomes was examined. The fibrillar substructure of premelanosomes was not measurably different between those of red and control skin, with two possible exceptions. Fibrils of all skins were regularly oriented parallel, were the same distances apart and were cross-linked at the same distances. In each skin, some melanosomes were found in which fibrils were cross-linked and separated with a periodicity of about 8 nm and in others these dimensions were about 16 nm. The latter appeared to represent a stage of melanization of single fibrils into pairs, as is seen in figure 1E. One possible exception was that rare premelanosomes with very fine fibrils only 4 nm apart were found in red skin, but one cannot be certain that such premelanosomes might not have been found in control skin were they not so well melanized. The second possible exception is that the premelanosomes of red skin often appeared to be coarsely granular, but this appearance could well have been due to cross-sectioning of fibrils 16 nm apart.

One possibly significant difference between red and control skins was in the dimensions of single melanosomes. In red skin, the largest single melanosomes measured no greater than 420×160 nm, whereas those of control skin regularly measured up to 600×300 nm (table I). The overall dimensions of melanosome complexes were larger still in all types of skin and reached 800×500 nm in red skin, but of course the individual melanosomes within complexes were small. For comparison, the larger, more evenly melanized melanosomes of dark brown control skin are shown in figure 1F.

Fig. 1. Electron micrographs of New Guinean skins. *A* Melanosomes of red skin are found more frequently in melanocytes and their dendrites than in keratinocytes. *B* Melanosomes in dendrite between keratinocytes of red skin. *C* Melanocytes of red skin actively oxidize dopa to melanin. *D* and *E* Melanosomes in keratinocytes of red skin. *F* Melanosomes of keratinocyte of dark brown control skin.

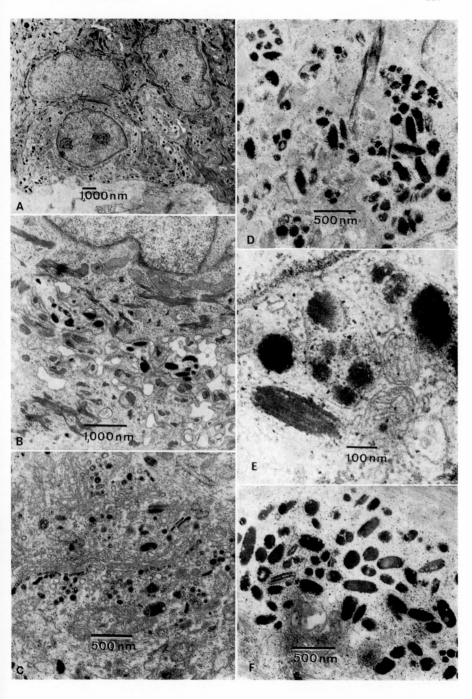

Table I. Electron microscopic findings in dark brown, pale brown and red skin

Structural feature	Dark brown	Pale brown	Red
Melanocyte dendrites	not obvious	obvious	obvious and loaded with melanosomes
Dopa oxidation by melanocytes	+	+	+
Melanosome distribution			
Number in melanocytes/ number in keratinocytes	1/99	40/60	60/40
Melanocyte melanosomes			
Fraction as premelanosomes, %	40	90	50
Fraction in complexes, %	0	0	0
Dimensions of largest, nm	420×240	400×150	420×160
Keratinocyte melanosomes			
Fraction as premelanosomes, %	$5-25$	50	$5-30$
Fraction in complexes, %	$5-40$	50	$50-90$
Dimensions largest singles, nm	600×300	600×250	410×150
Dimensions largest complexes, nm	700×550	750×450	800×500
All melanosomes			
Fibril orientation	regular	regular	regular
Distance between fibrils, nm	8 and 16	–	4, 8 and 16
Distance between fibril cross-links, nm	8 and 16	8	8

Table I summarizes the above electron microscopic findings for red, pale brown and dark brown skin. While many findings were identical for skin of all types, red skin differed from control skin most obviously in two respects: (1) thicker melanocyte dendrites more loaded with melanosomes, and (2) smaller maximum size of single melanosomes. Since melanosomes are of such dimensions as to interfere with the transmission of light in the visible range, it appears to be possible that differences in the size of melanosomes might be responsible for differences in their color and, in turn, in skin color. Thus the small size of the melanosomes of red skin could be responsible for its redness, and the large size of the melanosomes found in the hair follicles in the Chediak-Higashi syndrome could be responsible for the blue coloration of that hair [3]. These ultrastructural studies cannot indicate why the melanosomes of red skin are smaller than those of brown skin and do not exclude the possibility that the red melanin of red skin might be chemically different from that of brown skin, just as hair and feather phaeomelanins are chemically different from eumelanins.

We have also measured the concentrations of melanin precursors and related compounds in urine from our subjects. In the urine of all red subjects, the concentration of cysteinyldopa was low (0–0.04 μg/ml, like Caucasians), whereas it ranged up to high values (0.74 μg/ml) in the urine of dark brown subjects. The concentrations of dopa in the urine of those red subjects who also exhibited nystagmus varied widely from low to very high, giving high values for both the mean and the standard deviation. Pale brown subjects who also had nystagmus excreted similar amounts of dopa in their urine and both groups also had high urine concentrations of another aromatic amino acid, tyrosine, as well as the non-aromatic amino acid alanine. The concentration of dihydroxyphenylacetic acid appeared to be similar in the urine of all subjects. The excretion of dopamine in the urine of those red subjects who had nystagmus was consistently and significantly elevated at least 3-fold above that of other subjects. These differences in urine concentrations of aromatic amino acids and catecholamines suggest that they might be metabolized differently by controls and red-skinned subjects, but the significance of these differences is presently elusive.

Red or yellow melanins have been frequently described in hair and feathers of man, birds and animals, but this is the first description of red melanin in non-follicular melanocytes of skin. Our future studies will be directed at finding a chemical marker characteristic of the melanin of red skin.

It does appear that the inherited red skin color is associated: (1) with red-toned melanin granules in the skin; (2) with diminished transfer of melanosomes from melanocytes to keratinocytes, and (3) with smaller melanosomes. It remains to be seen whether or not the pathways of biosynthesis of the melanins of red and brown and other human skins are different and what is the precise site of the mutation which apparently results in red skin melanin.

Summary

New Guinea highlanders are normally dark brown, but skin color phenotype variations are relatively frequent. The 'red-skinned' phenotype is apparently inherited as an autosomal recessive. It is distinguished by a red quality, lightening of the skin color and sometimes by nystagmus. Light microscopic studies have shown that the melanocytes of red skin are distinguished by numerous thick dendrites.

On microspectrophotometric analysis, the pigment granules of red skin absorbed more light in the region 400–450 nm than did controls, consistent with the pigment granules being the site of the red skin color.

The melanosomes of red skin were most frequently small and packaged in complexes although some were single and normal in size. More than half the melanosomes of red skin were found in melanocyte dendrites, whereas most melanosomes of control skin were in keratinocytes. The fine structure of red skin melanosomes did not differ markedly from that of controls.

Compared to other phenotypes, New Guineans with red skin and nystagmus excreted significantly more dopamine in the urine. Some of those with nystagmus and either red or pale brown skin had increased amounts of dopa in the urine, but there appeared to be little significant difference between the groups. Urine cysteinyldopa content was low or undectable in those with red skin.

References

1   NIXON, P. F.: The 'red-skinned' New Guinean: distinctive melanocytes. Pigment Cell, vol. 1, pp. 6–13 (Karger, Basel 1973).
2   WALSH, R. J.: A distinctive pigment of the skin in New Guinea indigenes. Ann. hum. Genet. *34:* 379–385 (1971).
3   WINDHORST, D. B.; ZELICKSEN, A. S., and GOOD, R. A.: A human pigmentary dilution based on a heritable subcellular structural defect – the Chediak-Higashi syndrome. J. invest. Derm. *50:* 9–18 (1968).

Dr. P. F. NIXON, Department of Biochemistry, University of Queensland, *Brisbane* (Australia)

Pigment Cell, vol. 3, pp. 191–200 (Karger, Basel 1976)

Electron Microscopy of Pigment Cells in Variegated and Nonvariegated, Piebald-Spotted Dogs

ROBERT H. SCHAIBLE and JOHN A. BRUMBAUGH

Department of Medical Genetics, Indiana University School of Medicine, Indianapolis, Ind., and School of Life Sciences, University of Nebraska, Lincoln, Nebr.

Dalmatian and merle *(M)* dogs have been proposed as animal models of Waardenburg syndrome in man primarily because deafness and incomplete pigmentation of the skin, hair and eyes occurs in all three types [2, 10]. With regard to skin and hair pigmentation, all three types appear to be piebald in that the forehead and midventral regions are often unpigmented [4, 8, 9]. Waardenburg syndrome explicitly fits the piebald classification because electron micrographs of hair follicles of the white forelock fail to reveal any pigment cells [12].

SCHAIBLE [9] proposed that piebald mutants be subdivided into variegated and nonvariegated classes. ARIAS [1] seems to be the first to emphasize the occurrence of variegation in skin and hair pigmentation of Waardenburg syndrome. Because of the clonal appearance of spots on Dalmatian dogs, BURNET [3] urged that the development of the pattern be investigated to determine whether or not the spots formed as a result of somatic mutation. SCHAIBLE [9], presented preliminary evidence for a mutation rate of about 3% in the germ cells of merle homozygotes. If that rate is confirmed by additional data, it would be the highest spontaneous mutation rate known [6]. Such a high germinal mutation rate makes somatic mutation a reasonable mechanism for the variegated nature of the hair, skin, and eye pigmentation.

If merle and Waardenburg syndrome are comparable, the black forelock in ARIAS' [1] case 1 may represent 'normal' pigmentation rather than hyperpigmentation. 'Normal' or expected pigmentation is obvious in breeds of dogs such as the Shetland sheepdog in this study. The normal color is usually black over most of the body as determined by the mutant gene, *(a^t)* bicolor [10]. The merle gene reduces the black color to gray except for reverted patches of black. In most human families, there are so many intergrades of hair pigmentation that it would be difficult to predict the shade of nonmutant hair in a case of Waardenburg syndrome.

Although somatic mutation has not previously been seriously considered as the basis for variation in expression of Waardenburg syndrome within families [1], the variability among families led BROWN et al. [2] to propose heterogeneity of the major gene. Indeed, WAARDENBURG [11] believed the responsible locus to have a high mutation rate; 5 of his 16 probands appeared to be new mutations.

New mutant forms of merle are often the subject of rumors among breeders of purebred dogs. One such mutant having the pattern of a harlequin Great Dane has been documented as occurring in collies [5]. Apparently, no breeding records of the variant forms have been reported prior to this presentation.

Although the Waardenburg, Dalmatian and merle patterns all appear to have some characteristics of variegated piebald types, electron microscopy of the pigment cells in each of the levels of pigment intensity in all three types would determine whether or not there is actually variegation at the cellular level. Since the variegated nature of pigmentation in Waardenburg syndrome has been verified by electron microscopy [1], this investigation is concerned primarily with the electron microscopy of hair pigmentation in the two proposed animal models, Dalmatian and merle.

Materials and Methods

Subjects for electron microscopy were three AKC registered Shetland sheepdogs ('shelties', fig. 1–3), donated or loaned by breeders, and an AKC registered, black-spotted Dalmatian bitch owned by one of us (SCHAIBLE). From breeding records and appearances, all three Shelties are assumed to be homozygous for bicolor (a^t) and piebald (s) (See SEARLE [10] for more complete descriptions of mutants.) The bitch in figure 2 is also heterozygous for merle (M). The bitch in figure 3 is a harlequin modification of merle similar to the merle variant reported by FORD [5]. The Dalmatian (fig. 4), like all others of the breed, is assumed to be homozygous for piebald (s), dominant black (specific locus not established) and ticking (T). In addition, she is known to be heterozygous for brown (b) because her dam was brown-spotted.

The harlequin modification of merle (hereafter referred to as 'harlequin-merle') occurred spontaneously in a bitch puppy in a litter of two, the other sib being nonmerle. Their sire was a heterozygous merle and their dam was nonmerle. When bred to nonmerle males, the original harlequin-merle and a similar harlequin-merle granddaughter, together, have produced 5 harlequin-merle and 6 nonmerle (but no

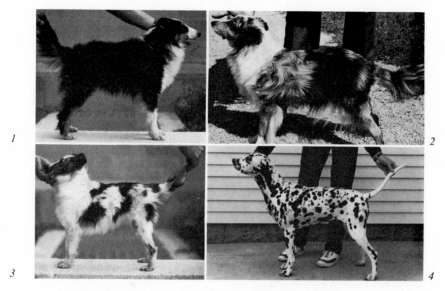

Fig. 1. Nonvariegated, piebald Sheltie.
Fig. 2. Variegated (heterozygous merle), piebald Sheltie.
Fig. 3. Variegated (heterozygous harlequin-merle), piebald Sheltie.
Fig. 4. Nonvariegated, piebald Dalmatian.

typical merle) progenies. Although more data is needed, the absence of typical merle offspring indicates that harlequin-merle is either the effect of a new allele of merle or a mutation at another locus.

One daughter of a cross of the original harlequin-merle to a heterozygous merle mate appears to be typical of merle homozygotes: being partially deaf, showing very little development of the eyes and showing pigment in very limited areas of the coat. When bred to nonmerle mates, she produced a total of 13 merle, 8 harlequin-merle (including bitch in fig. 3) and 1 nonmerle (fig. 1) progenies. These data indicate that harlequin-merle is a new allele of merle (provisional symbol, M^h) rather than a mutation at another locus. Hence, the dam of the Shelties in figures 1 and 3 will hereafter be referred to as a compound merle heterozygote rather than a merle homozygote. The exceptional nonmerle offspring (fig. 1) produced 6 nonmerle and no merle offspring when bred to a nonmerle bitch. Therefore, he is considered to be the result of a back mutation in a germ cell of his dam, the compound merle heterozygote.

Except for the observation of the birth of one litter of 2 merle and 3 harlequin-merle pups from the compound merle heterozygote, all of the breeding data given above on Shelties was submitted by breeders. To check the mode of genetic transmission of harlequin-merle, the compound merle heterozygote was subsequently bred to an AKC registered, agouti-colored (wild type) German shepherd by artificial insemination. As a check on the validity of germinal back mutation of the merle gene, the exceptional nonmerle offspring of the homozygous merle collie × Dalmatian cross reported by SCHAIBLE [9] was bred to a nonmerle mate (backcross to his Dalmatian dam).

In preparation for obtaining hair bulbs for electron microscopy, hairs were plucked clean from areas about 1 inch in diameter in the pigmented area of the lateral aspect of the thigh and the unpigmented chest region of the nonmerle Sheltie (fig. 1) and in a pigmented spot and an unpigmented region of the lateral aspect of the thigh of the Dalmatian (fig. 4). 10–14 days later, growing hair bulbs were plucked from the previously plucked areas and retained for processing. By the same procedure, hairs were also plucked from a gray area in a ventro-lateral, costal location in the merle heterozygote (fig. 2) and from a 'white hypopigmented' area in a dorso-lateral costal location in the harlequin-merle heterozygote (fig. 3). Areas referred to as 'white hypopigmented' in the harlequin-merle correspond in location to gray areas in merle heterozygotes.

Hair bulbs were fixed in 3% gluteraldehyde in 0.1 M phosphate buffer (pH 7.2), osmicated for 1 h (2% OsO_4) in phosphate buffer, dehydrated and embedded in Epon 812. Ultrathin sections were mounted on formvar coated grids and stained with uranyl acetate and lead citrate. Sections were viewed with an RCA EMU 3-B (modified) electron microscope.

Results

The exceptional nonmerle pup from the homozygous merle Collie × Dalmatian cross produced 11 nonmerle and no merle offspring when he was mated to nonmerle. This result confirms back mutation of a germ cell in the homozygous merle sire of the exceptional nonmerle pup.

In two litters sired by the agouti German shepherd, the compound merle heterozygote produced a total of 5 bicolor and 6 agouti progenies. Two of the bicolor type were merle and 3 were harlequin-merle. The gray background color on the harlequin-merle, bicolor pups was not reduced to white as in the purebred, harlequin Shelties described above, but the background was definitely a light enough shade to distinguish them from the typical merle, bicolor types. Also the size of individual back-mutated areas and the total amount of back-mutated area in each individual were much greater in the harlequin-merle, bicolor than in the merle, bicolor pups. The coats of the agouti segregates contained much yellow pigmentation which is not visibly affected by the merle alleles. Although it was possible to classify all of the agouti pups as merle, it was not possible to distinguish the harlequin-merle from the typical merle type.

These litters from the compound merle heterozygote raise her total number of progeny by nonmerle mates to 33 (32 merle or harlequin-

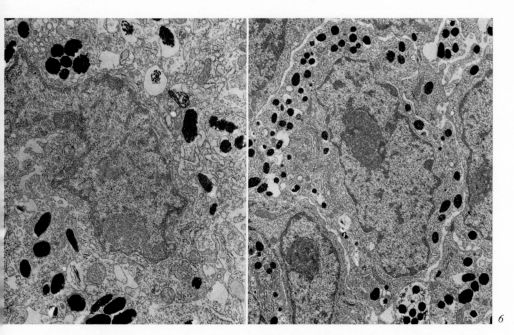

Fig. 5. Normal melanocyte in hair bulb from pigmented spot of Dalmatian. × 10,800.

Fig. 6. Normal melanocyte in hair bulb from pigmented area of nonmerle Sheltie in figure 1. × 6,800.

merle and one nonmerle exception). The average germinal mutation rate for her and the two merle homozygotes reported by SCHAIBLE [9] is 3.2%.

Electron microscopy revealed no definitive pigment cells in hair bulbs plucked from the white chest of the nonmerle Sheltie (fig. 1) or from the white region of the thigh of the Dalmatian. Typical productive melanocytes were found in hair bulbs plucked from pigmented areas on the thighs of both breeds (fig. 5, 6).

The gray background of the merle heterozygote (fig. 2) was composed of both black hairs and lightly pigmented hairs. Electron micrographs of the black hairs (fig. 7) appear the same as the black hairs from the Dalmatian and the nonmerle Sheltie. Melanosomes in the melanocytes of lightly pigmented hairs are smaller, rounder and less melanized (fig. 8). The condensed chromatin material in the nucleus suggests that the cells are fairly old. Thus, incomplete melanization is not due to an immature state of the cell.

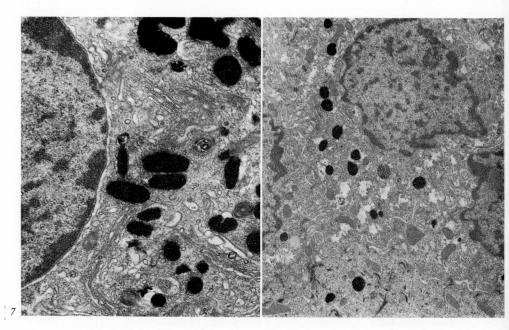

Fig. 7. Normal melanocyte in black hair bulb from gray area of heterozygous merle Sheltie in figure 2. × 18,400.

Fig. 8. Melanocyte in lightly pigmented hair bulb from gray area of heterozygous merle Sheltie in figure 2. Melanosomes are rounder and fewer in number than in normal melanocytes. × 9,200.

No mature melanosomes could be found in the pigment cells of hair bulbs from the white hypopigmented background of the harlequin-merle heterozygote (fig. 3). Organelles containing granular material inside a unit membrane can be seen in the electron micrograph in figure 9 (arrows). These organelles and similar ones in other cells appear to be 'abortive', early premelanosomes.

Discussion

The absence of pigment cells in the white regions of the nonmerle Sheltie (fig. 1) and the Dalmatian, as determined by electron microscopy, provides a firmer basis for the classification of the pigment defect in both animal models along with that of the Waardenburg syndrome as forms of piebaldism.

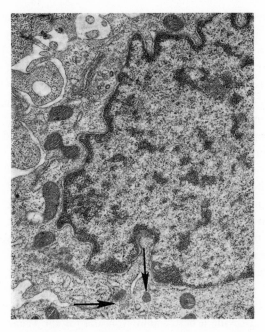

Fig. 9. Melanocyte showing only abortive, early premelanosomes (arrows) in white hair bulb from 'white hypopigmented' area of heterozygous harlequin-merle Sheltie in figure 3. × 15,400.

The absence of pigment cells in the white background and the uniform normalcy of the melanocytes in the pigmented spots of the Dalmatian indicate that its phenotype should be classified as nonvariegated piebald. Apparently, there are no amelanotic pigment cells in the skin which could back mutate and form the pigmented spots. The Dalmatian is born with pure white coat as a result of selection against the occurrence of large primary pigment areas. Possibly the direct migration of melanoblasts from the neural crest to the skin has been suppressed in favor of a more circuitous internal route via nervous or circulatory pathways to the skin. The small spots which develop postnatally appear to be distributed as though pigment cells had migrated off the endings of nerve fibers or blood vessels. REAMS [7] has concluded that melanoblasts do take an internal migratory pathway to the mesoderm ventral to the neural tube in addition to the pathway directly to the epidermis, as they are dispersed from the neural crest.

The decreased number and rounder shape of melanosomes in the melanocytes of lightly pigmented hairs versus black hairs in the gray areas of the heterozygous merle Sheltie (fig. 2) verifies its variegated nature at the cellular level. Because the ultrastructure of the melanocytes in black hair bulbs from gray areas of the merle heterozygote, from black areas of the exceptional, back-mutated Sheltie (fig. 1) and from the black spots of the Dalmatian (control, fig. 4) all appear the same, the conclusion can be drawn that back-mutation is a likely mechanism for the variegation.

The spontaneous appearance of the harlequin-merle mutant and its transmission to succeeding generations in the same form are evidence of a germinal, forward mutation of the merle gene. The immature state of the melanosomes in the white, hypopigmented areas (which are not expected to be white by the action of the *s* gene) is evidence of a more exterme form of variegation than is found in the typical merle mutant. White hypopigmented areas that breeders claim occasionally occur in merle heterozygotes may well be the result of similar somatic, forward mutations.

Because Waardenburg syndrome and both forms of the merle mutant all show evidence of variegation at the cellular level, all of them should be classified as variegated piebald. Thus, with respect to pigmentation patterns, the merle forms provide a better animal model for the Waardenburg syndrome than does the Dalmatian.

When biopsies for electron microscopy are taken from white regions in cases of Waardenburg syndrome or merle mutants of dogs, absence of pigment cells indicates the piebald effect in that region, but presence of melanocytes having immature melanosomes or reduced numbers of melanosomes indicates that the region is white because of variegation. Different findings for white regions in different locations on the same individual no longer need be considered as contradictory, but rather can be used as critera for diagnosing the case as one of variegated, piebald mutant types.

The high degree of interfamily and intrafamily variation of Waardenburg syndrome, as discussed by BROWN *et al.* [2], could be expected if the gene responsible for the variation is subject to as high a frequency of germinal and somatic mutation as appears to be true of merle mutants. Spontaneous germinal mutation to different alleles would establish families showing different combinations of the possible array of pleiotropic effects. Within families, the high rate of somatic back mutation to normal tissues in each afflicted individual probably would suppress the expression of one or more of the pleiotropic effects expected for all afflicted members of that particular family.

Summary

The Dalmatian and merle patterns in dogs and the Waardenburg syndrome in man can all be classified as piebald types, in that no pigment cells can be identified by electron microscopy in certain white regions of the skin and hair. Merle and Waardenburg syndrome can be further specified as variegated piebald because they both show areas having different shades of pigment. Electron micrographs reveal differences in the numbers of melanosomes in melanocytes taken from those areas. The spots are of uniform shade and the melanocytes are uniformly normal in the Dalmatian. With respect to pigmentation, the merle mutant is therefore better than the Dalmatian as an animal model for the Waardenburg syndrome.

Acknowledgments

This investigation was supported by NIH Research Grant GM 19241 from NIGMS to the senior author and by NIH Research Grant GM 18969 from NIGMS and PHS Research Career Development Award GM 42355 from NIGMS to the junior author. We are grateful for the technical assistance of Dr. K. W. LEE, CATHERINE A. SCHAIBLE and SYLVIA BONNET. We thank LIBBY BABIN, M. J. MAYFIELD, PATRICIA SEIPEL and Mr. and Mrs. MARVIN KEITH for donating Shelties and breeding records. We thank ANN ADLER for permission to pluck hairs from her heterozygous merle Sheltie.

References

1 ARIAS, S.: Genetic heterogeneity in the Waardenburg syndrome. Birth Defects Orig. Art. Ser. 7: 87–101 (1971).
2 BROWN, K. S.; BERGSMA, D. R., and BARROW, M. V.: Animal models of pigment and hearing abnormalities in man. Birth Defects Orig. Art. Ser. 7: 102–109 (1971).
3 BURNET, F. M.: Immunological surveillance (Pergamon Press, Oxford 1970).
4 FITZPATRICK, T. B. and QUEVEDO, W. C., jr.: Biological processes underlying melanin pigmentation and pigmentary disorders; in BORRIE Modern trends in dermatology, vol. 4, pp. 122–149 (Appleton Century Crofts, New York 1971).
5 FORD, L.: Defective collie dogs with heterozygous merling. J. Canine Genet. 1955: January, pp. 24–28.
6 MELVOLD, R. W.: Spontaneous somatic reversion in mice. Effects of parental genotypes on stability of the p-locus. Mutation Res. 12: 171–174 (1971).
7 REAMS, W. M., jr.: Pigment cell population pressure within the skin and its role in the pigment cell invasion of extraepidermal tissues; in MONTAGNA and HU Advances in biology of skin, the pigmentary system, vol. 8, pp. 489–501 (Pergamon Press, Oxford 1967).

8 SCHAIBLE, R. H.: Comparative effects of piebald-spotting genes on clones of melanocytes in different vertebrate species; in RILEY Pigmentation: its genesis and control, pp. 343–357 (Appleton Century Crofts, New York 1972).

9 SCHAIBLE, R. H.: Identification of variegated and piebald-spotted effects in dominant autosomal mutants. Pigment Cell, vol. 1, pp. 14–19 (Karger, Basel 1973).

10 SEARLE, A. G.: Comparative genetics of coat colour in mammals (Logos Press/Academic Press, London/New York (1968).

11 WAARDENBURG, P. J.: A new syndrome combining developmental anomalies of the eyelids, eyebrows and nose root with pigmentary defects of the iris and head hair and with congenital deafness. Am. J. hum. Genet. 3: 195–253 (1951).

12 WITKOP, C. J., jr.: Personal commun. Address: Division of Human and Oral Genetics, School of Dentistry, University of Minnesota, Minneapolis 1975.

Dr. ROBERT H. SCHAIBLE, Department of Medical Genetics, Indiana University School of Medicine, 1100 W. Michigan St., *Indianapolis, IN 46202* (USA)

Pigment Cell, vol. 3, pp. 201–210 (Karger, Basel 1976)

The Abnormal Albino Animal[1]

Carl J. Witkop, jr., Richard A. King and Donnell J. Creel

School of Dentistry, University of Minnesota, Minneapolis, Minn.

It has long been recognized that various mutations affecting the pigment system in animals are often associated with abnormalities in other biologic systems. Among numerous examples that could be mentioned are convulsive seizures in mice homozygous for dilute lethal mutation d^1, abnormalities of Auerbach's plexus leading to megacolon in certain piebald mice, microphthalmia found in mock-albino mice homozygous for the microphthalmia gene mi and abnormalities of membranes of lysosomal-like granules in cells of mink homozygous for the Aleutian gene a and the various homologs of this gene in other species such as Cesar-Chediak-Higashi syndrome in man [13]. The experimental use of animals with these types of mutations have made major contributions to our understanding of genetic control and regulation of various biologic systems including pigment regulation.

While these facts are well known, over the years the dichotomous situation has arisen wherein the most frequently used research animals have been albino and hypomelanotic strains of mice, rats, guinea pigs, and rabbits. Albino and other hypopigmented strains such as belted, chinchilla and Siamese animals among others, have been used as standard laboratory animals in numerous studies which have contributed heavily to basic theory development in such diverse fields as educational psychology, neuroanatomy, biochemistry, orthoptics, and drug testing to name only a few. The basic assumption in many of these studies was that the features of albinism were related to what might be termed first order effects of lack of pigment such as photophobia and susceptibility to epidermal carcinoma. Except for hypopigmentation, these animals were assumed to be normal,

1   Supported by NIH PHS DHEW Grant AM-15317.

had normal behavior patterns, normal response to drugs and intact neural pathways. Indeed, catalogs of animal supply houses still list albino mice as having normal vision [6].

This paper presents evidence that a variety of mutations resulting in hypopigmented phenotypes in man and animals are associated with abnormal optic neural pathways provided the mutation results in hypopigmentation of the retina and that various albino animals and humans have abnormal responses to some drugs when compared with their pigmented counterparts.

Neuronal Pathways in Albino Animals and Man

Vertebrates with laterally placed eyes such as most fish, amphibians and birds, have panoramic vision and for the most part there is complete decussation of optic neuronal fibers at the chiasm. With the phylogenetic shift of eyes to a frontal position and binocular vision, the proportion of fibers that originate for the most part in the temporal retina and do not cross the midline increases. Thus, the proportion of fibers ipsilateral to the eye of origin are approximately 10% in rat, 20% in dog and horse, 30–40% in cat and 40–50% in higher primates and man (fig. 1) [11]. In 1965, studies by SHERIDAN [15] and LUND [10] showed that the albino rat had reduced or absent ipsilateral fibers. Since that time, various investigators such as GIOLLI and GUTHRIE [5], GUILLERY [7] and CREEEL [2] demonstrated by anatomic, electrophysiologic or electroencephalographic means that albino animals such as rat, guinea pig, ferret, cat and mink have abnormal ipsilateral optic tracts. Up to 1973, all animals reported to show the anomaly had been mutations at the C or tyrosinase locus and included cc- albino guinea pig, rat, rabbit, mink and ferret; c^hc^h - himalayan or siamese (c^sc^s) cat; and $c^{ch}c^{ch}$ - chinchilla white tiger. It was postulated by others that because all of these animals had mutations at the C-locus controlling tyrosinase and because the optic neurons do not contain pigment, the decussation defect was associated with a non-pigmentary effect of an abnormality in the enzyme tyrosinase.

The present investigators asked the question: 'If the abnormal retinal → geniculate → visual cortex pathway is associated with an extra-pigmentary function of altered tyrosinase, why do our human albinos with tyrosinase-positive (ty-pos), yellow mutant (ym) and Hermansky-Pudlak syndrome (HPS) [18] mutations which are non-allelic with the tyrosinase-

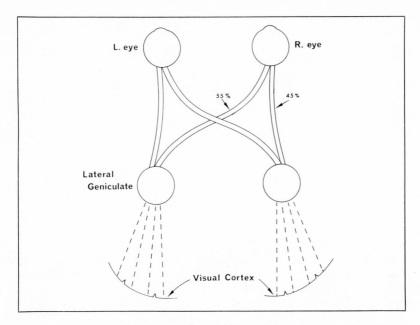

Fig. 1. Schematic drawing of the retinal → geniculate → visual cortex neuronal pathway in man. The major portions of fibers arising from the temporal retina course to the geniculate ganglion on the same (ipsilateral) side as the eye of orign, while those from the nasal retina cross at the midline to the opposite geniculate ganglion. This provides the anatomic mechanism for fusion of similar fields of vision. In primates and man, the proportion of fibers that cross the midline to non-crossed fibers is approximately 55:45. Approximately symmetrical visually evoked EEG responses would be expected from monocular photic stimulated subjects using occipital leads.

negative (most likely homologous with C-locus in animals) albinism and who have tyrosinase activity have ophthalmologic findings similar to the ty-neg albino?' Is it possible that any mutation resulting in lack of retinal pigment would also have abnormal optic pathways? One eye of mice homozygous for pink eye which is non-allelic with the C-locus was enucleated and degenerated fibers studied. These showed abnormal distribution similar to albino animals. 21 human albinos including 8 ty-neg, 9 ty-pos, 2 ym and 2 HPS albinos were tested for photic stimulated electroencephalographic responses using occipital leads over the area of visual cortex. If albinos had a paucity of ipsilateral fibers, then one would expect symmetrical responses on binocular stimulation but asymmetrical respon-

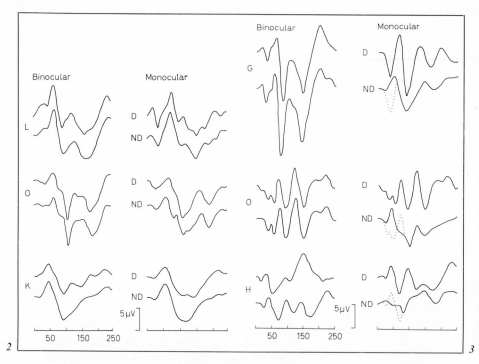

Fig. 2. Representative visually evoked potentials from normal brown-eyed subjects under conditions of binocular and monocular illumination. Recordings were
made from both hemispheres (O_1-A_1 and O_2-A_2). Monocularly evoked potentials
from the hemisphere receiving the decussated optic fibers (D) are similar to the
evoked potentials from the hemisphere receiving the nondecussated optic fibers
(ND). Horizontal base time is 250 msec. Negative is up.

Fig. 3. Representative visually evoked potentials from albino subjects under
conditions of binocular and monocular stimulation. Recordings were made from
both hemispheres (O_1-A_1 and O_2-A_2). Binocularly evoked potentials are nearly symmetrical, but monocularly evoked potentials are asymmetrical. Monocular recordings from the decussated fibers (D) compared with the nondecussated fibers (ND)
show components missing (dotted line) on the nondecussated side. Horizontal time
base 250 msec. Negative is up.

ses on monocular stimulation with reduced waves on the ipsilateral side.
Further, if the abnormality were due to an extrapigment effect of tyrosinase, then ty-neg albinos only would show the defect while ty-pos, ym and
HPS albinos who have tyrosinase activity would not. Ten normal brown-
eyed controls and 21 albinos including ty-neg, ty-pos, ym and PHS sub-

jects were tested using photically stimulated EEG responses recorded from occipital leads. There was no asymmetry in either the binocular or monocular stimulation of the 10 controls (fig. 2). There was no asymmetry in the binocular stimulated recordings of the 21 albino patients (fig. 3, left). However, 15 of the albino subjects showed definite asymmetrical responses on the ipsilateral side on monocular stimulation (fig. 3, right). Asymmetrical responses were found in 6 ty-neg, 7 ty-pos, and 2 HPS albinos. Two ty-neg, 2 ty-pos and 2 ym albinos did not show significant asymmetry. The absence of asymmetry in some albinos was expected, as dissection studies of animals show that the decussation anomaly is not an all-or-none phenomena in that 2 of 8 albino animals had no detectible abnormalities of optic tract.

The question was then asked: 'Are the ipsilateral fibers completely gone or are they misrouted possibly going to the opposite instead of the ipsilateral side?' If the temporal innervation were missing, then there should be a field defect. If the fibers were misrouted to the opposite side, reverting to a more primitive pattern, then there should be no field defect but a lack of binocular vision. Tests of the visual fields of all types of albinos show no field defect. Orthoptic studies of binocular vision showed that all albinos, including those subjects who had symmetrical EEG responses, had essentially monocular vision.

These studies suggest three conclusions: (1) the retinal optic fibers are present but misrouted; (2) that patients with congenital hypopigmentation of fundus would be expected to have essentially monocular vision; (3) that any mutation resulting in hypopigmentation of retina (optic cup) results in misdirection of retinal $\rightarrow$ geniculate $\rightarrow$ visual cortex pathways rather than an extrapigmentary effect of tyrosinase.

GUILLERY et al. [8] have now demonstrated that the Siamese cat not only has disorganization in the lateral geniculate but also anomalous pathways to the optic cortex. Briefly, two of his major findings are: (1) that the temporal retinal originated ipsilateral fibers do not form a complete A_1 layer but most cross over and terminate in the geniculate of the opposite side, and (2) that the projections of these fibers to the visual cortex resulted in an ordered sequence of the visual field projections but with abnormal fusion of binocularly similar fields. Recently, SANDERSON et al. [12] have shown that 8 different combinations of pigment mutants in mink, many of which involve genes other than of the albinism locus, result in hypopigmentation of the fundus and have anomalous optic pathways.

Abnormal Drug Responses in Albino Animals and Man

COLLINS and LOTT [1] were among early workers to report that albino rats of the Wistar strain were more affected by a single large dose of pentobarbital sodium than were pigmented rats of the Long-Evans strain. During the course of experiments mapping the electrophysiologic responses in the lateral geniculate on albino and pigmented rats anesthesized with pentobarbital sodium, one of the present investigators (CREEL) noted that the albino animals frequently died. This led SHEARER et al. [14] to compare the LD_{50} and LD_{100} dose of pentobarbital sodium among various albino and pigmented strains. The results are shown in table I. Note that the LD_{100} dose for all albino strains tested are milligrams less than the LD_{50} dose for the pigmented strains.

The question arises whether the albino gene is related to this difference or whether in the selection of albino strains some other linked genetic locus has been selected which could account for these differences. The use of congenic strains of animals in which the genome in the pigmented and albino animals differ only at the albino locus would be one method for attacking this problem.

This approach has been used by KING and RUSH [9], and is reported in detail elsewhere in this conference. Briefly, KING noted that human albino patients consistently gave a medical history indicating an intolerance to ethanol. RUSH [19] had noted that albino and pigmented congenic mice of the C57BL/6J and C57BL/6cJ strain had significantly different alcohol consumption ratios. Sleep times were then tested for homozygous black, heterozygous black, and homozygous albino mice following a standard per kilogram dose of injected ethanol. Table II summarizes these results. Liver alcohol dehydrogenase levels were not significantly different in these strains.

The basis for the differences in optic tract abnormalities, pentobarbital sodium and ethanol responses is as yet unclear. However, at a somewhat different level, it is now known that the abnormal bleeding response following aspirin ingestion by a certain type of human albino is the result of a platelet storage defect. A number of patients with Hermansky-Pudlak syndrome have had severe bleeding episodes following ingestion of aspirin following minor surgery, such as tooth extraction, and several of our patients' affected relatives have died from exsanguination under similar circumstances. Platelets from these patients lack normal dense bodies which are the storage organelles for ADP and serotonin which is normally

Table I. LD$_{50}$ and LD$_{100}$ of pentobarbital sodium for rat strains

Strain	LD$_{50}$ mg/kg	LD$_{100}$ mg/kg
Albino		
Fischer, F344/Sim	70	80
Holtzman, Aca: HOT (SD)	60	70
Sprague-Dawley, Sim: (SD)	60	80
Wistar, Sim: (WI)	70	80
Pigmented		
ACI, ACI/Sim	120	140
Black Long-Evans, Blu: (LE) BR	110	130
Brown Norway, NB/Mai	90	110

Table II. Sleep times

Strain	c-Alleles	N	Median, min
C57BL/6J	CC	15	55
C57BL/6J	Cc	17	81
C57BL/6cJ	cc	10	175

Comparisons	p<
CC+Cc	0.005
CC+cc	0.001
Cc+cc	0.001

released providing the massive secondary wave of irreversible aggregation. HPS platelets contain less than 10% of the normal amounts of ADP and serotonin (fig. 4) as found in normal platelets. Administration of aspirin blocks the synthesis of endoperoxides, the intermediate in the synthesis of prostaglandins from arachidonate. The labile aggregation-stimulating substance (LASS) has been found to be two closely linked endoperoxide intermediates of prostaglandin synthesis and is the substance blocked by aspirin [17]. Hence, blocking the production of LASS in the HPS platelets inhibits the release of the already reduced stored ADP and serotonin [4]. In addition to the platelet defect, HPS patients also have a lipid storage defect in that a ceroidlike substance accumulates in reticuloendothelial cells, urine, and oral mucosa [18].

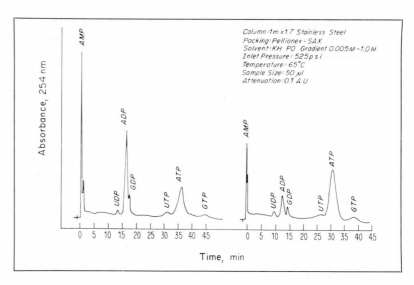

Fig. 4. High pressure liquid chromatographic analysis of nucleotides from platelets of normal subjects (left) and patients with Hermansky-Pudlak syndrome (right) show that ADP is the major nucleotide deficient in HPS platelets.

A similar, if not identical, platelet defect occurs in some strains of fawn-hooded rats [16].

There are numerous studies in the fields of neuropsychology, learning psychology, ophthalmology and drug metabolism, to name a few, where controversies have been extant concerning findings and interpretation of results of experiments on laboratory animals. In reviewing some of these, we find that one group of investigators were using albino animals and the other pigmented strains. In some of these, we can definitely point to the now known differences in the two types of animals used, while in others we suspect that the differences found were ascribable to the animal model used [3].

The dichotomy of using albino laboratory animals as a standard reference animal for normative data can be placed in another perspective. It would as if we collected normative data on humans by using albino patients, a design which if proposed by an investigator, certainly would meet overwhelming criticism. However, the value of this knowledge is not so much to criticize previous work, but to use these mutations as genetic tools to determine the relationship of normal chemistry, structure and function.

Summary

Albino animals have been used as 'standard' laboratory animals in research. However, studies indicate that albino animals, including human albinos, have abnormal optic neural pathways and abnormal responses to drugs. Abnormal ipsilateral optic-geniculate-visual cortex pathways were shown by Creel, Guillery and others, in many species with C-locus mutations cc, c^hc^h, $c^{ch}c^{ch}$, leading to the hypothesis that a nonpigment effect of altered tyrosinase was involved. Present studies of non-C-locus 'albino' animals, human ty-neg, ty-pos, ym and HP albinos show evidence for visual neural disorganization associated with any mutation resulting in retinal hypopigmentation. Ten normal subjects' EEGs compared with those of 20 albino patients showed reduced ipsilateral response on monocular stimulation in the albino but not normal subjects ($\chi^2 \cdot p < 0.001$). Orthoptic studies showed normal fields, but monocular vision in albinos. Deaths of albino animals anesthetized during electrophysiologic brain mapping led to studies showing that in common albino rat strains the LD_{50} and LD_{100} doses of pentabarbital are lower than in four pigmented strains. Coisogenic mice show ethanol sleep time differences related to genotype.

HP human albinos can convert to serious bleeders after blocking of release of storage pool-deficient platelet arachidonic endoperoxide by aspirin, some fatalities resulting.

References

1 COLLINS, T. B. and LOTT, D. F.: Stock and sex specificity in the response of rats to pentobarbital sodium. Lab Anim. Care *18:* 192–194 (1968).

2 CREEL, D. J.: Visual system anomaly associated with albinism in the cat. Nature, Lond. *231:* 465–466 (1971).

3 CREEL, D.; WITKOP, C. J., jr., and KING, R. A.: Asymmetric visually evoked potentials in human albinos. Evidence for visual system anomalies. Investve Ophthal. *13:* 430–440 (1974).

4 GERRARD, J. M.; WHITE, J. G.; RAO, G. H. R.; KRIVIT, W., and WITKOP, C. J., jr.: Labile aggregation stimulating substance (LASS): The factor from storage pool-deficient platelets correcting defective aggregation and release of aspirin-treated normal platelets. Br. J. Haemat. *29:* 657–665 (1975).

5 GIOLLI, R. A. and GUTHRIE, M. D.: The primary optic projections in the rabbit. An experimental degeneration study. J. comp. Neurol. *136:* 99–126 (1969).

6 GREEN, E. L. (ed.): Handbook on genetically standardized JAX mice. 2nd ed. (The Jackson Laboratory, Bar Harbor 1971).

7 GUILLERY, R. W.: An abnormal retinogeniculate projection in Siamese cats. Brain Res. *14:* 739–741 (1969).

8 GUILLERY, R. W.; CASAGRANDE, V. A., and OBERDORFER, M. D.: Congenitally abnormal vision in Siamese cats. Nature, Lond. *252:* 195–199 (1974).

9 KING, R. A. and RUSH, W. A.: Alcohol sensitivity in the albino mouse. Proc. 9th Int. Pigment Cell Conf. (in press).

10 LUND, R. D.: Uncrossed visual pathways of hooded and albino rats. Science *149:* 1506–1507 (1965).

11 POLYAK, S.: The vertebrate visual system; in KLÜVER (University of Chicago Press, Chicago 1957).

12 SANDERSON, K. J.; GUILLERY, R. W., and SHACKELFORD, R. M.: Congenitally abnormal visual pathways in mink *(Mustela vison)* with reduced retinal pigment. J. comp. Neurol. *34:* 223–248 (1974).

13 SEARLE, A. G.: Comparative genetics of coat colour in mammals (Logos Press, London 1968).

14 SHEARER, D.; CREEL, D., and WILSON, C. E.: Strain differences in the response of rats to repeated injections of pentobarbital sodium. Lab. Anim. Sci. *23:* 662–664 (1973).

15 SHERIDAN, C. L.: Interocular transfer of brightness and pattern discriminations in normal and corpus callosum-sectioned rats. J. comp. physiol. Psychol. *59:* 292–294 (1965).

16 TSCHOPP, T. B. and ZUKER, M. B.: Hereditary defect in platelet function in rats. Blood *40:* 217–226 (1972).

17 WILLIS, A. L. and KUHN, D. C.: A new potential mediator of arterial thrombosis whose biosynthesis is inhibited by aspirin. Prostaglandins *4:* 12 (1973).

18 WITKOP, C. J., jr.; WHITE, J. G., and KING, R. A.: Oculocutaneous albinism; in NYHAN Heritable disorders of amino acid metabolism. (Wiley & Sons, Chichester 1974).

19 RUSH, W. A.: Albinism and alcohol sensitivity in the house mouse. Ph. D. thesis. University of Minnesota, Minneapolis (1974).

20 WITKOP, C. J., jr. *et al.:* Hermansky-Pudlak syndrome (HPS). A proposed block in glutathione peroxidase. Oral Surg. *35:* 790–806 (1973).

Dr. CARL J. WITKOP, jr., School of Dentistry, University of Minnesota, *Minneapolis, MN 55455* (USA)

Pigment Cell, vol. 3, pp. 211–219 (Karger, Basel 1976)

Alcohol Sensitivity in the Albino Mouse[1]

RICHARD A. KING and WILLIAM A. RUSH

Division of Human and Oral Genetics, School of Dentistry, and Department of Medicine, School of Medicine, University of Minnesota, Minneapolis, Minn.

Introduction

Response to alcohol has been investigated extensively in inbred strains of mice. Alcohol consumption in choice situations varies considerably between different inbred strains [7]; for example, C57 mice are high consumers, and BALB/c are low consumers. Sleep time following a parenteral dose of alcohol has also been found to vary between inbred strains, tending to parallel the degree of alcohol consumption [6, 7]. High consumers generally sleep less than low consumers following a standard dose of alcohol. The mice used in these experiments have included both pigmented and albino strains, but for most pigment has not been evaluated as a variable in alcohol response. When these studies are reviewed with regard to coat color, all albino strains tested are low consumers. One study [5] has evaluated the effect of the albino locus on alcohol consumption using C57BL/6J congenic albino and pigmented mice. The albino animals consumed less alcohol than the pigmented, although no distinction was made between the homozygous and the heterozygous pigmented animal. A pilot study in our laboratory [8] confirmed this decreased alcohol consumption in the albino and suggested further investigation of the heterozygote.

Methods

Initial stocks of C57BL/6J albino and pigmented mice were obtained from the Jackson Laboratory. C57BL/6J (C/C) were produced from a cross of C57Bl/6J

1   This research was supported by Grants NIH AM 15317 and MH 10679.

(C/C) males and females. C57BL/6J (C/c) and (c/c) were produced from a cross of C57BL/6J (C/c) males and C57BL/6J (c/c) females. Since all mice are C57BL/6J and vary only at the c locus, they will be referred to only by their c locus genotype throughout the paper (C/C, C/c, c/c).

As a control for possible maternal effects in the previous matings and as another test for the differences between (C/C) and (C/c), C57BL/6J (C/C) males were crossed with C57BL/6J (C/c) females to produce a population of pigmented mice consisting of homozygous (C/C) and heterozygous (C/c) genotypes. These pigmented mice are referred to as the ?C57BL/6J, or ?(C/C) and ?(C/c), because they were tested for consumption and sleep time before their specific genotype was known. After completion of the sleep time testing, the genotype was determined by mating these mice to albinos.

The young were weaned at 21 days and housed with their siblings. At 40 days of age, they were separated by sex and housed in groups of 2–6 until consumption testing. Two days prior to consumption testing, they were individually placed in the experimental cages for familiarization. Immediately prior to testing they were weighed. Testing commenced when the mice were 70–80 days of age. During the 6-day consumption test, the mice had a choice between a 10% solution of ethyl alcohol in distilled water and plain distilled water, contained in 25-ml graduated cylinders with sipper tubes. The fluids were refilled every day, and at the beginning of the fourth day their position was switched. There were 4 unoccupied cages with cylinders that were treated in the same manner. The mean values from these four cages were used as daily controls for evaporation and drip. After consumption testing was completed, the mice were again weighed and returned to their housing cages to await sleep time testing.

The (C/C), (C/c) and (c/c) mice were tested for sleep time at 18 weeks of age. The ?(C/C) and ?(C/c) mice were tested at 15 weeks of age. On the day of sleep time testing, food was removed 3–4 h prior to testing. Each mouse was taken from its cage, weighed to the nearest 0.1 g and injected with 0.5 ml of ethyl alcohol per 100 g body weight, the alcohol in a 10% v/v solution in normal saline. The time of injection was time zero. The mice were placed on their backs in a shallow trough while unconscious. When the mouse could roll over twice within 1 min, it was considered to have regained the righting reflex, and the sleep time was the difference between the time of injection and the return of the righting reflex.

Consumption scores were analyzed by standard analysis of variance (unweighted means), and sleep times were analyzed by the Mann-Whitney test.

Results

The consumption ratio is defined as the ratio of 10% alcohol consumed to total fluid consumed. The mean consumption ratios of the (C/C), (C/c) and (c/c) mice are given in table I. There is a significant genotype and sex effect, although the genotype effect is due mainly to the low consumption by the (c/c) mice. When the (C/C) and (C/c) mice are com-

Table I. Mean consumption ratios, by sex, of C/C, C/c and c/c mice

Genotype	Sex	
	male	female
C/C		
Consumption ratio	0.63	0.73
SE	0.04	0.03
N	30	34
C/c		
Consumption ratio	0.71	0.74
SE	0.03	0.03
N	44	39
c/c		
Consumption ratio	0.27[1]	0.42[1]
SE	0.05	0.06
N	37	26

1 This group of mice appeared to show a bimodal distribution on this measure. Genotype, $p<0.01$; sex, $p<0.05$.

Table II. Means of alcohol consumed per unit of body weight per day (ml/100 g wt/day), by sex, for C/C, C/c and c/c mice

Genotype	Sex	
	male	female
C/C		
ml/100 g wt/day	1.44	2.01
SE	0.08	0.07
N	30	34
C/c		
ml/100 g wt/day	1.53	1.84
SE	0.07	0.07
N	44	39
c/c		
ml/100 g wt/day	0.60[1]	1.03[1]
SE	0.10	0.15
N	37	26

1 This group of mice appeared to show a bimodal distribution on this measure. Genotype, $p<0.01$; sex, $p<0.01$.

Table III. Mean consumption ratios, by sex, of ?C/C and ?C/c mice

Genotype	Sex	
	male	female
?C/C		
Consumption ratio	0.69	0.67
SE	0.03	0.02
N	29	38
?C/c		
Consumption ratio	0.58	0.64
SE	0.03	0.04
N	37	29

Genotype, $p < 0.05$.

Table IV. Means of alcohol consumed per unit of body weight per day (ml/100 g wt/day), by sex, for ?C/C and ?C/c mice

Genotype	Sex	
	male	female
?C/C		
ml/100 g wt/day	1.39	1.75
SE	0.08	0.06
N	29	38
?C/c		
ml/100 g wt/day	1.27	1.68
SE	0.07	0.11
N	37	29

Sex, $p < 0.01$.

pared without the (c/c) mice, there is no significant difference. The means of alcohol consumed per unit of body weight (ml/100 g weight/day) for the same groups are given in table II. The results are essentially the same with a slight increase in the significance of the sex effect.

The mean consumption ratios for the ?(C/C) and ?(C/c) mice are given in table III. The consumption ratios for these pigmented mice were determined before the genotype was known. There is a slight genotype effect

Table V. Mean consumption ratios, by sex, for ?C/c mice with maternal genotype C/c and C/c mice with maternal genotype c/c

Maternal genotype	Sex	
	male	female
c/c		
Consumption ratio	0.71	0.74
SE	0.03	0.03
N	44	39
C/c		
Consumption ratio	0.58	0.64
SE	0.03	0.04
N	37	29

Maternal genotype, p<0.01.

Table VI. Means of alcohol consumed per unit of body weight per day (ml/100 g wt/day), by sex, for ?C/c mice with maternal genotype C/c and C/c mice with maternal genotype c/c

Maternal genotype	Sex	
	male	female
c/c		
ml/100 g wt /day	1.53	1.84
SE	0.07	0.07
N	44	39
C/c		
ml/100 g wt/day	1.27	1.68
SE	0.07	0.11
N	37	29

Maternal genotype, p<0.01; sex, p<0.01.

and no sex effect for this measure. When alcohol consumed per unit of body weight (ml/100 g/day) is analyzed, given in table IV, there is no significant genotype effect but a significant sex difference. This is consistent with our impression that the consumption ratio is more sensitive to genotype differences, while the measure of alcohol consumed per unit of body weight is more sensitive to sex differences.

Because there was a significant difference between the ?(C/C) and

Table VII. Median sleep times, in minutes, by sex, for C/C, C/c and c/c mice

Genotype	Sex	
	male	female
C/C		
Median sleep time	56	57
N	9	6
C/c		
Median sleep time	89	87
N	10	7
c/c		
Median sleep time	178	170
N	5	5

Table VIII. Median sleep times, in minutes, by sex, for ?C/C and ?C/c mice

Genotype	Sex	
	male	female
?C/C		
Median sleep time	66	64.5
N	9	16
?C/c		
Median sleep time	96.5	62
N	14	10

?(C/c) mice (table III) while there was no significant difference between the (C/C) and (C/c) mice (table I), the possibility of this being due to differences in maternal genotype was investigated by looking at the (C/c) and the ?(C/c) mice with regard to the maternal genotype. The (C/c) mice had albino (c/c) mothers, whereas the ?(C/c) mice had heterozygous (C/c) mothers. Table V gives the mean consumption ratios for these heterozygous mice listed by the maternal genotype. There is a significant effect of the maternal genotype. Alcohol consumed per unit of body weight (ml/100 g/day) for the same group, table VI, has a significant maternal genotype effect, and again a significant sex effect.

Sleep times determined on (C/C), (C/c) and (c/c) mice are given in table VII. Although there were no significant sex differences, there were

significant differences between genotypes. The (C/C) males awoke significantly sooner than the (C/c) males (p<0.025), while the (C/C) females
did not differ significantly from the (C/c) females, although the trend was
in the same direction as the males. The (C/C) males and females awoke
significantly sooner than the (c/c) males and females (p<0.001 for males,
p<0.005 for females). The (C/c) males and females slept significantly less
than the (c/c) males and females (p<0.005 for both sexes).

Sleep times determined on ?(C/C) and ?(C/c) mice are given in table
VIII. The ?(C/C) males did tend to sleep longer than the ?(C/c) males,
but the difference is not significant. There was no difference in sleep time
between ?(C/C) and ?(C/c) females.

Discussion

The results of this study add to the increasing knowledge of the pleiotropic effects of pigment mutants. CREEL and co-workers [1–3] and GUIL-
LERY *et al.* [4] have shown that albinos or other c locus mutant animals
have a significant disorganization of their visual pathway, with a general
paucity of ipsilateral optic fibers to the lateral geniculate nuclei, pretectal
nuclei and superior colliculi. There is also disorganization of the laminae
of the lateral geniculate nucleus. SHEARER *et al.* [9] have shown that the
LD_{50} of pentobarbital is lower for albino rat strains than for pigmented
rat strains.

Behavioral research by WINSTON and LINDZEY [12] and by THIESSEN
et al. [10, 11] has shown that albino mice differ in their response in a
number of behavioral situations. Response to alcohol has been shown to
vary between mouse strains [6, 7], with albino strains tending to consume less alcohol and to sleep longer in response to alcohol than pigmented strains.

The present study has the feature of having evaluated alcohol response in a population of mice that are genetically identical at all but the
c locus. Our study shows that the albino mouse consumes less alcohol
than its pigmented counterpart, supporting the work of HENRY and
SCHLESINGER [5] and extends this line of investigation to sleep time,
where we find that the albino mouse sleeps significantly longer than its
pigmented counterpart.

The response of the heterozygote is one of the most intriguing aspects
of this study. For alcohol consumption, the (C/c) did not show a statisti-

cally significant difference from the (C/C), whereas the ?(C/c) did consume significantly less alcohol than the ?(C/C). The studies of maternal effects suggest that this disparity of results is due to the differences in the genotypes of the mothers. The genotype of the mothers of the ?(C/c) mice was (C/c), whereas that of the (C/c) mice was (c/c). Offspring of albino mothers consume significantly more alcohol than offspring of heterozygous mothers (table V), suggesting environmental influences on alcohol consumption.

The sleep time determinations show that the male (C/c) sleeps statistically longer than the male (C/C), with the trend being the same for the females although not quite significant. The male ?(C/c) tends to sleep longer than the ?(C/C), but the difference is not significant, and the female ?(C/C) and ?(C/c) do not differ. The explanation for this variance is not known, but we suspect that it is secondary to environmental factors. Between the consumption testing and sleep time determination the ?C57BL/6J mice were housed alone in small wire-bottom cages, while the C57BL/6J were housed in groups of 2–6 in plastic shoe-box cages. Furthermore, the sleep time was measured at 15 weeks for the ?C57BL/6J and at 18 weeks for the C57BL/6J.

While these results for alcohol consumption and sleep time in heterozygotes are not conclusive, the evidence suggests that the mouse heterozygous at the albino locus responds differently to alcohol than the homozygous pigmented mouse. Further investigation of this point is underway.

Summary

Alcohol consumption and sleep time following alcohol injection have been evaluated in congenic C57BL/6J (C/C), (C/c) and (c/c) mice. Albino mice (c/c) were found to consume significantly less alcohol and to sleep significantly longer than their pigmented counterparts (C/c, C/C). Heterozygous pigmented mice (C/c) tended to consume less alcohol and to sleep longer than homozygous pigmented mice (C/C), with some disparity in these results suggesting maternal and environmental influence.

References

1 CREEL, D. J.: Differences of ipsilateral and contralateral visually evoked responses in the cat: strains compared. J. comp. physiol. Psychol. 77: 161–165 (1971).

2   CREEL, D. J.: Visual system anomaly associated with albinism in the cat. Nature, Lond. *231:* 465–466 (1971).
3   CREEL, D. J.; WITKOP, C. J., and KING, R. A.: Asymmetric visually evoked potentials in human albinos: evidence for visual system anomalies. Investve Ophthal. *13:* 430–440 (1974).
4   GUILLERY, R. W.; CASAGRANDE, V. A., and OBERDORFER, M. D.: Congenitally abnormal vision in Siamese cats. Nature, Lond. *252:* 195–199 (1974).
5   HENRY, K. R. and SCHLESINGER, K.: Effects of the albino and dilute loci on mouse behavior. J. comp. physiol. Psychol. *63:* 320–323 (1967).
6   KAHIHANA, R.; BROWN, D. R.; McCLEARN, G. E., and TABERSHAW, I. R.: Brain sensitivity to alcohol in inbred mouse strains. Science *154:* 1574–1575 (1966).
7   RODGERS, D. A.: Factors underlying differences in alcohol preference among inbred strains of mice. Psychosom. Med. *28:* 498–513 (1966).
8   RUSH, W. A.: Albinism and alcohol sensitivity in the house mouse; Ph.D. thesis, Minneapolis (1974).
9   SHEARER, D.; CREEL, D., and WILSON, C. E.: Strain differences in the response of rats to repeated injections of pentobarbital sodium. Lab. Anim. Sci. *23:* 662–664 (1973).
10 THIESSEN, D. D.; LINDZEY, G., and OWEN, K.: Behavior and allelic variations in enzyme activity and coat color at the c locus of the mouse. Behav. Genet. *1:* 257–267 (1970).
11 THIESSEN, D. D.; OWEN, K., and WHITSETT, M.: Chromosomal mapping of behavioral activities; in LINDZEY and THIESSEN Contributions to behavior-genetic analysis: the mouse as a prototype. (Appleton Century Crofts, New York 1970).
12 WINSTON, H. and LINDZEY, G.: Albinism and water escape performance in the mouse. Science *144:* 189–191 (1964).

RICHARD A. KING, MD, PhD, Division of Human and Oral Genetics, School of Dentistry, University of Minnesota, *Minneapolis, MN 55455* (USA)

Pigment Cell, vol. 3, pp. 220–227 (Karger, Basel 1976)

Miniature Melanocytes

A Specific Cell Type in Murine Epidermis

W. M. Reams, jr., R. L. Salisbury, J. T. Earnhardt and
V. H. Howard, jr.

Department of Biology, University of Richmond, and Department of Dermatology, Medical College of Virginia, Richmond, Va.

Introduction

In the process of diagnosing a case of tuberous sclerosis by examination of a white leaf-shaped macule [2], we were especially intrigued with the diminutive size of the melanocytes of the lesion. During an earlier study, we had casually observed miniature melanocytes dispersed between the typical melanocytes in the epidermis of PET/Wmr mice, and we had assumed that they were early stages in the morphogenesis of typical-sized melanocytes. However, BREATHNACH [1] has described melanocytes smaller than normal in the marginal zone of a freckle covering a stretched scar and he has proposed that these, like the enlarged melanocytes of the freckle itself, breed true and have inherent differences representing distinct families of pigment cells. And, based on studies *in vitro*, KLAUS [5] has proposed that in the albino guinea pig the pigmentary system is a genetic mosaic of two distinct types of melanocytes.

With reexamination of dopa preparations of normal epidermis in PET mice, it became evident that their miniature melanocytes were smaller than typical not only with regard to general size, but the nucleus also was diminutive in size. Studies then were begun in attempts to determine the nature of these miniature melanocytes. This report embraces three experimental approaches, using morphogenetic impacts, which have led to the belief that the melanocyte system of the PET mouse is a mosaic and that the miniature melanocytes are a distinct cell type.

Materials and Methods

Mice employed in these studies were of the PET/Wmr strain maintained at the University of Richmond. These mice are dark black, non-agouti animals. To determine the normal state of the epidermal pigmentary system, samples of skin were removed from the dorsum of mice ranging in age from newborn to adult. Hair, when present, was removed with a commercial depilatory. The epidermis of the samples was removed with the aid of 2 M NaBr and then treated with dopa. Following mounting in balsam with the dermal side of the epidermis upwards, the state of the pigmentary system was examined with the light microscope. Counts and measurements were made with the aid of an ocular grid micrometer.

In order to insure that the structures we believed to be the nuclei of the melanocytes were nuclei indeed, samples of whole skin of both normal and experimental animals were treated with dopa after which the melanin was bleached to a light tan with hydrogen peroxide. The samples were paraffin-embedded, frontal sections were cut at 5 μm, the sections stained with hematoxylin, and then examined with the light microscope. The blue-stained, spheroidal nuclei could be easily seen as the bleached melanosomes offered little obstruction of view, yet gave specific identity to the melanocytes.

Chorioallantoic Membrane (CAM) Grafts

Fertile White Leghorn eggs were incubated at 38 °C for 12 days and then prepared in the traditional manner for CAM grafts. To prepare the grafts, newborn PET mice were killed by decapitation, a 5-mm square of skin was removed from the dorsum and placed in sterile saline containing 0.06 mg penicillin and 0.05 mg streptomycin per ml. Hypodermal fat was removed by scraping with a scapel blade. The grafts were transferred to the exposed CAM and positioned dermis-side-down in areas of good vascularization. The opening in the shell was covered with cellophane tape and the incubation was continued. Several grafts were recovered daily after 4–8 days cultivation on the CAM and the isolated epidermis was prepared for microscopic examination following treatment with dopa. A total of 107 grafts were done. The pigment cells of each graft were counted in five different areas and averaged. Then the average counts of the grafts recovered on a given day were averaged. In making the counts, score was kept of the typical and miniature melanocytes.

Ultraviolet Radiation

Three groups of newborn mice were irradiated daily with ultraviolet light (UVL) and each day, 3 mice of each group were killed, epidermal samples from the dorsum prepared with dopa, and the samples examined microscopically. Group 1 received UVL of 250 nm, group 2 received UVL of 300 nm, and group 3 received UVL of 360 nm. Preliminary tests had determined the exposure for each of the Westinghouse UV lamps which would give maximum pigment cell response with a minimum of tissue trauma. Also, a group of adult mice with the dorsum shaved were irradiated daily with 300 nm UVL for ten days and then the state of the epidermal melanocytes determined.

Nitrogen Mustard (NM)

In this study, 4 groups of mice were used. Group 1 started with newborn mice which received a daily topical application of 70% ethanol to the dorsum for 15 days. Group 2 started with newborn mice, but daily topical applications were given of 0.5 mg nitrogen mustard (NM) in 70% ethanol for 15 days. Group 3 had shaved adult mice which received applications of 70% ethanol, and group 4 was of adult mice treated with 0.5 mg NM in 70% ethanol daily, for 15 days. Each day, 3 mice from each group were killed and the dorsal epidermis prepared with dopa and examined.

Results and Discussion

Although the basis of melanocyte morphology is genetic, a number of environmental factors have been found to modify their expression. For example, melanocytes of mice with a dilute genotype lack extensive dendrites and appear small in comparison to the melanocytes of black genotypes. However, these small, nucleopetal melanocytes exhibit a non-dilute morphology if grown in the anterior chamber of the eye [6]. ROVEE [11] observed that with UV radiation, the greater the density of melanocytes, the smaller the size of the cells. Melanocytes have shown agility in changing their morphology and size *in vitro* [4]. All these differences in size and form have been related to differences in degree of dendrite formation [9] and therefore are primarily functions of the cytoplasm.

In general morphology, the miniature melanocytes of the PET mouse epidermis were considerably smaller than typical melanocytes and showed a reduction in the number and size of dendrites. Weakly, as well as strongly dopa-reactive cells were seen in both the miniature and typical melanocyte populations. But, of particular significance, the difference between the miniature and typical melanocytes was reflected primarily in the size of their nuclei. Whereas the typical melanocytes (fig. 1) of PET mouse epidermis have an average nuclear volume of 312 μm^3, the miniature melanocytes (fig. 2) have an average nuclear volume of 113 μm^3 – approximately one third the size of the typical.

As can be seen in figure 7, in the normal PET mouse epidermis the population of dopa-positive typical melanocytes increases rapidly from birth to day 3, then gradually declines. By postnatal day 21, only an occasional typical melanocyte can be demonstrated. Dopa-positive miniature melanocytes are present from birth, are among the last to be seen in the maturing mouse and, in comparison with the radically changing population of typical melanocytes, their population remains relatively constant.

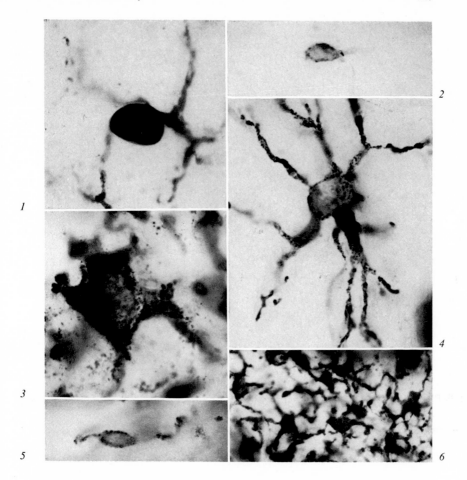

Fig. 1. Typical melanocyte in epidermis of 3-day PET mouse. × 1,000.

Fig. 2. Miniature melanocyte in same epidermis of 3-day PET mouse. × 1,000.

Fig. 3. Giant, nucleopetal-type melanocyte in epidermis treated for 8 days with NM. × 1,000.

Fig. 4. Enlarged melanocyte in epidermis treated for 5 days with NM. × 1,000.

Fig. 5. Miniature melanocyte in epidermis treated with NM. × 1,000.

Fig. 6. Melanocytes in epidermis treated 5 days with NM. × 450.

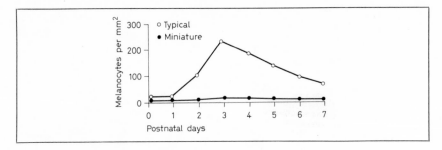

Fig. 7. Melanocyte population behavior in normal PET mouse epidermis.

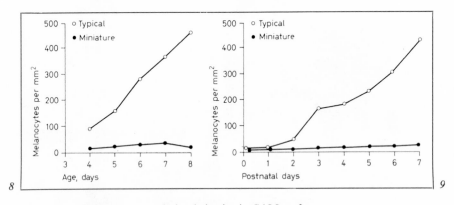

Fig. 8. Melanocyte population behavior in CAM grafts.

Fig. 9. Melanocyte population behavior in PET mouse epidermis with increasing dosages of 300 nm UVL radiation.

In an effort to ascertain whether the miniature melanocytes were immature stages of the typical melanocyte forms, or perhaps a distinct cell type, the melanocyte system of PET mouse epidermis was challenged with several morphogenetic stimuli. If the miniature melanocytes were immature forms, the stimuli should provoke their morphogenesis into typical melanocytes and the population of miniature melanocytes thereby would be reduced or eliminated. If, on the other hand, the miniature melanocytes remained resistant to the morphogenetic impacts, then one might conclude they are independent melanocyte forms.

REAMS [10] showed that the chick embryo produces a 'melanocyte morphogenetic factor' which reaches an effective titer by day 15 of incubation to bring about the maximum morphologic expression of the pigment cells. Further, it has been demonstrated that this factor of the chick was effective on mouse pigment cells grafted to host chick embryos [7]. By transplanting newborn mouse skin to the CAM of 12-day host chick embryos, the graft tissue had become vascularized and well established by the 15th day of host incubation. The recovered grafts represented skin equivalent in age to that of mice of from 4 to 8 days of age. Figure 8 shows that the typical pigment cells of the mouse epidermis responded fully to the chick influences with almost a doubling of the normal population of melanocytes by the end of 8 days cultivation. However, the population of miniature melanocytes in the grafts remained within the normal range. There was no evidence to suggest a significant transformation of miniature melanocytes into typical forms.

Inasmuch as the chick melanocyte morphogenetic factor had no measurable influence on the miniature melanocytes of the mouse, another approach to the problem was attempted. It is generally considered that most cells of an organism have a particular nuclear-cytoplasmic ratio specific to a given cell type. If the DNA of a cell can be increased, it should follow that the nucleus might show an increase in size and the cytoplasm might similarly respond. PATHAK et al. [8] demonstrated with guinea pigs that UV radiation in the 300 nm range promoted a significant increase in DNA synthesis, and SATO and KAWADA [12] showed such activity in a limited number of melanocytes in hairless mice with 253 nm UVL. Hence, we irradiated PET mice with UVL. UVL in the 360 nm range had virtually no effect on the pigment cell system while a modest tanning effect was evidenced with 250 nm UVL. Most pronounced was the effect of the 300 nm UVL (fig. 9). After a week of daily exposures to 300 nm UVL, the population of typical melanocytes had almost doubled. But, again, the population of miniature melanocytes remained essentially unchanged.

Recently, HILGER et al. [3] found that in hairless mice NM applications would induce a notable increase in the melanocyte population and a striking enlargement of the melanocyte cell size. We then applied NM to the dorsum of PET mice and, in comparison to the controls, were rewarded with a most spectacular pigmentary display. With each additional daily application of NM, the general pigment cells increased in number and in size and, as the 15th day of treatment was approached, the melanocyte number was more than double the maximum seen in the controls. By this time, counting of the melanocytes was hindered by the complex entanglement of the elaborate dendritic processes. Figure 4 shows the extensive dendrite formation (compare with fig. 1) after only 5 days treatment, and figure 6 shows the general melanocyte relationships at that time. Even though most of the melanocytes were enlarged due to extensive dendrite formation, their nuclei were of normal size.

After 8 days of treatment, a few melanocytes were seen of giant proportions, platelike with nucleopetal-type dendrites and with a nucleus three times the size of normal (fig. 3). But, throughout the series, whether with young mice or adults, there were the ever present miniature melanocytes. At best, the population of miniature melanocytes was doubled over normal, and their dendrites were more extensive (fig. 5), but the nuclei remained within the normal range.

As the typical melanocytes of PET mouse epidermis gave anticipated responses to the morphogenetic stimuli tested, but the population of miniature melanocytes remained relatively unaffected, it is tendered that the epidermal melanocyte system of the PET mouse is a genetic mosaic and that the miniature melanocytes constitute a specific form of pigment cell distinct from the typical.

Summary

In the epidermis of PET/Wmr mice, the population of melanocytes reaches a peak and begins to decline during the first postnatal week, and has disappeared within 4 weeks. Dispersed among the typical melanocytes are miniature melanocytes, which are generally weakly dopa-reactive and, based on nuclear volume as well as overall size, are less than one third the size of typical melanocytes. They appear early and are among the last to disappear.

Morphogenetic impacts have been employed to test whether these miniature melanocytes could be induced to differentiate into typical melanocytes. In one study, mice were exposed to UV radiation of 250, 300, and 360 nm, and the condition of the epidermal melanocytes determined. In another study, grafts of skin were cultivated on the chick chorioallantoic membrane where they would be subject to the melanocyte morphogenetic influences known to occur in older chick embryos. In a third study, nitrogen mustard was employed as a morphogenetic agent. The typical melanocytes have conformed to anticipated responses to the treatments. However, the populations of miniature melanocytes have shown no significant modification. It is proposed that the condition represents a genetic mosaic for pigmentation and that the miniature melanocytes constitute a form of melanocyte distinct from the typical.

Acknowledgements

This paper is dedicated to Dr. MARY RAWLES (Mrs. JOHN SPURBECK), a talented contributor to our knowledge of pigment cell biology, an inspiring teacher, and an endeared friend.

This study was supported by a grant from the University of Richmond Research Fund.

References

1   BREATHNACH, A. S.: Melanocyte pattern of an area of freckled epidermis covering a stretched scar. J. invest. Derm. *31:* 237–241 (1958).

2   FITZPATRICK, T. B.; SZABÓ, G.; HORI, Y.; SIMONE, A. A.; REED, W. B., and GREENBERG, M. H.: White leaf-shaped macules. Archs Derm. *98:* 1–6 (1968).

3   HILGER, R. G.; FUKUYAMA, K.; EPSTEIN, J., and ZACKHEIM, H.: Dynamics of increased active melanocytes following topical carmustine (BCNU) and nitrogen mustard (NM) in hairless mice. Clin. Res. *22:* 328A (1974).

4   KITANO, Y. and HU, F.: Morphological changes in the melanocytes of the giant bushbaby *in vitro;* in RILEY Pigmentation: its genesis and biologic control, pp. 77–88 (Appleton-Century-Crofts, New York 1972).

5   KLAUS, S. N.: Melanocytes of the albino guinea pig: identification of nucleopetal variants *in vitro.* J. invest. Derm. *50:* 268 (1968).

6   MARKERT, C. L. and SILVERS, W. K.: Effects of genotype and cellular environment on melanocyte morphology; in GORDON Pigment cell biology, pp. 241–248 (Academic Press, New York 1959).

7   NICHOLS, S. E. and REAMS, W. M., jr.: The occurrence and morphogenesis of melanocytes in the connective tissues of the PET/MCV mouse strain. J. Embryol. exp. Morph. *8:* 24–32 (1960).

8   PATHAK, M. A.; KRAMER, D., and GUNGERICH, U.: Formation of thymine dimers in epidermis by ultra-violet (290–320 nm) radiation *in vivo.* J. invest. Derm. *54:* 351 (1970).

9   QUEVEDO, W. C. and SMITH, J. A.: Studies on radiation-induced tanning of skin. Ann. N.Y. Acad. Sci. *100:* 364–388 (1963).

10 REAMS, W. M., jr.: An experimental study of the development of pigment cells in the coelomic lining of the chick embryo. J. Morph. *99:* 513–548 (1956).

11 ROVEE, D. T.: Relation of cell size to cell density in the melanocyte system of the mouse. A. S. B. Bull. *12:* 51 (1965).

12 SATO, T. and KAWADA, A.: Uptake of tritiated thymidine by epidermal melanocytes of hairless mice during ultraviolet light radiation. J. invest. Derm. *58:* 71–73 (1972).

Dr. WILLIE M. REAMS, jr., Department of Biology, University of Richmond, *Richmond, VA 23173* (USA)

Pigment Cell, vol. 3, pp. 228–236 (Karger, Basel 1976)

Effects of MSH on the Brain[1]

ABBA J. KASTIN, CURT A. SANDMAN and ANDREW V. SCHALLY

Veterans Administration Hospital and Tulane University School of Medicine,
New Orleans, La., and Ohio State University, Columbus, Ohio

Introduction

Much knowledge exists about the effects of melanocyte-stimulating hormone (MSH) on the skin, but very little is known about the actions of MSH on the brain. It is understandable that the primary interest of dermatologists studying MSH would be dermal pigment cells, but it is not so obvious why investigators from other disciplines would be so restrictive. Not only does pigmentation exist in many parts of the brain of several species of mammals, but the melanocytes of the skin and hair are derived from melanoblasts which migrate from the embryonic neural crest early in development.

In lower forms of vertebrates, such as amphibians, the change in skin color serves an adaptive function by permitting the organism to blend better with the environment and thereby escape predators. Such a role does not exist in mammals like man. Black people have essentially the same amount of MSH in their blood as white people, and pigmentation in the human being does not change as rapidly as it does in lower vertebrates. Therefore, it is likely that the main function of MSH in mammals is not the control of pigmentation. It is possible that MSH could serve no role at all in man, or during the course of evolution it could have acquired some extra-pigmentary functions.

1   Supported in part by grants from the Veterans Administration and NIH (NS 07664).

Now that data from several studies performed in man support the animal evidence for an effect of MSH on behavior, probably improving and sustaining the level of attention, it is incumbent on us to acquire the knowledge to better understand how and where it works.

Previous Work

Our approach to the actions of MSH on the central nervous system (CNS) has been twofold: first, to determine whether MSH has any effect on the CNS of man; second, to attempt to identify the behavioral systems which are involved by also studying animals. A notable part of this second aspect involves special attention to the role of MSH during development of the organism. Each part of this general approach is different from that taken by others. The superb early clinical studies of LERNER [19, 20] with MSH were concerned mainly with its pigmentary effects. Among the early animal studies of the effects of MSH on the nervous system, the group of KRIVOY [17, 18] looked only at the spinal cord and electric discharge. FERRARI's [5, 7] group, using a neurophysiologic approach, tested only stretching activity and yawning for several years. A more extensive behavioral effort was made by DE WIED [38, 39] and his collaborators but, for the most part, until recently [6] they almost exclusively restricted themselves to the conditioned avoidance response, and, like the earlier investigations of MURPHY and MILLER [24] and MILLER and OGAWA [22], initially approached the problem from a focus on ACTH rather than MSH itself. All of these excellent pioneering approaches contributed greatly to our knowledge in this area of study.

Animal Studies

Initially in our animal studies, all of which were conducted by investigators who did not know the identity of the solutions being injected, we examined the effects of MSH in appetitive tasks. In the first such study, hungry rats were placed in a T-maze and trained to run to the arm of the maze which contained food. After removal of the food, the animals which received MSH continued to run more often and faster to the goal box which previously had contained the food than did the rats injected with the diluent control solution [26]. Similarly, hungry rats trained to press a

lever in order to obtain food on a fixed ratio of reinforcement and injected with synthetic α-MSH were found to continue pressing the bar after
food was no longer available for a greater length of time than did control
rats [15]. Our findings with an appetitive task have been confirmed recently by GARRUD et al. [6]. Each of the appetitive tasks mentioned above
was performed in a relatively simple apparatus. Although the major effect
of MSH was observed during extinction when the reward was not present,
there was a tendency in one of these appetitive experiments toward facilitated learning (acquisition) of the task [26], and this was seen in an experiment involving avoidance of electric shock [29]. It seemed possible
[14] that the difficulty of the task might interact with the effects of MSH,
as we had found previously in a different type of study [35]. We reasoned
that perhaps a complex maze which could provide more incorrect choices
to the rat would make a slight effect of MSH on initial learning more
readily apparent. This possibility was tested with hungry rats placed in a
12-choice Warden maze. MSH was found to increase running speed as
well as reduce the variability and number of errors during acquisition of
the maze [37].

If it is possible that rats injected with MSH might be more active,
then this might account at least in part for delayed extinction of the conditioned avoidance response because the rat would continue to make the
same response, but it probably could not account for inhibition of a passive avoidance response in a two-chambered shuttle box [27]. We found
that rats which previously had received electric shock after entering the
second chamber remained longer in the first chamber if they had received
MSH than if they had received control solution.

Another situation in which the effects of MSH on perseveration
could be tested is in performance of a reversal discrimination task. Rats
were trained to escape [28] or avoid [29] shock in a Y-maze by running
to the door which was illuminated. After reaching the criterion of five out
of six trials for 2 successive days, the task was reversed so that escape
from shock was possible only by running to the arm of the Y-maze in
which the door was not illuminated. Rats injected with MSH reversed
faster than the animals injected with the control solution. This would not
be expected if MSH only caused perseveration of activity in this relatively
simple task.

The level of electric shock used in avoidance tasks is also an important variable. If rats were trained in a two-way shuttle box to avoid shock
presented at two levels of intensity, MSH was found to facilitate learning

at low but not at high levels of shock [36]. This finding emphasizes that MSH can affect facilitation of acquisition of avoidance tasks [29, 36] as well as appetitive tasks [37].

The stage of development of the rat may also influence its present and future response to MSH. Infant albino rats were injected with MSH once a day from the age of day 2 through 7 in two studies conducted at Ohio State University. In one of these studies [1], the rats were tested at the age of 33 days in a difficult 'DRL 20' operant task. In the second study involving different rats injected with MSH from the age of 2–7 days, a brightness discrimination type of task was used [32] when these animals were tested for the first time as 90-day-old adults. In both situations, rats injected with MSH as infants and tested as adults behaved differently from untreated adults [1, 32].

The effect of MSH administered to adult rats tested on an intradimensional shift to cues of the same type of visual problem previously had been tested in the Thompson-Bryant box. It was found that administration of MSH resulted in facilitation of the shift [29]. This pattern of improved performance on the intradimensional shift but deteriorated performance on the extradimensional shift after administration of MSH to rats [31] is similar to the pattern that we found in normal human beings tested with an active fragment of MSH (MSH 4-10) in intradimensional and extradimensional shifts [33].

Clinical Studies

MSH 4-10 was given to 10 healthy young men 21–30 years old and the results compared with those obtained from a similar group of 10 men given diluent in a 'double-blind' procedure in which neither the investigators nor the subjects knew the contents of the solution which were infused i.v. at a constant rate for 4 h. Since no significant difference in cortisol levels was noted between the two groups of subjects, it seemed reasonable to conclude that any changes found after infusion of MSH 4-10 were not due to an action of this peptide on the adrenal cortex. Earlier studies of the CNS actions of ACTH in animals and man usually were extremely difficult to interpret because they did not adequately take into consideration the secondary effects of ACTH stimulating the adrenal gland to release its hormones.

In our study [33], all the men were trained on a two choice discrimination problem in which color (e.g. red) was the relevant dimension of discrimination. This concept formation procedure involving visual discrimination is considered to be a very sensitive indicator of the state of attention of the subject [20, 21]. That MSH or its active component affects attention in normal men was further supported by the results from the Benton visual retention test in which a subject is instructed to reproduce geometric forms shown briefly a few seconds previously. After receiving MSH 4-10, the subjects improved significantly in this test. MSH also resulted in better performance in the Rod and Frame test, in which the subject is asked to align a vertical pole within a square frame which is placed in several different spatial configurations.

The improvement in the Benton visual retention test in man after MSH 4-10 confirmed our earlier finding of a similar improvement in normal as well as hypopituitary subjects after infusion of α-MSH [12]. No improvement in verbal retention as measured by the Wechsler memory scale was found in that study. In this investigation also, infusion for 4 h of 10 mg α-MSH, essentially equivalent to ACTH 1-13, did not stimulate the release of cortisol. The resulting increases in the averaged somatosensory evoked responses were so great that they could be seen directly on single trials of the EEG. They were greatest when the subjects were attentive to the electric stimulation. The changes in EEG frequency were not as dramatic as those seen in the first clinical study of the effects of MSH on the CNS. In that study performed in 1966 [10], half of the subjects showed EEG changes.

The effects of MSH on the EEG of normal men were examined more carefully in a study in which 10 mg MSH 4-10 was injected rapidly i.v. as a bolus [23]. The occipital EEG was analyzed in terms of the power output from four band-pass filters. The ten subjects who received the MSH 4-10 exhibited a statistically significant increase in the power output of the 12+ Hz and 7-12 Hz frequency bands as well as a slight decrease in the output of the 3–7 Hz band. They also showed significantly more 7–12 Hz activity than did controls. Whereas the subjects receiving diluent as a control showed habituation of the EEG response arousal pattern, the subjects receiving the MSH peptide did not habituate but persisted in the arousal pattern. ENDROCZI et al. [4] observed a similar effect with ACTH 1–10 and ACTH 1–24. We also found that injection of the MSH peptide resulted in improvement in the Benton visual retention test, as was observed in our other studies [12, 33]. In our study [23] in which MSH 4-10 was injected quickly as well as in our study in which it was infused for 4 h [33], decreased anxiety as measured by the state-trait anxiety inventory was found.

Future Considerations

It is not known whether the changes associated with the administration of exogenous MSH to rat and man represent exaggerations of physiological occurring responses and, at the moment, it does not seem crucial to determine this. Stress releases endogenous MSH [11], and this release can be 'conditioned' [30] and frequently separated from the release of ACTH [2, 9, 11, 13, 30]. Consideration of the physiologically adaptive role of MSH in the camouflage of lower vertebrates and its phylogenetic persistence makes it entirely reasonable for MSH to have an adaptive role in mammals. The fact that radioactive MSH is localized in certain areas of the brain [3, 25], that MSH affects blood flow differentially in the brain [8], or that MSH changes the turnover of certain biogenic amines in certain areas of the brain [16, 34] still does not identify the exact CNS function of MSH. Study of brain melanin and the enzymes involved in its formation might help in this matter. We believe that a logical investigative approach from several different directions by workers in many disciplines is most likely to enhance our understanding of the role(s) of MSH.

Summary

MSH or its active component was administered to rats and human beings in a series of studies. The behavioral and electrographic changes which were observed reinforce the concept that MSH has extra-pigmentary actions on the CNS of mammals.

References

1 BECKWITH, W. E.; SANDMAN, C. A.; HOTHERSALL, D., and KASTIN, A. J.: The effects of neonatal injections of melanocyte-stimulating hormone (MSH) on the DRL performance of juvenile rats (submitted).
2 DUNN, J. D.; KASTIN, A. J.; CARRILLO, A. J., and SCHALLY, A. V.: Additional evidence for dissociation of MSH and ACTH release. J. Endocr. 55: 463–464 (1972).

3   DUPONT, A.; KASTIN, A. J.; LABRIE, F.; PELLETIER, G.; PUVIANI, R., and SCHAL-
    LY, A. V.: Organ distribution of radioactivity after injection of (^{125}I) α-melano-
    cyte-stimulating hormone in rat and mouse. J. Endocr. *64:* 237–241 (1975).

4   ENDROCZI, E.; LISSAK, K.; FEKETE, T., and WIED, D. DE: Effects of ACTH on
    EEG habituation in human subjects. Prog. Brain Res. *32:* 254–262 (1970).

5   FERRARI, W.; GESSA, G. L., and VARGUI, L.: Stretching activity in dogs intracis-
    ternally injected with a synthetic melanocyte-stimulating hexapeptide. Exper-
    ientia *17:* 90 (1961).

6   GARRUD, P.; GRAY, J. A., and WIED, D. DE: Pituitary-adrenal hormones and ex-
    tinction of rewarded behaviour in the rat. Physiol. Behav. *12:* 109–119 (1974).

7   GESSA, G. L.; PISANO, M.; VARGUI, L.; CRABAI, F., and FERRARI, W.: Stretching
    and yawning movements after intracerebral injection of ACTH. Revue can.
    Biol. *26:* 229–236 (1967).

8   GOLDMAN, H.; SANDMAN, C. A.; KASTIN, A. J., and MURPHY, S.: MSH affects
    regional perfusion of the brain. Pharmac. Biochem. Behav. *3:* 661–664 (1975).

9   GOSBEE, J. L.; KRACIER, J.; KASTIN, A. J., and SCHALLY, A. V.: A functional re-
    lationship between the pars intermedia and ACTH secretion in the rat. Endo-
    crinology *86:* 560–567 (1970).

10 KASTIN, A. J.; KULLANDER, S.; BORGLIN, N. E.; DYSTER-AAS, K.; DAHLBERG, B.;
    INGVAR, D.; KRAKAU, C. E. T.; MILLER, M. C.; BOWERS, C. Y., and SCHALLY, A.
    V.: Extrapigmentary effects of MSH in amenorrheic women. Lancet *i:*
    1007–1010 (1968).

11 KASTIN, A. J.; SCHALLY, A. V.; VIOSCA, S., and MILLER, M. C.: MSH activity in
    plasma and pituitaries of rats after various treatments. Endocrinology *84:*
    20–27 (1969).

12 KASTIN, A. J.; MILLER, L. H.; GONZALES-BARCENA, D.; HAWLEY, W. D.; DYSTER-
    AAS, K.; SCHALLY, A. V.; VELASCO-PARRA, M. L., and VELASCO, M.: Psycho-
    physiologic correlates of MSH activity in man. Physiol. Behav. *7:* 893–896
    (1971).

13 KASTIN, A. J.; BEACH, G. D.; HAWLEY, W. D.; KENDALL, J. W.; EDWARDS, M.
    S., and SCHALLY, A. V.: Dissociation of MSH and ACTH release in man. J.
    clin. Endocr. Metab. *36:* 770–772 (1973).

14 KASTIN, A. J.; MILLER, L. H.; NOCKTON, R.; SANDMAN, C. A.; SCHALLY, A. V.,
    and STRATTON, L. O.: Behavioral aspects of melanocyte-stimulating hormone
    (MSH). Prog. Brain Res., vol. 39, pp. 461–470 (Elsevier, Amsterdam 1973).

15 KASTIN, A. J.; DEMPSEY, G. L.; BLANC, B. LE; DYSTER-AAS, K., and SCHALLY,
    A. V.: Extinction of an appetitive operant response after administration of
    MSH. Hormones Behav. *5:* 135–139 (1974).

16 KOSTRZEWA, R.; SPIRTES, M. A., and KASTIN, A. J.: α-MSH and MIF-I effects
    on catecholamine levels and synthesis in various rat brain areas. Pharmac.
    Biochem. Behav. *3:* 1017–1027 (1975).

17 KRIVOY, W. A. and GUILLEMIN, R.: On a possible role of β-melanocyte-
    stimulating hormone (β-MSH) in the central nervous system of mammalia: an
    effect of β-MSH in the spinal cord of the cat. Endocrinology *69:* 170–175
    (1961).

18 KRIVOY, W. A.; LANE, M.; CHILDERS, H. E., and GUILLEMIN, R.: On the action

of β-melanocyte-stimulating hormone (β-MSH) on spontaneous electric discharge of the transparent knife fish, G. *eigenmannia*. Experientia *18:* 521 (1962).

19 LERNER, A. B. and McGUIRE, J. S.: Effect of alpha- and beta-melanocyte-stimulating hormone on the skin colour of man. Nature, Lond. *189:* 176–179 (1961).

20 LERNER, A. B. and McGUIRE, J. S.: Melanocyte-stimulating hormone and adrenocorticotrophic hormone: their relation to pigmentation. New Engl. J. Med. *270:* 539–546 (1964).

21 MACKINTOSH, N. J.: Selective attention in animal discrimination learning. Psychol. Bull. *64:* 124–150 (1965).

22 MILLER, R. E. and OGAWA, N.: The effect of adrenocorticotrophic hormone (ACTH) on avoidance conditioning in the adrenalectomized rat. J. comp. physiol. Psychol. *55:* 211–213 (1962).

23 MILLER, L.; KASTIN, A. J.; SANDMAN, C. A.; FINK, M., and VEEN, W. J. VAN: Polypeptide influences on attention, memory and anxiety in man. Pharmacol. Biochem. Behav. *2:* 663–668 (1974).

24 MURPHY, A. V. and MILLER, R. E.: The effect of adrenocorticotrophic hormone (ACTH) on avoidance conditioning in the rat. J. comp. physiol. Psychol. *48:* 47–49 (1955).

25 PELLETIER, G.; LABRIE, F.; KASTIN, A. J., and SCHALLY, A. V.: Autoradiographic localization of MSH in the brain after intracarotid and intraventricular injection. Pharmac. Biochem. Behav. *3:* 671–674 (1975).

26 SANDMAN, C. A.; KASTIN, A. J., and SCHALLY, A. V.: Melanocyte-stimulating hormone and learned appetitive behavior. Experientia *25:* 1001–1002 (1969).

27 SANDMAN, C. A.; KASTIN, A. J., and SCHALLY, A. V.: Behavioral inhibition as modified by melanocyte-stimulating hormone (MSH) and light-dark conditions. Physiol. Behav. *6:* 45–48 (1971).

28 SANDMAN, C. A.; MILLER, L. H.; KASTIN, A. J., and SCHALLY, A. V.: A neuroendocrine influence on attention and memory. J. comp. physiol. Psychol. *80:* 54–58 (1972).

29 SANDMAN, C. A.; ALEXANDER, W. D., and KASTIN, A. J.: Neuroendocrine influences on visual discrimination and reversal learning in the albino and hooded rat. Physiol. Behav. *11:* 613–617 (1973).

30 SANDMAN, C. A.; KASTIN, A. J.; SCHALLY, A. V.; KENDALL, J. W., and MILLER, L. H.: Neuroendocrine responses to physical and psychological stress. J. comp. physiol. Psychol. *84:* 386–390 (1973).

31 SANDMAN, C. A.; BECKWITH, W.; GIDDIS, M. M., and KASTIN, A. J.: Melanocyte-stimulating hormone (MSH) and overtraining effects on extradimensional shift (EDS) learning. Physiol. Behav. *13:* 163–166 (1974).

32 SANDMAN, C. A.; BECKWITH, W. E., and KASTIN, A. J.: Effect of early injections of MSH on later adult discrimination learning in male and female rats (submitted).

33 SANDMAN, C. A.; GEORGE, J. M.; NOLAN, J. N.; RIEZEN, H. VAN, and KASTIN, A. J.: Enhancement of attention in man with ACTH/MSH 4-10. Physiol. Behav. *15:* 427–431 (1975).

34 SPIRTES, M. A.; KOSTRZEWA, R. M., and KASTIN, A. J.: MSH and MIF-I effects on serotonin levels and synthesis in various rat brain areas. Pharmac. Biochem. Behav. *3:* 1011–1015 (1975).

35 STRATTON, L. O. and KASTIN, A. J.: Melanocyte-stimulating hormone in learning and extinction of two problems. Physiol. Behav. *10:* 689–692 (1973).

36 STRATTON, L. O. and KASTIN, A. J.: Avoidance learning at two levels of motivation in rats receiving MSH. Hormones Behav. *5:* 149–155 (1974).

37 STRATTON, L. O. and KASTIN, A. J.: Increased acquisition of a complex appetitive task after MSH and MIF. Pharmacol. Biochem. Behav. *3:* 901–904 (1975).

38 WIED, D. DE: Opposite effects of ACTH and glucocorticoids on extinction of conditioned avoidance behavior. Proc. 2nd Int. Congr. Hormonal Steroids, Milan, No. 132, pp. 945–951 (Excerpta Medica, Amsterdam 1967).

39 WIED, D. DE: Effects of peptide hormones in behavior; in Frontiers in neuroendocrinology, pp. 97–140 (Oxford University Press, New York 1969).

Dr. ABBA J. KASTIN, Veterans Administration Hospital 1601 Perdido Street, *New Orleans, LA 70146* (USA)

Pigment Cell, vol. 3, pp. 237–243 (Karger, Basel 1976)

The Effect of Prostaglandin E_1 on Tissue-Cultured Embryonic Salamander Melanophores

R. R. NOVALES and B. J. NOVALES

Department of Biological Sciences, Northwestern University, Evanston, Ill.

Introduction

The prostaglandins are a family of biologically active lipids synthesized in many cell types in response to both physiological and pathological stimuli. Little is known about their effects on pigment cells, or any role they may play in pigment cell biology. However, they can darken frog skin in *Rana pipiens* [12, 14] and *Xenopus laevis* [15] and can disperse melanosomes in the melanophores of the black goldfish, *Carassius auratus* [1]. Although the mechanism of these actions is uncertain, it is likely that they result from an activation of the enzyme adenylate cyclase in the chromatophores, in view of the melanosome-dispersing action of adenosine $3',5'$-monophosphate (cyclic AMP) on frog [3] and teleost fish [10] melanophores, as well as the ability of cyclic AMP to aggregate reflecting platelets in *R. pipiens* iridophores [2]. Furthermore, PGE_1 (prostaglandin E_1) is a potent activator of adenylate cyclase in Cloudman mouse melanoma homogenates [6, 7]. Thus, it was felt desirable to determine the effect of PGE_1 on tissue-cultured melanophores of embryonic salamanders, since these cells respond to melanocyte-stimulating hormone (MSH) [8] or to cyclic AMP [9] by the formation of cellular processes (dendritogenesis) and melanosome dispersion. They thus are a good system for the study of melanophore control at the cellular level.

Materials and Methods

Developing embryos of *Ambystoma maculatum* were obtained commercially (Carolina Biological Supply Co.) and kept in the refrigerator until use. Hanging-drop cultures were then prepared according to methods previously described in detail [11]. Briefly, dorso-medial tissue containing neural crest was removed from Harrison stages No. 20–34 embryos, sterilized with penicillin and streptomycin and explanted in Niu-Twitty solution of the following composition in grams per liter: streptomycin, 0.05; NaCl, 3.4; KCl, 0.05; $Ca(NO_3)_2 \cdot 4H_2O$, 0.08; $MgSO_4$, 0.10; $NaHCO_3$, 0.20; Na_2HPO_4, 0.11; KH_2PO_4, 0.02 in double glass-distilled water. The culture medium also contained 100,000 units per liter Na penicillin G and was at pH 7.4. Cultures were incubated at 18 °C until melanophores appeared in the outgrowth zone. Coverslips were then transferred to perfusion chambers [4] for the experiments. PGE_1 (The Upjohn Co.) was prepared as a 1 mg/ml stock solution in 95% ethanol and diluted appropriately with Niu-Twitty solution for desired final concentrations, with controls consisting of 95% ethanol diluted the same way. The effect of the perfusions was observed through the microscope and recorded photomicrographically in most cases. A total of 7 perfusion experiments were performed. Synthetic alpha-MSH (K. Hofmann) was utilized as a lactose preparation [13] and cyclic AMP was obtained from Sigma Chemical Co.

Results

PGE_1 had a contracting action on the cultured melanophores at a concentration of 10^{-5} g/liter (3.1×10^{-7} M) in two experiments. Figures 1–4 show one of these experiments. A culture is shown in figure 1 immediately after being placed on the chamber. A fresh supply of Niu-Twitty solution was then perfused and a second photomicrograph taken after 15 min (fig. 2). No significant change occurred in any of the cells as a result of changing the medium or illumination. The melanophores show a condition of intermediate dendritogenesis and melanosome expansion. Figure 3 shows the culture after 20 min treatment with 10^{-5} g/liter PGE_1 in Niu-Twitty solution, which had an ethanol concentration of 9.5×10^{-4}%. Contraction has begun in the cell in the upper right-hand corner of the figure (arrow), as evidenced by a narrowing of the central region. Figure 4 is after a total PGE_1 treatment time of 50 min. The cell previously indicated has continued contracting its central region. Dendritic processes have narrowed and tended to lose their connection with the central region of the cell (clasmatosis). The cell on the left has also begun to round up. The effects continued after the PGE_1 medium was replaced with Niu-Twitty solution for a 30-min period, indicating that the effect is irreversible under these conditions.

The effect of PGE_1 was confirmed and the possible action of the ethanol controlled for in a second experiment (fig. 5–8). Figure 5 shows a

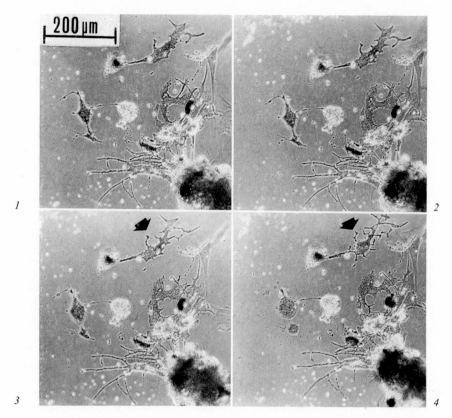

Fig. 1–4. The effect of PGE$_1$ on cultured melanophores of *Ambystoma maculatum*. The magnification scale is given in figure 1 (phase contrast). Fig. 1: A culture immediately after being mounted on the perfusion chamber. Three melanophores are present around the center of the figure. Fig. 2: The same culture after being perfused with fresh Niu-Twitty solution for 15 min. Fig. 3: After 20 min treatment with 10^{-5} g/liter PGE$_1$ in Niu-Twitty solution with an ethanol concentration of 9.5×10^{-40}/o. Responding cell indicated by arrow. Fig. 4: After a total PGE$_1$ treatment period of 50 min.

culture after 30 min on the chamber with fresh Niu-Twitty solution. The culture was then perfused with the control concentration of ethanol (9.5×10^{-40}/o) in Niu-Twitty solution for 30 min (fig. 6). Dendritogenesis occurred in 3 of the 5 large melanophores in the culture. The other 2 exhibited a somewhat more aggregated condition of their melanosomes. Thus, the effect of ethanol is somewhat variable. The PGE$_1$ solution was

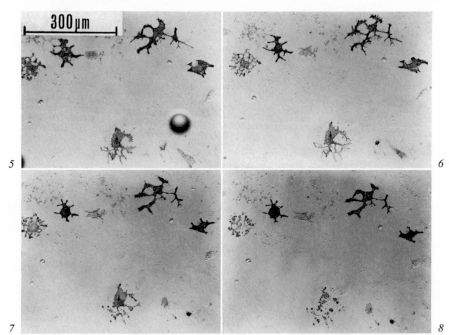

Fig. 5–8. The effect of ethanol and PGE$_1$ on cultured melanophores of *Ambystoma maculatum*. The magnification scale is given in figure 5 (Bright-field) Fig. 5: A culture after 30 min exposure to fresh Niu-Twitty solution for 30 min. Fig. 6: The same culture after treatment with the control concentration of ethanol (9.5×10^{-40}/o) in Niu-Twitty solution for 30 min. Fig. 7: After 45 min treatment with 10^{-5} g/l PGE$_1$ solution with an ethanol concentration of 9.5×10^{-40}/o. Fig. 8: After replacement of the PGE$_1$ solution with fresh Niu-Twitty solution for 15 min.

then perfused (10^{-5} g/liter) and a striking effect had taken place after 45 min (fig. 7). Clasmatosis and fragmentation occurred in several of the melanophores, whereas the other three exhibited a marked aggregation of their melanosomes and a withdrawal of dendritic processes. This effect continued in Niu-Twitty solution alone for 15 min (fig. 8) as in the previous experiment (fig. 1–4). Marked fragmentation occurred in two of the melanophores and the other three melanophores became even more 'rounded-up', with a dense condition of their melanosomes. Application of 10 U/ml synthetic alpha-MSH for 60 min to the culture was followed by melanosome dispersion in two of the intact 'rounded-up' cells, indicating some ability of MSH to reverse the PGE$_1$ effect.

PGE$_1$ was unable to produce any discernible effect at a lower concentration (3.1×10^{-8} M) in two experiments; thus 3.1×10^{-7} M is close to the minimal effective concentration. Furthermore, alpha-MSH (10 U/ml) produced its expected melanosome-dispersing and dendritogenic effects in the presence of the lower concentration of PGE$_1$ in a culture that had been pretreated with the PGE$_1$ for 50 min. This MSH effect was reversible with Niu-Twitty solution. However, 3.1×10^{-8} M PGE$_1$ was able to produce rounding up in melanophores pretreated with 10^{-2} M cyclic AMP in two experiments, indicating that cyclic AMP had sensitized the cells to the effect of the lower concentration of PGE$_1$.

Discussion

The observed effect was the opposite of the expected effect, in view of the ability of PGE$_1$ to disperse melanosomes in the melanophores of other amphibian species [12, 14, 15]. This melanosome-dispersing effect led us to expect a similar action on the cultured *Ambystoma* embryonic melanophores. However, a melanosome-*aggregating* action was observed. Furthermore, some withdrawal of dendritic processes took place, a manifestation of the shape changes that are known to occur in tissue cultured melanophores responding to stimuli [11], e.g. epinephrine or melatonin [8]. If PGE$_1$ were capable of enhancing melanophore cyclic AMP levels, a dendritogenic effect would have been produced, because cyclic AMP produces such an effect in these cells [9]. Thus, it is likely that PGE$_1$ is inactive on the adenylate cyclase of these melanophores. The observed effect is similar to the effect obtained with PGA$_2$ and cultured mouse fibroblasts [5]. In the latter case, cellular processes were withdrawn and the cells detached from the substrate, an effect similar to that seen in the present study. As a test of this, one experiment was conducted with PGA$_2$ at a concentration of 4×10^{-4} M, the maximally effective concentration in both fish [1] and frog [12] melanophores. PGA$_2$ had a pronounced contracting action over and beyond the effect of the ethanol control, suggesting that it has an action similar to PGE$_1$.

Since PGA$_2$ is poorly effective in stimulating adenylate cyclase [5], it is likely that the effects that we have observed with PGE$_1$ are unrelated to adenylate cyclase stimulation and may represent an action exerted on some other aspect of melanophore physiology. A toxic action seems to have occurred in those cells which fragmented in response to the PGE$_1$;

however, in cells which did not fragment, some ability of alpha-MSH was found to reverse the effect.

Summary

In view of the ability of prostaglandins to disperse the melanosomes in certain species of frog and teleost melanophores, their action on tissue-cultured embryonic melanophores of the salamander, *Ambystoma maculatum,* has been tested. PGE_1 at a concentration of 3.1×10^{-7} M produced a rounding up of a total of 7 cells accompanied by melanosome aggregation in two experiments. The rounding up was irreversible and sometimes accompanied by cellular fragmentation. However, synthetic alpha-MSH was capable of reversing the melanosome aggregation in cells which remained intact. The observed effect was the exact opposite of that expected, but bears a resemblance to the known action of PGA_2 on cultured fibroblasts, which probably does not involve cyclic AMP.

Acknowledgements

The authors would like to thank Dr. JOHN E. PIKE, The Upjohn Co., for prostaglandins, Dr. KLAUS HOFMANN, The University of Pittsburgh Medical School, for synthetic alpha-MSH, and Northwestern University for research support.

Research was supported by Biomedical Sciences Support Grant FR7028-05 to the Northwestern University from NIH.

References

1   ABRAMOWITZ, J. and CHAVIN, W.: *In vitro* effects of prostaglandins upon melanosome dispersion in the skin of black goldfish, *Carassius auratus* L. Prostaglandins *4:* 805–818 (1973).

2   BAGNARA, J. T. and HADLEY, M. E.: The control of bright colored pigment cells of fishes and amphibians. Am. Zoologist *9:* 465–478 (1969).

3   BITENSKY, M. W. and BURSTEIN, S. R.: Effects of cyclic adenosine monophosphate and melanocyte-stimulating hormone on frog skin *in vitro.* Nature, Lond. *208:* 1282–1284 (1965).

4   DICK, D. A. T.: An easily made tissue culture perfusion chamber. Q. J. Microscop. Sci. *96:* 363–369 (1955).

5   JOHNSON, G. S.; PASTAN, I.; PEERY, C. V.; OTTEN, J., and WILLINGHAM, M.: The role of prostaglandins in the regulation of growth and morphology of transformed fibroblasts; in RAMWELL and PHARRISS Prostaglandins in cellular biology, pp. 195–200 (Plenum Publishing, New York 1972).

6 KEIRNS, J. J.; KREINER, P. W.; BROCK, W. A.; FREEMAN, J., and BITENSKY, M. W.: Prostaglandins and the adenyl cyclase of the Cloudman melanoma; in SCHULTZ and GRATZNER The role of cyclic nucleotides in carcinogenesis, pp. 181–198 (Academic Press, New York 1973).

7 KREINER, P. W.; GOLD, C. J.; KEIRNS, J. J.; BROCK, W. A., and BITENSKY, M. W.: MSH-sensitive adenyl cyclase in the Cloudman melanoma. Yale J. Biol. Med. *46:* 583–591 (1973).

8 NOVALES, R. R.: Responses of cultured melanophores to the synthetic hormones α-MSH, melatonin and epinephrine. Ann. N.Y. Acad. Sci. *100:* 1035–1047 (1963).

9 NOVALES, R. R. and DAVIS, W. J.: Melanin-dispersing effect of adenosine 3′,5′-monophosphate on amphibian melanophores. Endocrinology *81:* 283–290 (1967).

10 NOVALES, R. R. and FUJII, R.: A melanin-dispersing effect of cyclic adenosine monophosphate on *Fundulus* melanophores. J. cell. Physiol. *75:* 133–136 (1970).

11 NOVALES, R. R. and NOVALES, B. J.: Sodium dependence of intermedin action on melanophores in tissue culture. Gen. comp. Endocr. *1:* 134–144 (1961).

12 NOVALES, R. R. and NOVALES, B. J.: Sodium-free and cytochalasin B inhibition of prostaglandin A$_2$ action on amphibian melanophores. Am. Zoologist *13:* 1277 (1973).

13 NOVALES, R. R.; NOVALES, B. J.; ZINNER, S. H., and STONER, J. A.: The effects of sodium, chloride, and calcium concentration on the response of melanophores to melanocyte-stimulating hormone (MSH). Gen. Comp. Endocr. *2:* 286–295 (1962).

14 PEASLEE, M. H.: Frog skin darkening effect of prostaglandins E$_1$, E$_2$ and F$_2\alpha$ Am. Zoologist *11:* 651 (1971).

15 VEERDONK, F. C. G. VAN DE and BROUWER, E.: Role of calcium and prostaglandin (PGE$_1$) in the MSH-induced activation of adenylate cyclase in *Xenopus laevis*. Biochem. biophys. Res. Commun. *52:* 130–136 (1973).

Erratum to Pigment Cell Vol. 1, 1973

In the article by R. R. NOVALES and BARBARA J. NOVALES: The Effect of Various Drugs on the Response of Isolated Frog Skin Melanophores to Melanocyte-Stimulation Hormone (MSH) and Adenosine 3′,5′-Monophosphate (Cyclic AMP), Table II should be changed:
Line 4, last column should read 37 ± 3 (5)
Line 5, last column should read 35 ± 5 (4)

Dr. RONALD R. NOVALES, Department of Biological Sciences, Northwestern University, *Evanston, IL 60201* (USA)

Pigment Cell, vol. 3, pp. 244–253 (Karger, Basel 1976)

The Action of Prostaglandins, Precursor, and Prostaglandin Endoperoxide on Melanocyte-Keratinocytes during Anagen Stage of Human Pigmented and Albino Hair

J. J. SAUK, jr., J. G. WHITE and C. J. WITKOP, jr.

Departments of Human and Oral Genetics, School of Dentistry, and School of Pediatrics, University of Minnesota Health Sciences Center, Minneapolis, Minn.

Activation of the melanocyte-keratinocyte complex for the production and dispersion of melanin pigment in man is dependent on a number of factors. Melanocyte-stimulating hormone (MSH) controls adenylate cyclase activity in melanocytes [1, 9, 11]. Adenylate cyclase regulates the production of cyclic AMP, which has been shown to regulate levels of tyrosinase [7]. In addition, cyclic AMP has been shown to promote dispersion of melanosomes into dendritic processes of the melanocyte and facilitate pigment transfer between mammalian melanocytes and keratinocytes [17].

Recently, PGs have been implicated as potent agents which significantly influence melanin pigmentation. PGs have been noted to darken frog skin [13]. Specifically, PGE_1 darkened frog skin at the same rate and final optical density as MSH and produced a concomitant increase in levels of cyclic AMP [9]. Additionally, PGE_1 significantly increased adenylate cyclase activity in Cloudman melanoma to a level greater than that produced by either porcine MSH or PGE_2 [9]. When PGE_1 and MSH are used together as stimulating agents, they produce an additive effect on melanoma adenylate cyclase levels [9]. ABRAMOWITZ and CHAVIN [2] reported that PGs caused melanosome dispersion in black goldfish and suggested that PGs evoked melanophore responses by dissociating calcium-ATP complexes in the melanophore membrane, thereby allowing ATP to serve as a substrate for adenylate cyclase. SAUK et al. [14] noted that arachidonate, the precursor of PGs, was more potent than PGs in evoking melanosomal responses in melanocytes and keratinocytes of human anagen hair bulbs *in vitro* and suggested that these effects may be mediated by endoperoxide intermediates of PG.

The purpose of the present study was to compare the effects of exogenous PGE_1, PGE_2, arachidonate, and endoperoxide intermediates of PG generated by vesicular gland microsomes as active components of melanin pigmentation. Additionally, the effects of these various compounds were investigated with anagen hair bulbs of tyrosinase-negative, tyrosinase-positive, Hermansky-Pudlak, and yellow mutant oculocutaneous albinos.

Materials and Methods

Hair bulbs were obtained from normally pigmented Caucasian human volunteers with brown hair and tyrosinase-negative, tyrosinase-positive, Hermansky-Pudlak, and yellow mutant oculocutaneous albinism, as previously described by Sauk *et al.* [14]. Only anagen hair bulbs were selected. Immediately after harvesting, the samples were placed in 5 ml of Dulbecco's modified media (7 mg% tyrosine) and maintained at 37 °C in an atmosphere of 95% air and 5% CO_2.

Endoperoxide Intermediates

Rinsed microsomal pellets were obtained from sheep vesicular gland suspended and homogenized in 20 ml of 92 mM potassium phosphate buffer, pH 7.4, containing 7.2 mg 1 mM of sodium *p*-hydroxymercuribenzoate (Sigma Chemical Co.). The mixture was kept at 37 °C for 2 min and subsequently incubated for 30 sec with 5 mg of arachidonic acid (NuChek Prep) in 0.1 ml of ethanol. The mixture was acidified with 25 mM HCl and extracted twice with diethyl ether. The ether phases were washed twice with water and dried over 75 g of anhydrous Mg SO_4, thus yielding endoperoxide intermediates. The endoperoxides were diluted with acetone and used subsequently in concentrations of 5-100 ng in 1-1.5 µl of acetone.

The hair bulbs were stabilized for 1 h in culture media at the above temperature and atmospheric conditions [1], PGE_1, PGE_2 (courtesy Dr. John Pike, Upjohn Co.), sodium arachidonate (Sigma) and endoperoxide intermediates were added to individual cultures in concentrations from 5 ng/ml to 100 µg/ml. The hair bulbs were incubated for periods of 5, 10, and 30 min, 1 and 24 h. Control incubations without PG or arachidonate were also performed. Albino hair bulbs were also incubated at similar time intervals with 1% Triton X-100 and culture media to study the effects of the detergent on the degree and rate of hair bulb melanization.

In each instance, the experiment was terminated by fixation in 3% cacodylate-buffered gluteraldehyde containing 0.1% $CaCl_2$ at 30 °C for 90 min. Hair bulbs were then washed in cacodylate buffer with 0.1% $CaCl_2$ three times and post-fixed with 2% osmium tetroxide. Specimens were dehydrated in an increasing series of acetone 25–100% and embedded in Epon 812. Thin sections were prepared on an LKB ultramicrotome and stained with uranyl acetate and Venable's lead citrate. All sections were examined in a Phillips 200 transmission electron microscope at 80 kV.

Table I. Summary of intermediate endoperoxide, arachidonate and PG effects on anagen hair bulbs

	5 ng/ml	30 ng/ml	50 ng/ml	100 ng/ml	5 μg/ml	10 μg/ml	50 μg/ml	100 μg/ml
Control	−	−	−	−	−	−	−	−
Intermediate endoperoxides	−	+	+ +	+ +	+ +	0	0	0
Arachidonate	−	−	+	+ +	+ +	0	0	0
PGE₁	−	−	−	−	−	+	+	+ +
PGE₂	−	−	−	−	−	−	−	+

+ = Positive effect of agent on cellular events after; + + = toxic or exaggerated effects; − = negative effect; 0 = not tested.

Results

The results of PG, arachidonate, and endoperoxide effects on pigment hair bulbs are presented in table I.

Normally Pigmented Hair Bulbs

Untreated controls. Untreated controls revealed normal morphology. Large numbers of melanocytes were seen in the melanocytic zone of the hair bulbs. Mitochondria were abundant and located throughout the cytoplasm. Golgi zones were easily recognized and located about the nucleus. Dendritic processes were noted extending from the cells. Melanosomes in different stages of maturity were often noted. Microfilaments (10 nm) were occasionally observed and were usually associated with dendritic processes. Keratinocytes of hair bulbs were recognized by their nondendritic nature, presence of tonofilaments, and joining desmosomes. Melanosomes could be noted distributed throughout the cytoplasm. Similar findings were observed at 5 and 10 min, 1 and 24 h of incubation in culture media.

Endoperoxide intermediates. Anagen hair bulbs, after 1 h incubation with 30 ng/ml sheep vesicular gland endoperoxides, showed all stages of melanosome development in melanocytes. There also appeared to be increased numbers of premelanosomes in melanocytes. In addition, a well-developed Golgi zone, endoplasmic reticulum and numerous mitochondria were present. Microtubules (25–75 nm) were prominent, as

Table II. Summary of intermediate endoperoxide, arachidonate and PG effects on pigmentation of albino hair bulbs

	Endoperoxide intermediates	Arachidonate	PGE$_2$	PGE$_1$	Control
Tyrosinase-positive	+ +	+ +	+	+ +	−
Tyrosinase-negative	−	−	−	−	−
Hermansky-Pudlak	−	−	−	−	−
Yellow mutant	−	−	−	−	−

+ = Weak pigmentation of hair bulb; + + = pigmentation of hair bulb; − = no change from control.

were microfilaments (10 nm) which were oriented parallel to each other primarily within dendritic processes. In addition, there was an enhanced appearance of microfilaments within the dendritic process and a loss of microfilaments from the perikaryon. After 1 h incubation, there appeared to be some scattering of mitochondria and melanosome complexes began to form. Keratinocytes revealed numerous microtubules, and melanosomes appeared aggregated in membrane bound complexes. 24 h incubation still revealed many well-developed cytoplasmic organelles in melanocytes and increased numbers of large melanosome complexes in keratinocytes (fig. 1).

When the concentration of endoperoxides was raised to 5 μg/ml or greater, larger complexes of melanosomes were noted in melanocytes, and degradation of melanosomes was evident (fig. 2). In addition, indentation of the nucleus was noted, and keratinocytes showed extreme degradation of melanosomes.

Arachidonate, PGE$_1$ and PGE$_2$. The actions of arachidonate, PGE$_1$ and PGE$_2$ were comparable to that of endoperoxide intermediates. However, it required 50 ng/ml of arachidonate, 10 μg/ml PGE$_1$, and 100 μg/ml PGE$_2$ to elicit the same responses at 30 ng/ml of the endoperoxide intermediates.

Albinism

The results of PG, arachidonate and endoperoxide effects on albino hair bulbs are presented in table II.

Tyrosinase-Positive Albinism

In general, tyrosinase-positive hair bulbs reacted similarly to pigmented controls. However, after 1 h of treatment of tyrosinase-positive hair bulbs with endoperoxide intermediates, formation of melanosome complexes and pigmentation of melanosomes were noted. Melanosomes were completely pigmented after 1.5 h of incubation (fig. 3). The lowest concentrations of endoperoxides that elicited these responses was 30 ng/ml. Incubations with endoperoxides for longer periods of time, 24 h, revealed extremely large pigmented melanosome complexes. Within keratinocytes, melanosomes did not reveal significant pigmentation after incubations to 1 h (fig. 4). However, after 24 h, both pigmented and non-pigmented melanosome complexes could be seen in keratinocytes (fig. 5). Dissolution of melanosome complexes was evident at 15 min and was persistent after 24 h of treatment with endoperoxides.

Arachidonate, PGE_1 and PGE_2. The action of arachidonate, PGE_1 and PGE_2 was comparable to that of the endoperoxide intermediates. However, the responses were concentration-dependent, requiring progressively greater concentrations of arachidonate (50 ng/ml), PGE_1 (50 μg/ ml) and PGE_2 (100 μg/ml), to evoke the response of melanosome pigmentation.

Triton X-100. The addition of 1% Triton X-100 to otherwise untreated tyrosinase-positive hair bulbs in culture media resulted in destruction of cellular and melanosome membranes. Only occasional partial pigmentation of the disrupted melanosome membranes was noted at 1 h with 7 mg% tyrosine concentrations used in the culture media. After 24 h, the amount of pigmentation was increased but not complete.

Fig. 1. Normally pigmented hair bulb after 24 h of endoperoxide (30 ng/ml) melanocyte contains numerous cellular organelles including Golgi systems, mitochondria, and developing melanosomes. × 16,600.

Fig. 2. 1 h treatment of anagen melanocyte with 5 μg/ml of arachidonate resulting in indentation of the nucleus and a large melanosome complex formation. × 10,000.

Fig. 3. Tyrosinase-positive albino hair bulb with completely pigmented melanosomes after treatment with arachidonate. × 9,400.

Fig. 4. Tyrosinase-positive albino hair bulb after 1 h of incubation reveals melanosome complexes which are in various stages of pigmentation. × 13,300.

Fig. 5. Tyrosinase-positive keratinocyte after 24 h of incubation and stimulation of endogenous PG synthesis. Both pigmented and unpigmented melanosomes are noted. × 6,270.

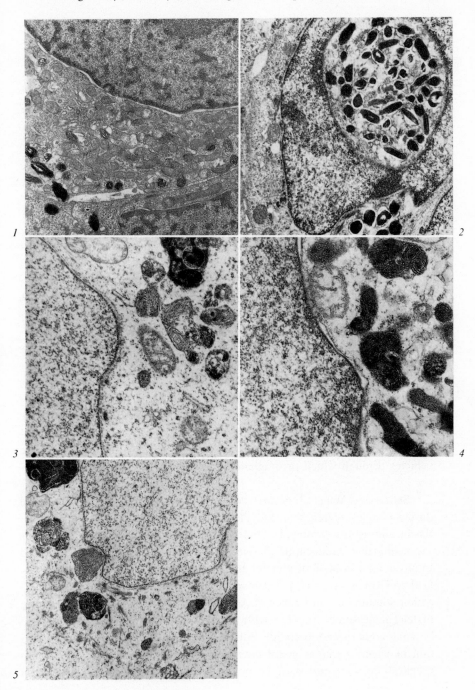

Tyrosinase-Negative, Hermansky-Pudlak, and
Yellow Mutant Albinism

The action of endoperoxides, arachidonate and PGs on tyrosinase-negative, Hermansky-Pudlak, and yellow mutant albinism gave morphologic changes similar to those obtained in tyrosinase-positive bulbs. Endoperoxide intermediates were most effective, followed by arachidonate, PGE_1 and PGE_2. However, unlike tyrosinase-positive hair bulbs, pigmentation could not be induced in any of the other forms of albinism.

Discussion

PGE_1, PGE_2, arachidonate, and endoperoxide intermediates stimulated a series of cellular events which appeared to be dependent upon the concentration and duration of exposure to these compounds. The greater effectiveness of PGE_1 compared with PGE_2 was in agreement with previous observations on the potency of one class of PG over another [9, 10]. The effectiveness of endoperoxide intermediates at nanogram levels as compared with microgram quantities necessary to elicit a similar response by exogenous PG revealed that in hair bulbs endoperoxide intermediates were significant mediators of PG-controlled cellular events.

The action of endoperoxides and arachidonate on maturation of melanosomes, orientation of microfilaments in dendritic processes, melanosome complexing, and ultimate dissolution of melanosomes paralleled the action of 3'5' cyclic AMP [17] and MSH [12]. The data suggest that intermediate products of endogenous PG synthesis are the most effective vehicles through which prostaglandins mediate adenylate cyclase responses.

SMITH and WILLIS [16] first demonstrated that PGs were synthesized during platelet aggregation. SILVER et al. [15] showed that both indomethacin and aspirin inhibited platelet aggregation and PG production, thus suggesting that endogenous platelet PG synthesis, was intimately related to physiologic control of platelet aggregation. Recently, WILLIS and KUHN [18] and GERRARD et al. [3] demonstrated the production of labile aggregation-stimulating substances (LASS) which were produced by reacting platelet microsomal fractions with arachidonate. The LASS was shown to be analogous to endoperoxide intermediates of PG formed from the action of sheep vesicular gland microsomes with arachidonate, since both preparations were noted to be potent mediators of platelet aggregation

[4]. Thus, the observed effects of arachidonate and endoperoxides on hair bulb melanocytes and keratinocytes parallel many of the findings on platelets.

Although arachidonate was almost as effective as endoperoxide intermediates generated from vesicular glands, it is difficult to explain these effects, since JONSSON and ANGGARD [8] demonstrated that only 2% of exogenous arachidonate was synthesized into PGs. However, recent studies in platelets by HAMBERG et al. [4–6] have revealed a novel transformation of arachidonate to endoperoxide intermediates by a lipoxygenase. The metabolic products of these intermediate compounds were nonprostonoate in nature. Whether these nonprostonoate intermediates are present in melanocytes or possess biologic activity is yet to be determined.

Albinism

In the present investigation, PGs and intermediate endoperoxides were able to cause pigmentation of tyrosinase-positive melanosomes. These effects were presumably due to stimulation of adenylate cyclase with subsequent activation of tyrosinase. Thus, if one accepts that MSH is a significant mediator of mammalian pigmentation, it would be possible that a defect of MSH-binding sites in tyrosinase-positive hair bulbs would not generate the necessary levels of arachidonic acid for PG synthesis and subsequent stimulation of adenylate cyclase. However, the present investigation showed that the events shared by MSH and cyclic AMP were operable in tyrosinase-positive hair bulbs, except for pigmentation. The latter is also supported by observations by WITKOP et al. [20, 21] demonstrating formation of melanosomes, peripheral orientation of microfilaments, melanosome transfer and ultimate degradation of melanosomes in untreated tyrosinase-positive hair bulbs. These apparent contradictions may be resolved, in part, by recent evidence that endogenous PGE_1 synthesis in Cloudman melanoma is independent of MSH stimulation [9].

However, the specific processes for the activation of melanocytic pigmentation of melanosomes in tyrosinase-positive hair bulbs by endoperoxide intermediates was not apparent in this investigation. The present study did note that endogenous PG effects could be generated by exogenous treatment with arachidonate and result in hair bulb pigmentation. Thus, a defect in melanocyte PG synthetase did not appear as the basis for the tyrosinase-positive phenotype.

In addition, the inability of endoperoxides, arachidonate and exogenous PGs to pigment Hermansky-Pudlak and yellow mutant hair bulbs supports clinical evidence that the tyrosinase-positive phenotype is heterogeneous and includes tyrosinase-positive albinism, Hermansky-Pudlak syndrome, and yellow mutant albinism as separate biochemical entities.

Summary

PGE$_1$, PGE$_2$, arachidonate, and endoperoxide intermediates of prostaglandin (PG) generated by sheep vesicular gland microsomes were tested on normally pigmented anagen hair bulbs and albino hair bulbs. PG-mediated responses were evoked at nanogram levels of endoperoxide intermediates, and arachidonate, while microgram quantities of PGE$_1$ and PGE$_2$ were necessary to evoke similar responses. These data suggest that intermediate products of endogenous PG synthesis are the most effective vehicles through which PGs mediate cellular responses in anagen hair bulbs.

References

1 ABE, K.; BUTCHER, R. W.; NICHOLSON, W. E.; BURD, W. E.; LIDDLE, R. A., and LIDDLE, G. W.: Adenosine 3',5' monophosphate (cyclic AMP) as the mediator of the action of melanocyte-stimulating hormone (MSH) and norepinephrine on the frog skin. Endocrinology 84: 362–368 (1969).

2 ABRAMOWITZ, J. and CHAVIN, W.: The melanosome dispersing activity of prostaglandins in black goldfish. Prostaglandins 4: 805–818 (1973).

3 GERRARD, J. M.; WHITE, J. G.; RAO, G. H. R.; KRIVIT, W., and WITKOP, C. J., jr.: Labile aggregation stimulating substance (LASS). The factor from storage pool-deficient platelets correcting defective aggregation and release of aspirin treated normal platelets. Br. J. Haemat. (in press).

4 HAMBERG, M.; SVENSSON, J.; WAKABAYASKI, T., and SAMUELSSON, B.: Isolation and structure of two prostaglandin endoperoxides that cause platelet aggregation. Proc. natn. Acad. Sci. USA 71: 345–349 (1974).

5 HAMBERG, M. and SAMUELSSON, B.: Prostaglandin endoperoxides. Novel transformation of arachidonic acid in human platelets. Proc. natn. Acad. Sci. USA 71: 3400–3404 (1974).

6 HAMBERG, M.; SVENSSON, J., and SAMUELSSON, B.: Prostaglandin endoperoxides. A new concept concerning the mode of action and release of prostaglandins. Proc. natn. Acad. Sci. USA 71: 3824–3828 (1974).

7 JOHNSON, G. S. and PASTON, I.: N^6,O^2-debutyryl adenosine 3',5'-monophosphate induces pigment production in melanoma cells. Nature new Biol. 237: 267–268 (1972).

8 JONSSON, C. E. and ANGGARD, E.: Biosynthesis and metabolism of prostaglandin E$_2$ in human skin. Scand. J. clin. Lab. Invest. 29: 289–296 (1972).

9 KREINER, P. W.; GOLD, C. J.; KEIRNS, J. J.; BROCK, W. A., and BITENSKY, M.

W.: MSH-sensitive adenyl cyclase in Cloudman melanoma. Yale J. Biol. Med. 46: 583–591 (1973).

10 KUEHL, F. A.; CIRILLO, V. J.; HAM, E. A., and HUMES, J. L.: The regulatory role of the prostaglandins on the cyclic 3′,5′-AMP system. Adv. Biol. Sci. 9: 155–172 (1972).

11 LEE, T. H. and LEE, M. S.: In vitro effects of MSH on tyrosinase and melanogenesis of pigmentary system. Yale J. Biol. Med. 46: 493–499 (1973).

12 MOELLMAN, G.; McGUIRE, J., and LERNER, A. B: Intracellular dynamics and the fine structure of melanocytes with special reference to the effects of MSH and cyclic AMP on microtubules and 10 nm filaments. Yale J. Biol. Med. 46: 337–360 (1973).

13 PEASLEE, M. H.: Frog skin darkening effect of prostaglandins E_1, E_2 and $F_2\alpha$. Am. Zoologist 11: 651 (1971).

14 SAUK, J. J.; WHITE, J. G., and WITKOP, C. J.: Influence of prostaglandins E_1, E_2 and arachidonate on melanosomes in melanocytes and keratinocytes of anagen hair bulbs in vitro. J. invest. Derm. (in press).

15 SILVER, J. J.; HERNANDOVITCH, J.; INGERMAN, C., et al.: Persistent inhibition by aspirin of collagen-induced platelet prostaglandin formation; in SHERRY and SCRIABINE Platelets and thrombosis, pp. 91–98 (University Park Press, Baltimore 1974).

16 SMITH, J. B. and WILLIS, A. L.: Formation and release of prostaglandins by platelets in response to thrombin. Br. J. Pharmacol. 40: 545 (1970).

17 WIKSWO, M. A.: Action of cyclic AMP on pigment donation between mammalian melanocytes and keratinocytes. Yale J. Biol. Med. 46: 592–601 (1973).

18 WILLIS, A. L. and KUHN, D. C.: A new potential mediator of arterial thrombosis whose biosynthesis is inhibited by aspirin. Prostaglandins 4: 127–130 (1973).

19 WILLIS, A. L.: Isolation of a chemical trigger for thrombosis. Prostaglandins 5: 1–25 (1974).

20 WITKOP, C. J., jr.; WHITE, J. G.; NANCE, W. E., and UMBER, R. E.: Mutations in the melanin pigment system in man resulting in features of oculocutaneous albinism; in RILEY Pigmentation: its genesis and biologic control, pp. 359–377 (Appleton Century Crofts, New York 1971).

21 WITKOP, C. J., jr.; WHITE, J. G.; NANCE, W. E., et al.: Classification of albinism in man; in Hair, skin, nails. Birth Defects Orig. Art. Ser. 7: 13–25 (1971).

Dr. JOHN J. SAUK, jr., Departments of Human and Oral Genetics, School of Dentistry, University of Minnesota Health Sciences Center, Minneapolis, MN 55455 (USA)

Pigment Cell, vol. 3, pp. 254–264 (Karger, Basel 1976)

An Analysis of the Mechanism of Pigment Migration in Fish Chromatophores

MASATAKA OBIKA

Department of Biology, Keio University, Yokohama

Introduction

In recent studies on the mechanism of pigment migration within vertebrate melanophores, attention has been concentrated upon the participation of contractile microfilaments and microtubules. Among hormone-controlled, slow-reacting amphibian melanophores, centrifugal melanosome movement appears to rely on microfilaments [8, 11–13, 15], while microtubules seem to be involved in centripetal movement [9, 10]. In nerve-controlled, rapid-reacting fish melanophores, the ubiquitous presence of a well-developed microtubule system has led to an assumption that microtubules rather than microfilaments provide the motive force for pigment migration [1, 14, 18, 20, 21]. Regarding the pigment translocation within bright-colored pigment cells, only limited knowledge has been obtained at present. PORTER [16] has suggested that the microtubule system is involved in pigment migration within the erythrophores of a fish, and ROHRLICH [17] has indicated that microfilaments are the possible mediator of iridophore responses. Change in cell shape during pigment migration is also a matter of controversy. Whether it is a passive consequence of pigment translocation within the cell, or is more actively concerned with chromatophore responses, remains to be determined.

The purpose of the present investigation is to analyze the mechanism of pigment migration in chromatophores, mainly in melanophores, of a freshwater teleost, *Oryzias latipes*. Chromatophore responses have been studied in conjunction with morphological changes, and the effects of cytochalasin B and colchicine on melanosome movement have also been examined.

Materials and Methods

Scale chromatophores of wild type fish (BBRR) were routinely used although in some instances a color mutant, BdmR, characteristic in having physiologically inactive, fully dispersed melanophores, was also employed. Scales were plucked from the antero-dorsal region of the fish.

Physiological methods. Epinephrine (Sigma, 10 μM), theophylline (Tokyo Kasei, 10 mM) and colchicine (Merck, 5 mM) were directly dissolved in Ringer's solution. Melatonin (Sigma, 1 μg/ml) was prepared after dissolving it in a small quantity of alcohol. Cytochalasin B (CB) (ICI, 10 μg/ml) was made by diluting a stock solution dissolved in dimethylsulfoxide (DMSO). At the concentrations employed, both alcohol and DMSO had no appreciable effect on chromatophore responses. The responses were observed under a light microscope and recorded by photomicrography. Each experiment contained at least 5 scales and was repeated at least 3 times. In some cases, overlying epidermis of the isolated scales was carefully removed by forceps in order to bring melanophores into direct contact with the perfusion media. Experiments were carried out at 18–22 °C.

Electron microscopy. For transmission electron microscopy, materials were fixed in 3% glutaraldehyde for 2 h at 20–22 °C and post-fixed with 1% OsO_4 for 2 h at 0 °C, each buffered with 0.1 M phosphate buffer at pH 7.3. They were dehydrated in a graded series of alcohol and embedded in Epon 812. Sections were made with a LKB ultramicrotome with glass knives, stained with uranyl acetate and lead citrate, and observed in a Hitachi HS-7 type electron microscope. Ruthenium red staining was carried out according to the method of Luft [7]. Fixatives were buffered with cacocylate, and the materials were fixed for 1 and 3 h, respectively, at room temperature. Each fixative contained commercial ruthenium red (Chroma) at a final concentration of 494 ppm. Sections were observed without further staining. For scanning electron microscopy, scales without overlying epidermal layer were fixed and dehydrated through a series of alcohol and amylacetate, dried in liquid CO_2 and observed in a JEOL 100 B type electron microscope with a scanning attachment.

Results

Melanophores of wild type fish. Melanophores of this strain are generally dispersed in Ringer's solution, and perfusion with epinephrine, melatonin or isotonic KCl solution (only effective up to 60–90 min following isolation) induces a rapid melanosome aggregation within a few minutes. KCl- or epinephrine-induced aggregation is inhibited by a 20 min pretreatment of the scales in an alpha adrenergic antagonist, dibenamine (Sigma, 10 μM) while the effect of melatonin is unaffected. Dibenamine-treated, melatonin-aggregated melanophores respond with dispersion to epinephrine, suggesting the presence of beta adrenergic receptors.

Dispersed melanophores are generally flat while in aggregated ones, collapse of the dendrites and compensatory swelling of the centrosphere are evident (fig. 1, 2). In dispersed cells, abundant microtubules are mostly in orderly array. In dendrites, they are arranged parallel to the long axis (fig. 3). Filamentous materials are rarely encountered. In aggregated melanophores, microtubules are very abundant in collapsed dendrites and in the melanosome-free area of the centrosphere. Filamentous structures, about 7 nm in diameter, are commonly found in collapsed dendrites (fig. 4, 5). Membranous elements, mitochondria and ribosomes are densely packed in the pigment-free area. When ruthenium red staining is applied immediately after (within 1 min) the administration of epinephrine, numerous vesicles in dendrites are deeply stained, while in the centrosphere, a few cortical pits are the only structures other than the plasma membrane which take up this specific dye. In contrast to this, ruthenium red-positive vesicles other than cortical pits are only rarely found in the dendrites of dispersed cells (fig. 6, 7).

When melanophores are brought into direct contact with CB, centrospheres and dendrite tips swell up within 10 min, thereby inducing a partial aggregation of melanosomes. Epinephrine induces aggregation under the presence of the drug, but redispersion by theophylline occurs to a limited extent, leaving a large cluster of melanosomes in the centrosphere (fig. 8a–c). The effect of CB is readily reversed by washing. The electron density of the matrix cytoplasm becomes uniformly high, somewhat granular, and occasionally filamentous (fig. 9).

When freshly excised specimens are immersed in an isotonic KCl solution containing colchicine, melanophores respond with a rapid, incomplete aggregation immediately followed by gradual redispersion. Epinephrine-induced aggregation, however, proceeds normally at first and the aggregated state persists as long as epinephrine is present in the medium

---

Fig. 1. Scanning electron micrograph of a dispersed melanophore. × 630.

Fig. 2. Scanning electron micrograph of an aggregated melanophore. × 1,860.

Fig. 3. Cross-sectional profile of a dendrite of a dispersed melanophore. Microtubules (arrows) are abundant at cortical area. × 36,400.

Fig. 4. Horizontal section of a dendrite portion of an aggregated melanophore. Numerous microtubules (arrows) and some filaments (arrowhead) are seen. × 24,300.

Fig. 5. Horizontal section of a dendrite of an aggregated melanophore. Microtubules (arrows) and filaments (arrowheads) are observed. × 45,000.

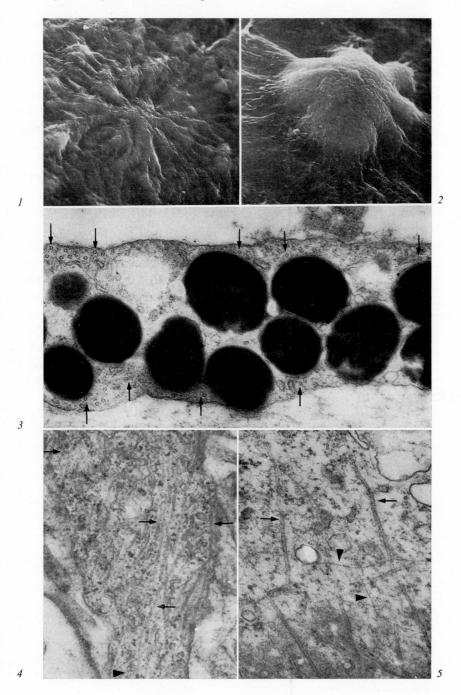

(up to 80 min in this experiment), and successive perfusion of theophylline gives rise to a rapid, full redispersion. In the specimens pretreated in the drug for longer than 30 min, slowing down of melanosome aggregation becomes evident. There is a latent period at the early phase of response movement and a slowing down of mass movement which is caused by an emphasized back-and-forth movement, is observed. Figure 10 shows a dendrite portion of an epinephrine-aggregated melanophore in the presence of colchicine. Some microtubules and numerous thin filaments, about 6 nm in diameter, are present.

Melanophores of BdmR strain. Melanophores of this mutant fish always remain dispersed although random back-and-forth movements of individual melanosomes are observed. Perfusion with epinephrine or melatonin causes very little effect, if any. When an extremely high dose of epinephrine (1 mM) is administered, melanophores respond with slight aggregation which is reversed by theophylline. Microtubule system is well developed both in dendrites and at the central area (fig. 11, 12) and filaments are seen around the nucleus (fig. 13). CB treatment up to 60 min has very little effect on these cells (fig. 14a, b).

Xanthophores and leukophores (iridophores) of wild type fish. Xanthophores of the present species respond to various stimuli as do melanophores and are apparently under the control of alpha adrenergic receptors. Light-reflecting pigment cells are predominantly under the control of

---

Fig. 6. Cross-sectional view of a dendrite of dispersed melanophore stained with ruthenium red. Plasma membrane (pm) is deeply stained. Some microtubules (small arrows) are seen. × 32,300.

Fig. 7. Cross-sectioned dendrite of an aggregating melanophore stained with ruthenium red. Plasma membrane and numerous vesicles (arrows) are stained. Abundant microtubules (small arrows) are present. 1e = Leukophore. × 32,300.

Fig. 8. Melanophore (without overlying epidermis) responses in CB solution: (a) melanophores preincubated in CB for 140 min; (b) after perfusion with epinephrine-CB (5 min); (c) after perfusion with theophylline-CB (5 min). × 270.

Fig. 9. Cross-sectioned dendrite of a CB-treated melanophore. Microtubules (arrows) and filamentous materials (arrowheads) are observed. × 36,000.

Fig. 10. Proximal portion of a dendrite of an aggregated melanophore in the presence of colchicine. Horizontal section. Some microtubules (arrows) and numerous filaments (arrowheads) are present. × 34,000.

Fig. 11. Cross-sectional profile of the central area of a BdmR melanophore showing well-developed microtubule system. n = Nucleus. × 36,400.

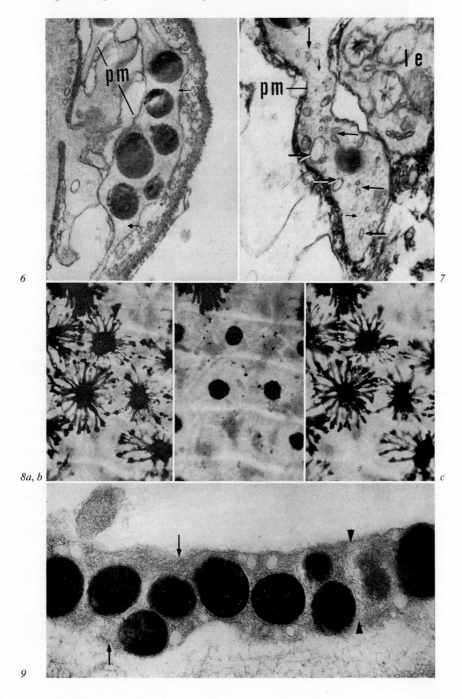

6

7

8a, b

c

9

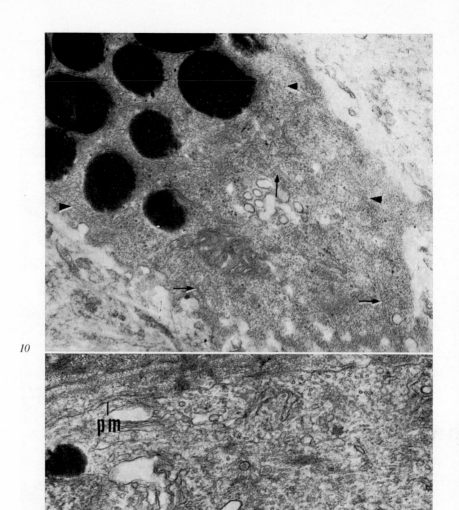

10

11

For legends see p. 258.

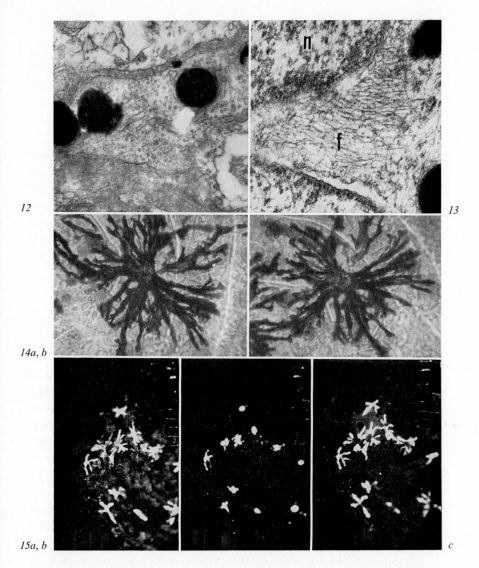

Fig. 12. A dendrite of BdmR melanophore. Cross section. Note the numerous microtubules. × 30,000.

Fig. 13. Filamentous materials (f) near the nucleus (n) of a BdmR melanophore. × 45,000.

Fig. 14. The effect of CB on BdmR melanophore: (a) in Ringer's solution; (b) the same melanophore treated in CB for 30 min. No appreciable effect of CB on cell shape. × 670.

Fig. 15. Responses of light-reflecting leukophores: (a) in Ringer's solution; (b) melatonin-induced aggregation (4 min); (c) theophylline-induced redispersion (5 min). × 65.

beta receptors. They respond to KCl and epinephrine with dispersion, but this response is completely inhibited by a 20-min pretreatment in a beta antagonist, propranolol (Sigma, 100 μM). Melatonin induces aggregation within a few minutes and theophylline causes a rapid redispersion (fig. 15a–c). Dibutylyl cyclic AMP (Sigma, 1 mM) also induces a slow dispersion.

Microtubule systems in these bright-colored pigment cells are less well-developed than in melanophores; however, filaments (6–8 nm) are abundant, especially in light-reflecting leukophores. Unlike those of typical iridophores, pigment granules of leukophores are spherical or somewhat irregularly shaped, possessing an electron-dense material in the center of the pigment vesicles in unstained sections. Ruthenium red-positive vesicles other than cortical pits are rare in xanthophores while they are frequently found in leukophores.

Discussion

This results of the present experiment suggest that the change in cell shape during pigment migration is not merely a passive event. CB induces a partial aggregation of melanosomes, and removal of the drug restores the cell shape and melanosome redistribution. The lack of this CB-sensitive system in BdmR melanophores is probably correlated to their physiological inertness. Melanosome movement is, however, not totally inhibited by CB, and there must be some mechanisms which prevent regurgitation of aggregated melanosomes. Whether this is solely interpreted by microtubule-granule interaction, or some other factors are also involved, as implicated by the dense arrays of microtubules and the appearance of numerous filaments and ruthenium red-positive vesicles, requires further clarification.

Response of leukophores of the present species are different from those described in the other iridophores (reviewed by BAGNARA and HADLEY [2]) containing purine platelets [3, 6, 19]. Structural characteristics of the leukophore have been described briefly [5], and the pigment contained is supposed to be uric acid [4]. ROHRLICH [17] has suggested that the thick (10 nm) filaments in iridophores function as cytoskeletal elements while thin (6 nm) filaments are iridophore actin. Studies on the participation of the filaments found in xanthophores and leukophores of the present species in pigment migration are in progress.

Summary

Chromatophore responses of a fresh water teleost, *Oryzias latipes,* have been studied with special reference to the morphological changes during pigment migration. Dense arrays of microtubules and microfilaments are observed in collapsed dendrites after melanosome aggregation. Continuity of some vesicles to the plasma membrane in collapsing dendrites is demonstrated by ruthenium red staining. Cytochalasin B reversibly induces swelling of the centrosphere and concomitant melanosome translocation. Physiologically inactive melanophores of a mutant, BdmR, have a well-developed microtubule system but are insensitive to cytochalasin B treatment. Leukophores are aggregated by melatonin and dispersed by theophylline or dibutyllyl cyclic AMP.

Acknowledgments

The author is deeply indebted to Dr. HIDEO TOMITA of Nagoya University for his generous supply of BdmR (f 9) mutant. Thanks are also extended to Dr. TANEAKI OIKAWA of Yamagata University for suggesting the use of this mutant strain. This investigation was supported in part by research grants from Keio University.

References

1   BIKLE, D.; TILNEY, L. G., and PORTER, K. R.: Microtubules and pigment migration in the melanophores of *Fundulus heteroclitus* L. Protoplasma *61:* 322–345 (1966).
2   BAGNARA, J. T. and HADLEY, M. E.: Chromatophores and color change (Prentice Hall, Englewood Cliffs 1973).
3   BAGNARA, J. T.; TAYLOR, J. D., and HADLEY, M. E.: The dermal chromatophore unit. J. Cell Biol. *38:* 67–79 (1968).
4   HAMA, T.: On the coexistence of drosopterin and purine (drosopterinosome) in the leucophore of *Oryzias latipes* (teleostean fish) and the effect of phenylthiourea and melamine; in Chemistry and biology of pteridines (Int. Acad. Print., Tokyo 1970).
5   KAMEI-TAKEUCHI, I.; EGUCHI, G., and HAMA, T.: Ultrastructure of the pteridine pigment granules of the larval xanthophore and leucophore in *Oryzias latipes* (teleostean fish). Proc. Jap. Acad. *44:* 959–963 (1968).
6   KAWAGUTI, S. and TAKEUCHI, T.: Electron microscopy on guanophores of the medaka, *Oryzias latipes.* Biol. J. Okayama Univ. *14:* 55–65 (1968).
7   LUFT, J. H.: Ruthenium red and violet. I. Chemistry, purification, methods of use for electron microscopy and mechanism of action. Anat. Rec. *171:* 347–368 (1971).
8   MAGUN, B.: Two actions of cyclic AMP on melanosome movement in frog skin. Dissection by cytochalasin B. J. Cell Biol. *57:* 845–858 (1973).

9 MALAWISTA, S. E.: On the action of colchicine. The melanocyte model. J. exp. Med. *122:* 361–384 (1965).

10 MALAWISTA, S. E.: The melanocyte model. Colchicine-like effects of other antimitotic agents. J. Cell Biol. *49:* 848–855 (1971).

11 MALAWISTA, S. E.: Cytochalasin B reversibly inhibits melanin granule movement in melanocytes. Nature, Lond. *234:* 354–355 (1971).

12 McGUIRE, J. and MOELLMANN, G.: Cytochalasin B. Effects on microfilaments and movement of melanin granules within melanocytes. Science *175:* 642–644 (1972).

13 McGUIRE, J.; MOELLMANN, G., and McKEON, F.: Cytochalasin B and pigment granule translocation. J. Cell Biol. *52:* 754–758 (1972).

14 MURPHY, D. B. and TILNEY, L. G.: The role of microtubules in the movement of pigment granules in teleost melanophores. J. Cell Biol. *61:* 757–779 (1974).

15 NOVALES, R. R. and NOVALES, B. J.: Effect of cytochalasin B on the response of the chromatophores of isolated frog skin to MSH, theophylline, and dibutyryl cyclic AMP. Gen. comp. Endocr. *19:* 363–366 (1972).

16 PORTER, K. R.: Microtubules in intracellular locomotion. Ciba Found. Symp. *14:* 149–166 (1973).

17 ROHRLICH, S. T.: Fine structural demonstration of ordered arrays of cytoplasmic filaments in vertebrate iridophores. J. Cell Biol. *62:* 295–304 (1974).

18 SCHLIWA, M. and BEREITER-HAHN, J.: Pigment movements in fish melanophores. Morphological and physiological studies. III. The effects of colchicine and vinblastine. Z. Zellforsch. *147:* 127–148 (1973).

19 SETOGUTI, T.: Ultrastructure of guanophores. J. Ultrastruct. Res. *18:* 324–332 (1967).

20 WIKSWO, M. A. and NOVALES, R. R.: The effect of colchicine on migration of pigment granules in the melanophores of *Fundulus heteroclitus.* Biol. Bull. *137:* 228–237 (1969).

21 WIKSWO, M. A. and NOVALES, R. R.: Effect of colchicine on microtubules in the melanophores of *Fundulus heteroclitus.* J. Ultrastruct. Res. *41:* 189–201 (1972).

Dr. M. OBIKA, Department of Biology, Keio University, *Yokohama-Hiyoshi 223* (Japan)

Pigment Cell, vol. 3, pp. 265–274 (Karger, Basel 1976)

Receptor-Specific Calcium Requirement for Melanophore-Stimulating Hormone

Control of Melanophores

DAVID L. VESELY and MAC E. HADLEY

College of Medicine, and Department of Biological Sciences,
University of Arizona, Tucson, Ariz.

Introduction

The calcium ion is clearly implicated in the mechanism of action of a number of peptide hormones [2, 10, 11]. The calcium ion is also required for the mechanism of action of melanophore-stimulating hormone (MSH) in dispersing melanosomes (melanin granules) within integumental melanophores of the lizard, *Anolis carolinensis* [16]. There are conflicting reports for either a divalent or monovalent cation dependency for MSH action in frogs [12, 13].

In the present report, we demonstrate a receptor specific Ca^{2+} ion requirement for MSH action in both the lizard, *Anolis carolinensis,* and the frog, *Scaphiopus couchi.* In addition, these results clearly illustrate a nonspecific monovalent requirement for hormone action. The possible locus of the Ca^{2+} ion requirement for MSH action is discussed.

Methods

Both sexes of the lizard, *Anolis carolinensis,* and the frog, *Scaphiopus couchi,* were used in these studies. The source and specific photometric reflectance methods for utilization of skins of these lizards [4] and frogs [5] have been described previously. In general, skins are prepared as described for the frog skin bioassay of MSH [14, 18]. Reflectance measurements are obtained from the outer surface of skins and involve color changes, lightening (melanosome aggregation) or darkening (melanosome dispersion), resulting from intracellular melanin granule movements within integumental dermal melanophores in response to hormonal or pharmacological stimulation.

Skins are placed in 50 ml beakers containing amphibian Ringer (NaCl, 111 mM; NaHCO$_3$, 2 mM; KCl, 2 mM; CaCl$_2$, 1 mM) at pH 7.3–7.5 for a 2-h pre-experimental equilibration period. During this time, there is a slow perinuclear aggregation of melanosomes within melanophores, resulting in the skins becoming quite light in color. The skins are then placed in control or experimental solutions and, after a number of fresh changes of the respective solutions, 20 ml of solution is allowed to remain in each beaker to cover the skin. All solutions are made with doubly glass-distilled water to insure ionic purity. All concentrations of hormonal and pharmacological agents used are expressed as the final concentration after addition to the skins.

Results

The calcium ion is required for the melanosome dispersing action of MSH on dermal melanophores of the lizard, *Anolis carolinensis* (table I) as previously demonstrated [16]. A similar Ca^{2+} requirement for MSH action is also demonstrated for the frog, *Scaphiopus couchi* (fig. 1). MSH darkens frog skins incubated in the Ringer solution but not skins residing in a Ca^{2+}-free Ringer solution or in an isotonic sodium chloride solution (with or without K$^+$). The response to MSH in isotonic NaCl containing Ca^{2+} is abolished by the Ca^{2+} chelator ethylenediaminetetraacetic acid (EDTA).

These results leave unanswered whether there is an additional and specific monovalent (sodium) cation requirement for the action of MSH. It was clearly shown in both the lizard (table II) and the frog (fig. 2) that neither the Na$^+$ or K$^+$ ion is required for the action of MSH in dispersing melanosomes within melanophores. Rubidium, cesium, and choline (table IIB) will also replace the Na$^+$ ion of the Ringer but, again, only if the calcium ion is present (table III).

Catecholamines, as well as MSH, darken the skins of *Anolis* [4] and *Scaphiopus* [5]. In contrast to its role in MSH darkening, the Ca^{2+} ion is not obligatory for melanosome dispersion in response to isoproterenol, a rather specific beta-receptor adrenergic catecholamine agonist (table IV). Again, as for MSH, substitution by Li$^+$ revealed that neither Na$^+$ nor K$^+$ are required for catecholamine stimulation of melanosome dispersion in *Anolis* (table V). Norepinephrine and other catecholamines have been shown to reverse the action of MSH and lighten MSH-darkened *Anolis* skins via stimulation of alpha-adrenergic receptors [4]. Norepinephrine will also lighten *Anolis* skins darkened by isoproterenol. This reversal of isoproterenol darkening is, also, not dependent upon the presence of the

Table I. Inhibition of MSH in Ca^{2+}-free media

Experimental solution	Number of skins	Decrease in reflectance[a], %	SE[b]
Ringer	8	39	±2.63
NaCl (120 mM)	8	6	±1.69
NaCl (120 mM) + EDTA (5 mM)	6	0	±0.67
NaCl (120 mM) + Ca+ (1 mM)	6	39	±3.69

[a] Values represent the maximal darkening response within 30 min after addition of 4×10^{-9} g/ml porcine alpha-MSH to *Anolis* skins.
[b] SE = Standard errors of the means.

Table II. Comparison of the MSH response of *Anolis* skins with various monovalent cations replacing the sodium ion

Experimental solution	Decrease in reflectance[a], %	SE[b]
A.		
Ringer	48	±1.41
LiCl (120 mM)	0	±0.85
LiCl (120 mM) + Na+ (2 mM)	0	±0.81
LiCl (120 mM) + K+ (2 mM)	0	±0.77
LiCl (120 mM) + Ca²⁺ (1 mM)	32	±2.72
B.		
Ringer	53	±1.50
Choline chloride (120 mM)	1	±2.58
Choline chloride (120 mM) + Na+ (2 mM)	7	±1.53
Choline chloride (120 mM) + K+ (2 mM)	9	±3.93
Choline chloride (120 mM) + Ca²⁺ (1 mM)	36	±3.66

[a] Values represent the maximal darkening response within 30 min after addition of 4×10^{-9} g/ml porcine alpha-MSH to the seven *Anolis* skins in each experimental group.
[b] SE = Standard errors of the means.

calcium ion. These results demonstrate that melanosome aggregation as mediated through alpha-adrenergic receptors is not dependent upon the presence of the Ca^{2+} ion. It was previously demonstrated that melanosome aggregation following removal of MSH from *Anolis* skins is independent of the Ca^{2+} ion [8, 16].

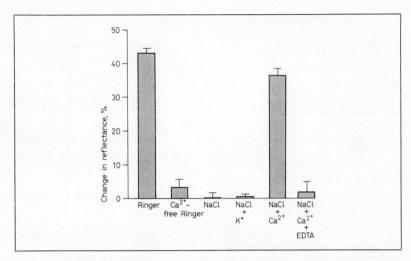

Fig. 1. Response of *Scaphiopus* skins to MSH in various experimental media: Ringer [15], Ca²⁺-free Ringer [8], isotonic NaCl, 120 mM, or isotonic NaCl containing either 2 mM of K⁺ [4] or 1 mM of Ca²⁺ [20] or 1 mM Ca²⁺ plus EDTA, 10^{-3} M [4]. Values represent the maximal responses within 60 min after the addition of porcine alpha-MSH (4×10^{-9} g/ml). The number of skins in each experimental group is indicated within the parenthesis following each experimental solution. Vertical lines indicate the standard error of the means.

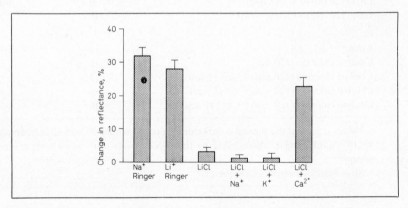

Fig. 2. In vitro response of *Scaphiopus* skins to MSH in amphibian Ringer [8] lithium Ringer [15], or isotonic LiCl, 120 mM [8], containing either 2 mM of Na⁺ [15] or K⁺ [15], or 1 mM of Ca²⁺ [15]. Lithium Ringer consists of LiCl, 111 mM; KCl, 2 mM; KHCO₃, 2 mM; and CaCl₂; 1 mM. Values represent the maximal darkening responses within 60 min after addition of 4×10^{-9} g/ml porcine alpha-MSH. The number of skins in each experimental group is indicated following each group. Vertical lines indicate the standard errors of the means.

Table III. Response of *Anolis* skins to MSH in media containing either rubidium or cesium replacing the sodium ion

Experimental solution[a]	Decrease in reflectance[b], %	SE[c]
Ringer	62	±1.21
Cesium chloride	5	±2.36
Cesium Ringer	57	±1.47
Rubidium chloride	6	±2.41
Rubidium Ringer	40	±3.52

[a] The rubidium and cesium chloride solution were isotonic solutions consisting of 120 mM of either cation. Cesium or rubidium Ringer consisted of 111 mM; of CsCl or RbCl; KHCO$_3$, 2 mM; KCl, 2 mM; CaCl$_2$, 1 mM.
[b] Values represent the maximal darkening response within 30 min after addition of 4×10^{-9} g/ml alpha-MSH to the eight *Anolis* skins in each group.
[c] SE = Standard errors of the means.

Table IV. Response of *Anolis* and *Scaphiopus* skins to isoproterenol

Experimental solution	Decrease in reflectance[a], %	SE[b]	p[c]
A. *Anolis carolinensis*			
Ringer	33	±1.55	
NaCl (120 mM)	42	±1.35	NS
NaCl (120 mM) + K$^+$ (2 mM)	42	±2.46	NS
NaCl 120 mM) + Ca^{2+} (1 mM)	38	±1.73	NS
B. *Scaphiopus couchi*			
Ringer	27	±2.25	
Ca^{2+}-free Ringer	35	±2.47	NS

[a] Values represent the maximal darkening responses within 60 min after addition of 10^{-5} M isoproterenol bitartrate to the eight skins in each experimental group.
[b] SE = Standard errors of the means.
[c] The differences between groups were evaluated with the Student's *t* test. NS = No significant difference at the $p > 0.05$ level between Ringer and the various groups. All these groups darkened equal to or better than the Ringer control with isoproterenol.

Table V. Response of *Anolis* skins to isoproterenol

Experimental solution	Decrease in reflectance[a], %	SE[b]	p[c]
Ringer	30	±2.96	
LiCl (120 mM)	31	±1.50	NS
LiCl (120 mM) + Na+ (2 mM)	32	±3.16	NS
LiCl (120 mM) + K+ (2 mM)	29	±1.55	NS
LiCl (120 mM) + Ca²+ (1 mM)	31	±3.09	NS

[a] Values represent the maximal darkening response within 30 min after the addition of 10^{-5} M isoproterenol bitartrate to the 7 *Anolis* skins in each group.
[b] SE = Standard errors of the means.
[c] The differences between groups were evaluated with the Student's *t* test. NS = No significant difference at the $p > 0.05$ level between Ringer control and the various groups.

These results further imply that melanosome movements *per se* are not dependent upon the Ca^{2+} ion. This is additionally borne out by the demonstration that either theophylline, a methylxanthine, or dibutyryl cyclic AMP darken *Anolis* skins in a Ca^{2+}-free isotonic NaCl solution [16]. Similarly, melanosome dispersion in response to theophylline has no specific monovalent cation requirement since either cesium or lithium ions will replace the sodium ion and allow skin darkening. Thus, although melanosome dispersion can be stimulated by either MSH, theophylline (methylxanthines), catecholamines (e.g. isoproterenol), or dibutyryl cyclic AMP, only MSH requires the calcium ion for its mechanism of action.

A Ca^{++} requirement for MSH dispersal of integumental melanophores of the frog, *Rana pipiens,* could also be demonstrated. Substitution of the lithium ion for the sodium ion inhibited MSH [12, 18], but not melanosome dispersion in response to theophylline (or caffeine [12]) or to isoproterenol. Theophylline and isoproterenol darken *R. pipiens* skins in the absence of the Ca^{2+} ion. These results reveal that melanosome movements *per se* are not dependent upon the specific presence of either sodium or calcium ions.

Discussion

Calcium is specifically required for the action of MSH on melanosome dispersion within lizard *(Anolis carolinensis)* and frog *(Scaphiopus couchi*) melanophores *in vitro*. The response to the hormone is directly related to the concentration of the calcium ion [16]. Calcium itself, in high concentrations, is hormone-mimetic in that it causes dispersion of melanosomes [3, 16]. Lithium, choline, rubidium, and cesium ions will replace the sodium and potassium of Ringer solution if calcium is present. The immediacy of the calcium requirement for MSH action is demonstrated by the rapid and maximal darkening of *Anolis* skins which follows addition of Ca^{2+} to skins residing in Ca^{2+}-free Ringer. Subsequent transfer of maximally darkened skins to a Ca^{2+}-free Ringer (but still containing MSH, as before) results in a rapid and complete reversal (lightening) of darkened skins [16]. Barium, beryllium and strontium could replace calcium and permit melanosome dispersion in response to MSH, but since these divalent ions are generally unavailable under normal conditions, they are of limited significance in the normal physiology of the pigment cell. The other divalent cations studied (Mg^{2+}, Zn^{2+}, Co^{2+}, Cd^{2+}, Cu^{2+}) either failed to substitute or were apparently lethal to melanophores.

Catecholamines, as well as MSH, darken *Anolis* skins by dispersing melanosomes within the dendritic processes of dermal melanophores. There is evidence that these hormones (first messengers) control melanosome movements by regulating the level of the intracellular second messenger, cyclic adenosine monophosphate (cyclic AMP). The receptors through which these structurally different hormones stimulate melanophore dispersion have been shown to be separate, as demonstrated by the preferential blockade of one receptor while the functional integrity of the other is maintained [6]. Catecholamines disperse melanosomes through stimulation of beta-adrenergic receptors, whereas MSH interacts with and disperses melanosomes through a different, but as yet undefined receptor. In addition, lightening of skins, resulting from melanosome aggregation, is controlled through catecholamine stimulation of alpha-adrenergic receptors.

Thus, at least three separate receptors are implicated in melanophore control. Further evidence for separate receptors of melanophores is demonstrated by the difference in ionic requirements for receptor stimulation by MSH from that of catecholamines on either the alpha- or beta-adrenergic receptor. Calcium, although necessary for MSH-mediated melanophore dispersion, is not necessary for adrenergic receptor stimulation. These results demonstrate a receptor-specific calcium requirement for melanosome dispersion within melanophores of both an amphibian and a reptile.

The calcium ion requirement for MSH action appears to be an early event in that calcium is not required for melanosome dispersion itself, since theophylline or dibutyryl cyclic AMP reversibly darken lizard skins in the absence of calcium. Calcium is needed for MSH action, but MSH is not necessary for the hormone-mimetic action of calcium. Therefore, the calcium effect may be distal to the MSH receptor, but necessary for increased cyclic AMP levels in response to MSH which are apparently a prerequisite for melanosome movement. If adenyl cyclase is stimulated by MSH and by isoproterenol to increase melanophore cyclic AMP levels, then, it is also clear that there is a Ca^{2+} requirement only for the MSH-adenyl cyclase interrelationship. As we have pointed out elsewhere, the Ca^{2+} requirement for MSH action on melanophores in consistent with a similar cation requirement for the lipolytic action of adrenocorticotropic hormone (ACTH) on isolated fat cells [10] or the stimulation of adenyl cyclase activity in adrenal cortical microsomal fractions [2]. The similarity in structure of these two hormones might suggest a similar mechanism of action.

These results complement those of GOLDMAN and HADLEY [7] who demonstrated a receptor-specific sulfhydryl requirement for MSH action on *Anolis* melanophores. A variety of sulfhydryl inhibitors were shown to inhibit melanosome dispersion in response to MSH, but were without such an inhibitory effect on catecholamine-induced melanosome dispersion as mediated through melanophore beta-adrenergic receptors. These results, then, point out the separate mechanisms by which first messengers mediate their effects at the cellular level.

The Ca^{2+} ion is not requisite for melanosome dispersion in response to beta-adrenergic stimulation by catecholamines. Indeed, it would appear from the analysis of the data from many experiments that melanosome dispersion proceeds to a greater extent in the absence of the Ca^{2+} ion. It is apparent, from a review of our data [17], that melanosome dispersion is physiologically analogous to smooth muscle relaxation. Smooth muscle relaxation apparently proceeds following an increase in cyclic AMP production and a sequestering of Ca^{2+} from the cytoplasm to the plasma membrane [1]. It would appear from our studies, then, that although Ca^{2+} is required for an initial mechanism specific to the MSH receptor, that melanosome dispersion itself proceeds in the absence of the Ca^{2+} ion, possibly by a mechanism involving a reuptake of Ca^{2+} ion from the cytoplasm. KREINER et al. [9] demonstrated that the Ca^{2+} ion was required for MSH activation of adenyl cyclase in melanoma cells, but was not a requirement of prostaglandin-induced melanoma cyclase activity.

In summary, then, these results clearly demonstrate the ionic requirements for melanosome movements within melanophores of a number of poikilotherm vertebrates. These results clearly do not support other investigations [12, 13, 15], suggesting a specific monovalent (sodium) cation requirement for MSH action.

Summary

The calcium ion is specifically required for the mechanism of action of melanophore stimulating hormone (MSH) in dispersing melanosomes within integumental melanophores of the lizard, *Anolis carolinensis,* and the frog, *Scaphiopus couchi.* This divalent cation is not required for melanophore dispersion or aggregation as mediated by catecholamines acting through beta- and alpha-adrenergic receptors, respectively. There is no Ca^{2+} ion requirement for melanosome movements *per se* since theophylline and dibutyryl cyclic AMP disperse melanin granules in Ca^{2+}-free media, thus further specifying the Ca^{2+} ion requirement for MSH action. Sodium and potassium ions are not required for melanosome dispersion induced by MSH, isoproterenol, theophylline, or dibutyryl cyclic AMP.

Acknowledgments

This research was supported by a biomedical sciences support grant FR 07002 from the General Research Resources, Bureau of Health Professions Education and Manpower Training, NIH, and National Institute of Dental Research Training Grant 5-T01DE00184, NIH.

References

1 ANDERSSON, R.; LUNDHOLM, L.; MOHME-LUNDHOLM, E., and NILSSON, K.: Role of cyclic AMP and Ca^{++} in metabolic and mechanical events in smooth muscle. Adv. cyclic Ncleotide Res. *1:* 213–229 (1972).

2 BÄR, H. P. and HECHTER, O.: Adenyl cyclase and hormone action. III. Calcium requirement for ACTH stimulation of adenyl cyclase. Biochem. biophys. Res. Commun. *35:* 681–686 (1969).

3 DIKSTEIN, S.; WELLER, C. P., and SULMAN, F. G.: Effect of calcium ions on melanophore dispersal. Nature, Lond. *200:* 1106 (1963).

4 GOLDMAN, J. M. and HADLEY, M. E.: *In vitro* demonstration of adrenergic receptors controlling melanophore responses of the lizard, *Anolis carolinensis.* J. Pharmacol. exp. Ther. *166:* 1–7 (1969).

5 GOLDMAN, J. M. and HADLEY, M. E.: The beta-adrenergic receptor and cyclic

3′,5′ adenosine monophosphate: possible roles in the regulation of melano-phore responses of the spadefoot toad, *Scaphiopus couchi*. Gen. comp. Endocr. *13:* 151–163 (1969).

6   GOLDMAN, J. M. and HADLEY, M. E.: Evidence for separate receptors for me-lanophore-stimulating hormone and catecholamine regulation of cyclic AMP in the control of melanophore responses. Br. J. Pharmacol. *39:* 160–166 (1970).

7   GOLDMAN, J. M. and HADLEY, M. E.: Sulfhydryl requirement for alpha-adre-nergic receptor activity and melanophore-stimulating hormone (MSH) action on melanophores. J. Pharmacol. exp. Ther. *182:* 93–100 (1972).

8   HOROWITZ, S. B.: Energy requirements of melanin granule aggregation and dis-persion in the melanophore of *Anolis carolinensis*. J. Cell. comp. Physiol. *51:* 341–357 (1958).

9   KREINER, P. W.; GOLD, C. J.; KEIRNS, J. J.; BROCK, W. A., and BITENSKY, M. W.: MSH-sensitive adenyl cyclase in the Cloudman melanoma. Yale J. Biol. Med. *46:* 483–591 (1973).

10 KUO, J. F.: Differential effects of Ca^{2+}, EDTA and adrenergic blocking agents on the action of some hormones in adenosine 3′,5′-monophosphate levels in isolated adipose cells as determined by prior labeling with $8\text{-}^{14}C$ adenine. Biochim. biophys. Acta *208:* 509–516 (1970).

11 LOPEZ, E.; WHITE, J. E., and ENGEL, F. L.: Contrasting requirements for the li-polytic action of corticotropin and epinephrine on adipose tissue *in vitro*. J. biol. Chem. *234:* 2254–2258 (1959).

12 NOVALES, R. R.: The effects of osmotic pressure and sodium concentration on the response of melanophores to intermedin. Physiol. Zool. *32:* 15–28 (1959).

13 NOVALES, R. R.: On the role of cyclic AMP in the function of skin melano-phores. Ann. N.Y. Acad. Sci. *185:* 494–506 (1971).

14 SHIZUME, K.; LERNER, A. B., and FITZPATRICK, T. B.: *In vitro* bioassay for mel-anocyte-stimulating hormone. Endocrinology *54:* 553–560 (1954).

15 TERCAFS, R. R.: Chromatophores and permeability characteristics of frog skin. Comp. Biochem. Physiol. *17:* 937–951 (1966).

16 VESELY, D. L. and HADLEY, M. E.: Calcium requirement for melanophore-stimulating hormone action on melanophores. Science *173:* 923–925 (1971).

17 VESELY, D. L. and HADLEY, M. E.: Unpublished data.

18 WRIGHT, M. R. and LERNER, A. B.: On the movement of pigment granules in frog melanocytes. Endocrinology *66:* 599–609 (1960).

MAC E. HADLEY, PhD, Department of Biological Sciences, University of Arizo-na, *Tucson, AZ 85721* (USA)

Pigment Cell, vol. 3, pp. 275–283 (Karger, Basel 1976)

The Activation of Adenylate Cyclase by MSH in the Skin of *Xenopus laevis*

F. C. G. van de Veerdonk[1]

Zoological Laboratory, University of Utrecht, Utrecht

Like many invertebrate species, cold-blooded vertebrates are able to change their skin color dependent on the color of their background. This color change is caused by a dispersing and aggregating movement of pigment granules within the chromatophore cells. In amphibians, several types of chromatophores are involved cooperating in the chromatophore unit [5, 28]. The most investigated of these are the melanophores containing the black-brown pigment melanin in granules, which are called melanosomes. Whereas in other species the stimulus may be hormonal and/or neural, in amphibians only hormonal stimulation occurs [3, 16, 29]. The hormone responsible for the dispersing pigment migration is MSH, which is secreted from the intermediate lobe of the pituitary gland. Like many other peptide hormones, MSH initiates the dispersion reaction by activating the enzyme adenylate cyclase, which is located in the plasma membrane of the melanophores. Activation of adenylate cyclase results in an increased intracellular level of cyclic AMP, as was demonstrated for *Rana pipiens* by Bitensky and Burstein [8] and Abe *et al.* [1], and for *Xenopus laevis* by van de Veerdonk and Konijn [33]. The way in which the increased cyclic AMP amount initiates the melanosome movement is still unknown and is currently under investigation. A possible involvement of microtubules and/or microfilaments has been suggested [20–22].

The molecular mechanism by which hormones are capable of activating the membranous enzyme adenylate cyclase is subject of investigation in many other hormonal processes. Formation of a hormone-receptor complex is generally assumed to be the first step in a sequence of events. This has been demonstrated in a number of systems [14, 19, 37], but in

1   The author is grateful to Mrs. A. W. Vink-van Wijngaarden for invaluable assistance, to Mr. J. J. van der Vlis for the drawings, and to Prof. Dr. J. C. van de Kamer for continuous interest and encouragement.

melanophores it still awaits experimental confirmation. The process or processes occurring between the formation of the hormone-receptor complex and the activation of the catalytic site of the enzyme adenylate cyclase, is generally defined as the 'transducer' chain of reactions [27]. This paper deals with the transducer reactions taking place in the plasma membrane of the melanophores of *Xenopus laevis*, between the supposed formation of the MSH-receptor complex and the ultimate formation of cyclic AMP.

It should be kept in mind that results obtained cannot be generalized to all amphibian melanophores. There is a difference between *Xenopus laevis* and various *Rana* species as to the function of catecholamines in pigment migration. In *Rana*, catecholamines are lowering the cyclic AMP level [1, 2], resulting in pigment aggregation; in *Xenopus*, however, catecholamines increase the amount of intracellular cyclic AMP [33], resulting in pigment dispersion. In this respect, *Xenopus*' melanophores behave like most other hormone-induced systems, where also catecholamines are mimicking the hormonal action.

The first part of this paper is concerned with the determination of the sequence of events taking place in the transducer chain of *Xenopus*' melanophores. In the second part, a hypothesis will be presented situating the successive reactions in a more or less logical mechanism, which is open to further investigation. Melanophore dispersing activity was determined *in vivo* by injection of agents and inhibitors into the dorsal lymphatic sac, as well as *in vitro* using excised webs of the hindlegs of adult *Xenopus laevis*. The well-known HOGBEN and SLOME index [17] was used to evaluate the dispersion state.

Older investigations revealed a dispersing activity of MSH, catecholamines (of which norepinephrine, NE, was most frequently used) and cyclic AMP. The dispersing activity of MSH and NE proved to be sensi-

Table I. The influence of the adrenergic β-blocking agent, propranolol, on the melanophore dispersing activities of MSH, NE, and cyclic AMP

	Ringer solution	Propranolol, 0.5 mM
MSH, 0.01 μg/ml	+	−
NE, 0.1 mM	+	−
cAMP, 10 mM	+	+
Ringer solution	−	−

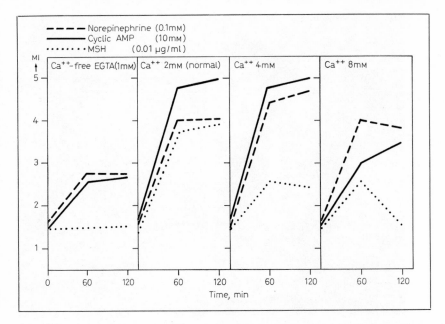

Fig. 1. Melanophore dispersion, induced by α-MSH (0.1 μg/ml), NE (10^{-4} M), and cyclic AMP (10^{-2} M) in amphibian Ringer solution, containing various Ca^{++} concentrations.

tive to the β-blocking agent propranolol [9, 10, 33]. Table I summarizes the results. The conclusion was drawn that in this system a β-adrenergic receptor was involved in the hormonal action of MSH. In this respect, melanophores differ from other target cells where the β-adrenergic receptor and the peptide-hormone receptor are independently capable of activating the enzyme adenylate cyclase [6]. Thus, the preliminary sequence of active substances operating in the transducer chain of *Xenopus'* melanophores is:

MSH — catecholamines — cyclic AMP.

The function of Ca^{++} in a number of stimulus-response reactions, including hormonal stimulation, has been studied [26], and is generally accepted at present. In pigment migration a role of Ca^{++} has been demonstrated [24, 35]. We studied the influence of Ca^{++} on the dispersion reaction in the melanophores of *Xenopus*, induced by MSH, NE, and cyclic AMP. Ca^{++} concentrations ranging from 0 up to 32 mM were used. The result is shown in figure 1. Compared to normal (2 mM Ca^{++}), higher Ca^{++}

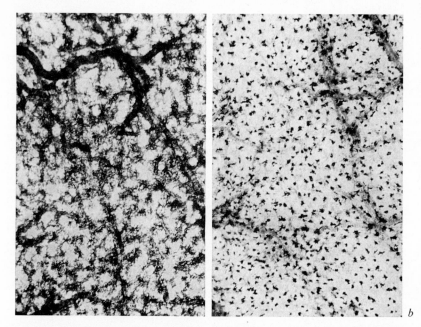

a   b

Fig. 2. Melanophores in the web of a hindleg of *Xenopus laevis,* adapted to a black background, during 3.75 h: (a) control animal; (b) animal after three hourly injections of indomethacin (each 24 mg/kg).

concentrations gradually suppress the dispersing activity of MSH, NE and cyclic AMP. The same counts for lower Ca^{++} concentrations with the exception of a medium which is absolutely devoid of Ca^{++} (with addition of EGTA, 1 mM). In this Ca-free medium, MSH does not produce any dispersion at all. This result suggests an absolute Ca^{++} indispensibility for MSH, whereas Ca^{++} play a minor (though definite) role in NE and cyclic AMP activities. Therefore, in the transducer chain Ca^{++} are suggested to be situated between MSH and NE:

MSH – Ca^{++} – catecholamines – cyclic AMP.

Apart from Ca^{++}, prostaglandins are concerned with membrane activity, especially as modulators of cyclic AMP formation [7, 11, 25]. This prostaglandin influence may result in either an increase or a decrease of the intracellular cyclic AMP level [15, 31]. PGE_1 and PGF_1 showed a dispersing activity on the melanophores of *Xenopus laevis in vitro*. The fol-

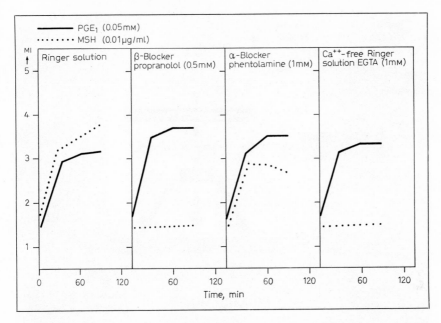

Fig. 3. Melanophore dispersion, induced by α-MSH (0.03 μg/ml) and PGE₁ (5.10⁻⁵ M) in amphibian Ringer solution, in the α-blocking agent phentolamine (10⁻⁴ M), in the β-blocking agent propranolol (10⁻⁴ M), and in a Ca-free medium containing EGTA (10⁻³ M).

lowing experiments have been performed with PGE₁ only. First of all, a physiological role of prostaglandins had to be determined. For this reason, a black background-adapted *Xenopus* was injected with indomethacin, an inhibitor of prostaglandin synthesis [34]. The result (fig. 2) indicates a function of PGE₁ in the MSH-induced dispersion reaction. In order to situate PGE₁ in the transducer reactions, the dispersing activity of PGE₁ was studied in amphibian Ringer in the presence of adrenergic α- and β-blocking substances, and in a Ca-free medium. The result is shown in figure 3. Absence of Ca⁺⁺ and presence of β-blockers do not influence PGE₁ activity, whereas MSH activity is influenced as described before. These data suggest a localization of prostaglandins in the transducer chain after catecholamines. The sequence of events in the transducer chain of *Xenopus'* melanophores, so far demonstrated, is proposed to be:

MSH – Ca⁺⁺ – catecholamines – prostaglandins – cyclic AMP.

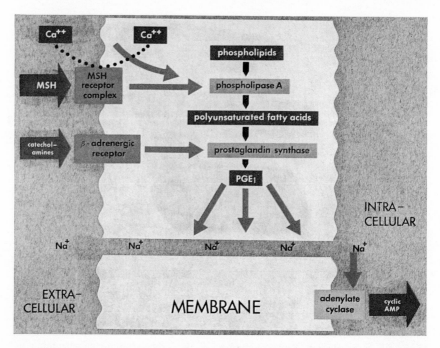

Fig. 4. Hypothetical model of the reactions taking place in the transducer chain in the melanophores of *Xenopus laevis*.

What reasonable mechanism can be supposed, underlying the above demonstrated sequence of reactions in the transducer chain? The following hypothesis (fig. 4) is presented, which is open to further investigations:

The first step in the transducer chain, the formation of the MSH-receptor complex, is suggested to activate membranous phospholipase A. Experimental evidence for this suggestion is lacking, but the structural resemblance between the fat mobilizing factor and MSH [13] may support the presumptive lipolytic activity of MSH. Furthermore, the absolute Ca requirement of phospholipase A [4, 12, 32] is in accordance with the Ca requirement early in the transducer chain. The proposed lipolytic activity may result in the release of polyunsaturated fatty acids necessary for prostaglandin biosynthesis [18]. We suggest catecholamines to play a role as coenzymes in this prostaglandin synthesis in *Xenopus'* skin. A similar role of catecholamines in the mechanism of PGE_1 biosynthesis by ovine seminal vesicle preparations has been suggested earlier by SIH *et al.* [30].

A number of different coenzymes for prostaglandin synthase has been described, which may account for the species differences as to the function of catecholamines in the dispersion mechanisms of *Xenopus* and *Rana* species. In accordance with the suggestion of RAMWELL and SHAW [25], we suggest an influx of Na^+ to be the result of prostaglandin activity, opening in one way or another the Na^+ pores in the plasma membrane, by which a passive entry of this ion may occur. A sodium influx coupled to pigment dispersion has already been described in 1959 by NOVALES [23]. The last step in the transducer chain, the activation of the catalytic site of adenylate cyclase resulting in an increase in the intracellular cyclic AMP level, may be brought about by this increased amount of sodium ions. A similar suggestion had been presented by RAMWELL and SHAW [25] in 1970, in the action of hormones regulating the permeability of frog skin.

The way in which the increased intracellular cyclic AMP level induces the melanosomes to start moving is beyond the scope of this paper. This field as well as various steps of the proposed mechanism need further investigation.

Summary

MSH-induced pigment dispersion in *Xenopus laevis* is mediated by cyclic AMP. The series of reactions by which MSH induces the enzyme adenylate cyclase to increase cAMP synthesis is called the transducer chain. By means of pharmacological techniques the sequence of active substances subsequently playing a role in the transducer chain, is proposed to be:

MSH – Ca^{++} – catecholamines – prostaglandins – cyclic AMP.

A mechanism underlying this sequence of active compounds has been presented as a working hypothesis.

References

1   ABE, K.; BUTCHER, R. W.; NICHOLSON, W. E.; BAIRD, C. E.; LIDDLE, R. A., and LIDDLE, G. W.: Adenosine 3',5'-monophosphate (cyclic AMP) as the mediator of the actions of melanocyte-stimulating hormone (MSH) and norepinephrine on the frog skin. Endocrinology 84: 362–368 (1969).
2   ABE, K.; ROBISON, G. A.; LIDDLE, G. W.; BUTCHER, R. W.; NICHOLSON, W. E., and BAIRD, C. E.: Role of cyclic AMP in mediating the effects of MSH, norepinephrine and melatonin on frog skin color. Endocrinology 85: 674–682 (1969).

3   ALLEN, B. M.: The results of extirpation of the anterior lobe of the hypophysis and the thyroid of *Rana pipiens* larvae. Science *44:* 755–757 (1916).

4   ARNESJO, B. and GRUBB, A.: The activation, purification and properties of rat pancreatic juice phospholipase A. Acta chem. scand. *25:* 577–589 (1971).

5   BAGNARA, J. T.; TAYLOR, J. D., and HADLEY, M. E.: The dermal chromatophore unit. J. Cell Biol. *38:* 67–79 (1968).

6   BÄR, H. P. and HECHTER, O.: Adenyl cyclase and hormone action. I. Effects of adrenocorticotropic hormone, glucagon and epinephrine on the plasma membrane of the rat fat cells. Proc. natn. Acad. Sci. USA *63:* 350–355 (1969).

7   BERGSTRÖM, S.: Prostaglandins: members of a new hormonal system. Science *157:* 382–391 (1967).

8   BITENSKY, M. W. and BURSTEIN, S. R.: Effects of cyclic adenosine monophosphate and MSH on frog skin *in vitro*. Nature, Lond. *208:* 1282–1284 (1965).

9   BROUWER, E.: The involvement of catecholamines in the dispersion reaction of the melanophores of *Xenopus laevis* resulting from black background adaptation; diss., Utrecht (1973).

10   BROUWER, E. and VEERDONK, F. C. G. VAN DE: Possible involvement of α- and β-receptors in the natural colour change and the MSH-induced dispersion in *Xenopus laevis in vivo*. Eur. J. Pharmacol. *171:* 234–239 (1972).

11   BUTCHER, R. W. and SUTHERLAND, E. W.: The effects of the catecholamines, adrenergic blocking agents, prostaglandin E_1, and insulin on cyclic AMP levels in the rat epididymal fat pad *in vitro*. Ann. N.Y. Acad. Sci. *139:* 849–859 (1967).

12   HAAS, G. H. DE; POSTEMA, N. M.; NIEUWENHUIZEN, W., and DEENEN, L. L. M. VAN: Purification and properties of phospholipase A from porcine pancreas. Biochim. biophys. Acta *159:* 103–117 (1968).

13   GRÁF, L.; BARÁT, E.; CSEH, G., and SAJGÓ: Amino acid sequence of porcine γ-lipotropic hormone. Acta biochim. biophys. hung. *5:* 305–307 (1970).

14   GOLDFINE, I. D.; ROTH, J., and BIRNBAUMER, L.: Glucagon receptors in β-cells. Binding of ^{125}I-glucagon and activation of adenylate cyclase. J. biol. Chem. *247:* 1211–1218 (1972).

15   HARWOOD, J. P.; MOSKOWITZ, J., and KRISHNA, G.: Dynamic interaction of prostaglandin and norepinephrine in the formation of adenosine 3′,5′-monophosphate in human and rabbit platelets. Biochim. biophys. Acta *261:* 444–456 (1972).

16   HOGBEN, L. T. and WINTON, F. R.: Studies on the pituitary. I. The melanophore stimulant in posterior lobe extracts. Biochem. J. *16:* 619–630 (1922).

17   HOGBEN, L. T. and SLOME, D.: The pigmentary effector system. VI. The dual character of endocrine co-ordination in amphibian colour change. Proc. R. Soc. B *108:* 10–53 (1931).

18   LANDS, W. E. M. and SAMUELSSON, B.: Phospholipid precursors of prostaglandins. Biochim. biophys. Acta *164:* 426–429 (1968).

19   LEFKOWITZ, R. J. and HABER, E.: A fraction of the ventricular myocardium that has the specificity of the cardiac β-adrenergic receptor. Proc. natn. Acad. Sci. USA *68:* 1773–1777 (1971).

20   MALAWISTA, S. E.: Cytochalasin B reversibly inhibits melanin granule movement in melanocytes. Nature, Lond. *234:* 354–355 (1971).

21   McGUIRE, J. and MOELLMANN, G.: Cytochalasin B. Effects on microfilaments

and movement of melanin granules within melanocytes. Science *175:* 642–644 (1972).

22 MOELLMANN, G.; McGUIRE, J., and LERNER, A. B.: Intracellular dynamics and the fine structure of melanocytes. With special reference to the effects of MSH and cyclic AMP on microtubules and 10-nm filaments. Yale J. Biol. Med. *46:* 337–360 (1973).

23 NOVALES, R. R.: The effects of osmotic pressure and sodium concentration on the response of melanophores to intermedin. Physiol. Zool. *32:* 15–28 (1959).

24 NOVALES, R. R. and NOVALES, B. J.: The effects of osmotic pressure and calcium deficiency on the response of tissue-cultured melanophores to melanocyte-stimulating hormone. Gen. comp. Endocr. *5:* 568–576 (1965).

25 RAMWELL, P. W. and SHAW, J. E.: Biological significance of the prostaglandins. Recent Prog. Horm. Res. *26:* 139–187 (1970).

26 RASMUSSEN, H. and TENENHOUSE, A.: Cyclic adenosine monophosphate, Ca^{++}, and membranes. Proc. natn. Acad. Sci. USA *59:* 1364–1370 (1968).

27 RODBELL, M.; LIN, M. C.; SALOMON, Y.; LONDOS, C.; HARWOOD, J. P.; MARTIN, B. R.; RENDELL, M., and BERMAN, M.: The role of adenine and guanine nucleotides in the activity and response of adenylate cyclase systems to hormones: evidence for multi-site transition states. Acta endocr., Copenh. *77:* suppl. 191, pp. 11–37 (1974).

28 SCHMIDT, W. J.: Über das Verhalten der verschiedenartigen Chromatophoren beim Farbwechsel des Laubfrosches. Arch. mikr. Anat. *93:* 414–472 (1919).

29 SMITH, P. E.: Experimental ablation of the hypophysis in the frog embryo. Science *44:* 280–282 (1916).

30 SIH, C. J.; TAKEGUCHI, C., and FOSS, P.: Mechanism of prostaglandin biosynthesis. III. Catecholamines and serotonin as coenzymes. J. Am. Chem. Soc. *92:* 6670 (1970).

31 STEINBERG, D.: Prostaglandins as adrenergic antagonists. Ann. N.Y. Acad. Sci. *139:* 897–909 (1967).

32 UTHE, J. F. and MAGEE, W. L.: Phospholipase A_2: action on purified phospholipids as affected by deoxycholate and divalent cations. Can. J. Biochem. *49:* 776–784 (1971).

33 VEERDONK, F. C. G. VAN DE and KONIJN, T. M.: The role of adenosine 3′,5′-cyclic monophosphate and catecholamines in the pigment migration process in *Xenopus laevis*. Acta endocr., Copenh. *64:* 364–376 (1970).

34 VANE, J. R.: Inhibition of prostaglandin synthesis as a mechanism of action for aspirin-like drugs. Nature new Biol. *231:* 232–235 (1971).

35 VESELY, D. L. and HADLEY, M. E.: Calcium requirement for melanophore-stimulating hormone action on melanophores. Science *173:* 923–925 (1971).

36 VONKEMAN, H. and DORP, D. A. VAN: The action of prostaglandin synthetase on 2-arachidonyl-lecithin. Biochim. biophys. Acta *164:* 430–432 (1968).

37 WOHLTMANN, H. J. and NARAHARA, H. T.: Binding of insulin-^{131}I by isolated frog sartorius muscles. Relationship to changes in permeability to sugar caused by insulin. J. biol. Chem. *241:* 4931–4939 (1966).

Dr. F. C. G. VAN DE VEERDONK, Zoological Laboratory, Section of Histology and Cell Biology, Transitorium III, Padualaan 8 (De Uithof) *Utrecht* (The Netherlands)

Pigment Cell, vol. 3, pp. 284–290 (Karger, Basel 1976)

MSH, c-AMP and Embryonic Melanophore Development in Amphibians

Harvey L. Wahn, John D. Taylor and T. T. Tchen

Departments of Biology, Chemistry and Comparative Medicine, Wayne State University, Detroit, Mich.

Introduction

The pigment cells, particularly the melanophores, have been a favorite subject for studying cellular differentiation due to their built-in histochemical markers – the pigments. The development of early embryonic melanophores has the additional importance that, as they are derived from the neural crest, their development may be taken as an indicator of the processes of primary induction and neurulation. We reasoned that the primary inductor(s) is (are) similar to hormones in that they are intercellular messengers. Since the primary inductor(s) appear(s) to be protein(s) in nature, they are not likely to penetrate the target cells, but would most likely act on the cell membrane, possibly via an intracellular second messenger such as c-AMP. We undertook two approaches: test the effects of c-AMP and its derivatives on whole embryos and on cultures of small explants of undetermined presumptive epidermis. We shall present here the results and speculate on their significance.

Results and Discussion

1. Cultures of Small Explants of Undetermined Presumptive Epidermis

Using the culture technique developed by Barth and Barth [1], we have shown that derivatives of c-AMP in combination with theophylline, can induce neurodifferentiation in cultures of presumptive epidermis from three amphibian species: *Pleurodeles waltlii*, *Serodon mexicanam,* and *Xenopus laevis*. In this technique, small explants of a few hundred cells were removed from presumptive epidermal area as soon as the dorsal lip becomes visible. These explants were placed in Falcon Cooper dishes and incubated with Niu-Twitty solution with or without the addition of various nucleotides. In the absence of additional nucleotides, or in the presence of 10^{-3} M 5'-AMP, 2',3'-c-AMP, or dibutyryl-c-GMP, little or no neurodifferentiation was observed. In the presence of 10^{-3} M 8-Br-c-AMP, dibutyryl-c-AMP, or c-AMP, or c-AMP with theophylline, extensive neurodifferentiation was observed after 3 (in the case of *Xenopus laevis*) or 7–10 (in the case of the two other species) days. Simple neurons appeared first, followed by astrocytes, melanophores, complex neurons, and oligodendroglial cells [4]. The melanophores produced may be amorphous or highly dendritic in structure (fig. 1).

2. Intact Embryos

When whole embryos of *Xenopus laevis* or *Pleurodeles waltlii* were treated with dibutyryl-c-AMP (varying from 10^{-6}–10^{-3} M), no gross abnormality of development was observed. In other words, the presumptive epidermis does not appear to undergo neurodifferentiation. There is, however, a reproducible change in the rate of melanophore development. In both species, melanophores appeared two stages earlier than in control embryos. The location (or distribution), morphology, and the ultimate number of melanophores per embryo were not altered. This is illustrated in figure 2.

Besides dibutyryl-c-AMP, the following agents produced exactly the same response: α-MSH ($>10^{-14}$ g/ml), β-MSH (10^{-9} g/ml), ACTH (0.25 IU/ml), and theophylline (10^{-3} M). 5'-AMP (10^{-3} M) and 2',3'-c-AMP (10^{-3} M) are totally without effect. From these results, we concluded that the observed effect on melanophore development is due to increase in intracellular c-AMP in melanoblasts (or immature amelanotic melanophores) which can be achieved by: (1) flooding with dibutyryl-c-AMP added externally; (2) activation of hormone (MSH)-dependent adenyl cyclase, or (3) inhibition of intracellular c-AMP phosphodiesterase by theophylline (this will be discussed in detail elsewhere).

3. Cultures of Large Explants of Presumptive Neural Ectoderm

The entire region of presumptive neural ectoderm was removed at different stages of embryonic development and incubated in Niu-Twitty solution with or without the addition of α-MSH (10^{-9} g/ml) or dibutyryl-c-AMP (10^{-3} M). The results obtained in the absence of MSH or dibutyr-

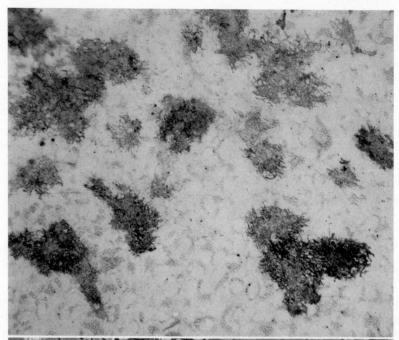

A

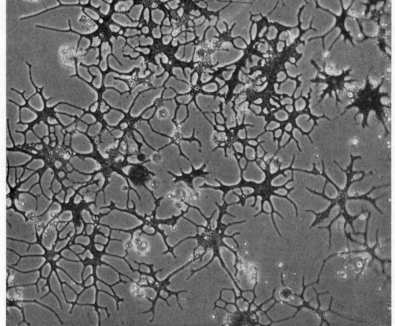

B

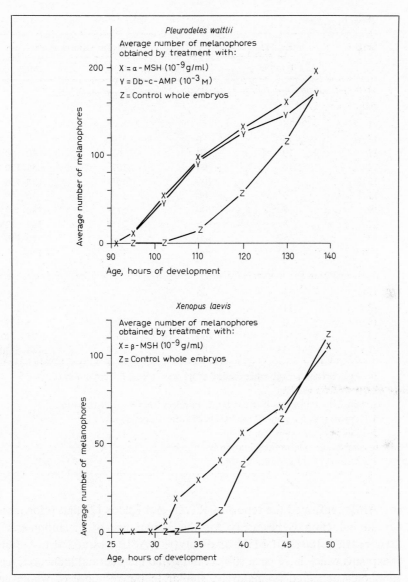

Fig. 2. Melanophore development following treatment of whole embryos with either MSH or dibutyryl-c-AMP (Db-c-AMP).

Fig. 1. Photomicrographs of *Pleurodeles waltlii* cell cultures with (A) a bright field image of melanophores exhibiting amorphous structure and (B) a phase contrast image of melanophore with highly dendritic structure. × 97.

Table I

Stage[1]	Explants		Melanophores in explants	
	number	% responding	mean	range

Melanophore differentiation in isolated neural plates without underlying chordo-mesoderm[2]

11	14	0	–	–
12	14	0	–	–
13	10	60	63	30–100
14	10	90	109	59–170
15	5	100	101	25–138
17	9	100	156	70–205
19	8	100	225[3]	180–>250[3]
21	8	100	225[3]	185–>255[3]
28[4]	5[5]	100	90	70–110
29a[4]	5[5]	100	170	150–>220[3]

Melanophore differentiation in isolated neural plates with underlying chordo-mesoderm[1]

11[6]	8	0	–	–
12	11	64	52	20–150
13	8	75	78	45–120
14	10	100	137[3]	75–>170[3]
29a[7]	5[5]	100	180[3]	143–>200[3]

1 Developmental stage when neural plate was removed from embryo.
2 *Pleurodeles waltlii.*
3 Approximate figures because large numbers were difficult to count.
4 Control (28) for stages 11–15 and (29a) for stages 17–21.
5 Whole embryo controls.
6 Chordo-mesoderm invagination incomplete.
7 Control (29a) for stages 11–14.

yl-c-AMP confirmed the report of RAVEN and KLOOS [2] that prior mesodermal induction is necessary for the appearance of melanophores in these organ cultures. If MSH or dibutyryl-c-AMP was added to cultures of explants which have been subject to *in vivo* mesodermal induction, melanophores appeared prematurely, similar to the response of whole embryos to these agents (table I).

From these results, it may be concluded that only the mesodermal primary inductor(s) can induce the determination of melanophores whereas elevation of intracellular c-AMP can stimulate and accelerate the cytodifferentiation of 'determined immature amelanotic melanophores'.

4. The Paradox

It is clear that the effects of c-AMP vary with the experimental conditions. If one were to divide somewhat arbitrarily the development of differentiated cells into two stages: determination (or commitment) and cytodifferentiation, the results obtained with small explants indicate that c-AMP can cause determination and may stimulate cytodifferentiation, whereas the results obtained with large explants and with whole embryos indicate that c-AMP cannot cause determination, but can only stimulate cytodifferentiation of certain cells.

5. Rationalization

In an attempt to resolve the above-mentioned paradox, we considered the differences in the experimental conditions employed. The most striking difference is that the small explants attach to the plastic surface, flatten out, and become monolayers. Eventually, individual cells migrate away from the explant and lose contact with other cells. In the case of whole embryos or large explants which invariably roll into balls of cells, the cells remain in intimate contact with adjacent cells throughout the experiment. In the literature, one finds abundant examples where cellular contact causes profound changes in cellular activities, e.g. contact inhibition. It thus seems reasonable to assume that the difference observed with small explants versus large explants and whole embryos may be due to some inhibitory action of adjacent cells. Indeed, there is available evidence in the classical literature of embryology to support this view. When, after the first cleavage of a fertilized egg, the two cells were mechanically separated, each cell will develop into a complete embryo. In contrast, if one of the two cells was killed mechanically, but the residual membrane not removed from the surviving cell, this cell will develop partially into a half embryo [3]. It is well known that primary induction and neurulation involve not only induction but also morphogenic movement. The embryonic development of melanophores is particularly well documented to involve induction, migration, and cytodifferentiation. It is possible that in the normal case of whole embryos and in the 'semi-normal' case of large explants, the primary inductor not only induces the determination of certain cells, but also proper morphogenic movements, so that these cells can proceed with cytodifferentiation. In the abnormal case of small explants, the latter requirement for morphogenic movement is relieved by the migration of the cells on the plastic surface. According to this view, c-AMP should have induced determination (to form neural fold-derived cells) in large explants and in presumptive epidermal regions of whole embryos, but cytodifferentiation could not take place because of inhibitory action of certain adjacent cells.

The above rationalization is not the only possible explanation of the paradox. However, it is reasonable and, more importantly, amenable to experimental verification or refute, and we hope that current and future work will prove or disprove its validity.

Summary

Whole *Pleurodeles waltlii* embryos or organ cultures of the neural fold of these embryos were treated with MSH, ACTH, dibutyryl-c-AMP, c-AMP plus theophylline, theophilline, c-AMP, 5'-AMP, or 2',3'-c-AMP. The development of melanophores were accelerated (appearing two stages earlier than in control embryos or explants) by MSH ($\geq 10^{-14}$ g/ml), ACTH (≥ 0.25 IU), dibutyryl-c-AMP ($\geq 10^{-6}$ M), c-AMP plus theophylline (both at 10^{-3} M), or theophylline alone (10^{-3} M). By the time the embryos developed to stage 28, the control and treated embryos were indistinguishable in the number, distribution, and general morphology of their melanophores; c-AMP alone (10^{-3} M), 5'-AMP (10^{-3} M), or 2',3'-c-AMP (10^{-3} M) were ineffective. This effect on neural fold explants apparently requires preinduction by the invaginating mesoderm as explants of presumptive neural ectoderm excised at stage 12 or earlier failed to produce any melanophores with or without MSH or dibutyryl-c-AMP. Similar results were also obtained with *Xenopus laevis*.

References

1   BARTH, L. G. and BARTH, L. J.: J. Embryol. exp. Morph. *7:* 210 (1959).
2   RAVEN, C. P. and KLOOS, J.: Acta neerl. morph. *4:* 348 (1945).
3   SAXEN, L. and TOIVONEN, S.: Primary embryonic induction, p. 271 (Logos Press, London 1962).
4   WAHN, H. L.; LIGHTBODY, L.; TAYLOR, J. D., and TCHEN, T. T.: Science *188:* 336 (1975).

Dr. T. T. TCHEN, Departments of Biology, Chemistry and Comparative Medicine, Wayne State University, *Detroit, MI 48202* (USA)

Pigment Cell Photobiology and Control Mechanisms

Pigment Cell, vol. 3, pp. 291–298 (Karger, Basel 1976)

Effect of UV-A, UV-B, and Psoralen on *in vivo* Human Melanin Pigmentation

Cellular and Subcellular Characterization on Delayed Tanning Reactions Induced by Single or Multiple Exposures to UV-A, UV-B or UV-A plus 8-Methoxypsoralen[1]

M. A. Pathak, K. Jimbow, J. A. Parrish, K. H. Kaidbey, A. L. Kligman and T. B. Fitzpatrick

Department of Dermatology, Massachusetts General Hospital, Harvard Medical School, Boston, Mass., and Department of Dermatology, University of Pennsylvania, Philadelphia, Pa.

Introduction

Tanning of the human skin stimulated by solar radiation involves two distinct photobiological processes of melanin pigmentation: (1) immediate tanning (IT), and (2) delayed tanning (DT) [1]. In this paper, the sequential light and electron microscopic changes that occur in human skin during DT reactions after single and multiple exposures to ultraviolet radiation or UV-A (320–400 nm), UV-B (290–320 nm) and UV-A plus 8-methoxypsoralen (8-MOP) will be presented. Our findings concerning IT reaction were reported at the Yale Conference on Pigment Cell Biology [2].

Materials and Methods

Eight normal Caucasoid adults volunteered for this study. Irradiation with UV-A, UV-B, and UV-A plus 8-MOP was carried out as outlined in tables I and II. Exposure to UV radiation was carried out either on the buttock or on the back region. Biopsies were obtained either after a single exposure or after repeated multiple exposures (6–21 times) on days 0, 1, 4, 7, and 60 after irradiation. Biopsy specimens

1   This study was supported by Grants USPHS CA-21208 and CA-05003.

were divided into two parts for both light microscopic and electron microscopic studies. The specimens for light microscopy were treated with routine hematoxylin and eosin stain, PAS stain, Fontana's silver stain, and 'split-dopa [3]. Split-dopa preparations were obtained after immersing the biopsy specimens into 2N NaBr for 2 h at 37 °C and then incubating them in 0.1% dopa (L-3,4-dihydroxyphenylalanine) solution made in 0.1 M sodium phosphate buffer (pH 7.4) at 37 °C for 4–5 h. The specimens for electron microscopy were fixed with 2.5% glutaraldehyde-2.5% paraformaldehyde solution made in cacodylate buffer (0.1 M, pH 7.4) solutions at room temperature [4]. They were dehydrated by ethyl alcohol solutions, mounted in epoxy resins, sectioned by LKB microtome, and observed under a Siemens Elmiskop I electron microscope.

Results

Macroscopic Degree of Medium Pigmentation
After a Single Exposure to either UV-A, UV-B, or
UV-A plus 8-MOP
UV-A exposure with and without 8-MOP resulted in IT which was related to exposure dose and preexisting pigment content of the skin. Exposure of skin to high energy dose (225 J/cm^2) resulted in intense darkening which persisted for more than 48 h and, in fact, blended imperceptibly into DT or new melanogenesis. Low energy dose of UV-A (46 J/cm^2) caused modest IT which faded over 24–48 h. UV-B exposures caused minimal IT. All exposures resulted in DT which was greatest for UV-A plus 8-MOP and could be seen within 72 h after exposure.

After Repeated Multiple Exposures to either UV-A (21 times),
UV-B (6 times), or UV-A plus 8-MOP (6 times)
All four subjects showed basically similar patterns of increased melanin pigmentation after each type of UV exposure. Of the three different types of UV exposures, multiple repeated exposures (twice weekly for 3 weeks) to UV-A (5–7.5 J/cm^2/day) plus 8-MOP (60 mg orally) caused the most noticeable skin pigmentation. Multiple repeated exposures (21 times in 3 weeks) to a moderate dose of UV-A (15 J/cm^2/day) were not preceded by any obvious erythema or scaling, but caused marked new melanogenesis. This was distinctive since multiple repeated exposures (twice weekly for 3 weeks) to UV-B (2 MED, 30 mJ/cm^2/day) always caused erythema and scaling and the degree of new melanogenesis was appreciably less than UV-A alone.

Table I. Effect of a single exposure of UV-A, UV-B, and UV-A plus 8-MOP on the population of human melanocytes

Subject	Site of biopsy	Biopsy time	Control	Number of melanocytes/mm²		UV-A + 8-MOP
				UV-A	UV-B	
I	buttock	day 4	986 ± 36	997 ± 24	1,007 ± 36	970 ± 42
(A.M.)	buttock	day 7		1,037 ± 48	1,027 ± 54	1,072 ± 31
II	buttock	day 4	985 ± 12	995 ± 24	1,002 ± 12	948 ± 36
(D.M.)	buttock	day 7		993 ± 30	951 ± 18	1,068 ± 27
III	back	day 1	1,435 ± 24	1,493 ± 42	1,438 ± 66	
(V.R.)		day 7		1,633 ± 96	1,585 ± 48	
	buttock	day 1	1,168 ± 30			1,086 ± 48
		day 7				1,137 ± 126

Irradiance. Subjects I and II: UV-A = USHIO 500 W, λ 365 nm, 225 J/cm²; UV-B = Westinghouse FS-40, 121 mJ/cm² (3MED); UV-A + 8-MOP = Sylvania black light 7.5 J/cm², 40 mg 8-MOP (orally). Subject III: UV-A = Westinghouse high intensity 400 W, 46 J/cm²; UV-B = Westinghouse FS-20, 45 mJ/cm² (3MED); UV-A + 8-MOP = Sylvania black light, 4 J/cm², 40 mg 8-MOP (orally).

Light Microscopical Findings

After a Single Exposure to either UV-A, UV-B, or UV-A plus 8-MOP

Examination of split-dopa preparations revealed that the increase in the visual degree of skin pigmentation after a single exposure was primarily due to the changes in the functional activity of the melanocytes and not due to the numerical increase in the population density of the melanocytes. A single exposure to either UV-A, UV-B, or UV-A plus 8-MOP did not cause any obvious and statistically significant increase in the population of the dopa-positive melanocytes, even in situations when a high dose of UV-A (225 J/cm²) was used (table I). A prominent change was reflected by arborization of the dendritic processes and hypertrophy of the perikaryon of the melanocytes. These two changes became obvious at 48–72 h after exposure with UV-A or UV-B, whereas with UV-A (4–7.5 J/cm²) plus 8-MOP (40 mg orally), they were not obvious until days 7–14.

After Repeated Multiple Exposures to either UV-A (21 times),

UV-B (6 times), or UV-A plus 8-MOP (6 times)

Repeated multiple exposures to UV-A, UV-B, or UV-A plus 8-MOP resulted in a marked increase in the number of the dopa-positive melano-

Table II. Changes in human melanocyte system following single and multiple exposures of UV-A, UV-B and UV-A plus 8-MOP

Subject	Number of exposures	Type of UV exposure	Number of melanocytes per mm²	Visual degree of pigmentation	Size of melanosomes nm	Ratio of single melanosomes in keratinocytes $\left(\frac{S}{S+MC}\right) \times 100$	Number of melanosomes per melanosome complex
I	0	control	1,435 ± 24	±	427 ± 41	23.1 ± 2.1	3.5 ± 1.1
(V.R.)	1	UV-A	1,633 ± 96	+ +	468 ± 18	21.6 ± 12.5	4.5 ± 1.1
	1	UV-B	1,585 ± 48	+ +	443 ± 41	26.4 ± 10.1	3.5 ± 1.0
	0	control	1,168 ± 30	±	383 ± 41	21.7 ± 9.3	3.6 ± 0.9
	1	UV-A + 8-MOP	1,137 ± 126	+ +	398 ± 55	27.4 ± 9.1	5.1 ± 2.9
II	0	control	952 ± 67	±	421 ± 29	11.3 ± 5.5	4.4 ± 1.5
(T.F.)	21	UV-A	1,918 ± 90	+ + +	499 ± 39	25.1 ± 12.2	3.6 ± 1.4
	6	UV-B	1,916 ± 50	+ +	452 ± 46	24.8 ± 13.3	3.7 ± 2.1
	6	UV-A + 8-MOP	2,026 ± 31	+ + + +	505 ± 46	27.4 ± 4.3	3.4 ± 0.9
III	0	control	716 ± 42	±	415 ± 40	18.7 ± 9.6	4.5 ± 1.5
(S.L.)	21	UV-A	1,928 ± 38	+ + + +	546 ± 57	34.0 ± 11.9	3.5 ± 1.0
	6	UV-B	1,514 ± 40	+ +	548 ± 25	24.7 ± 10.3	4.1 ± 1.5
	6	UV-A + 8-MOP	1,924 ± 60	+ + + +	545 ± 30	29.9 ± 10.7	2.8 ± 1.4
IV	0	control	882 ± 34	±	469 ± 52	10.0 ± 3.5	4.6 ± 1.0
(W.D.)	21	UV-A	1,842 ± 86	+ + + +	–	–	–
	6	UV-B	1,794 ± 75	+ +	574 ± 74	29.1 ± 8.1	2.8 ± 1.0
	6	UV-A + 8-MOP	1,960 ± 30	+ + + +	578 ± 60	29.4 ± 14.7	3.0 ± 0.7
V	0	control	872 ± 48	±	424.9 ± 30	10.2 ± 7.5	6.1 ± 2.6
(D.M.)	21	UV-A	1,916 ± 30	+ + + +	481 ± 65	30.0 ± 10.6	3.4 ± 1.3
	6	UV-B	1,749 ± 45	+ +	460 ± 22	23.0 ± 9.4	3.4 ± 1.0
	6	UV-A + 8-MOP	2,142 ± 75	+ + + +	516 ± 31	29.5 ± 7.9	3.1 ± 0.8

S = Single, non-aggregated melanosomes in keratinocytes; MC = melanosome complexes in keratinocytes (group of 2 or more melanosomes surrounded by a membrane).
Irradiance. UV-A = Westinghouse high intensity 400 W (320–400 nm); subject I received 46 J/cm²; subjects II-V received 15 J/cm²/day for a total of 21 exposures in 3 weeks. UV-B = Westinghouse FS-20 (290–320 nm); subject I received 45 mJ/cm² equivalent to 3 MED; subjects II-V received 30 mJ/cm²/day equivalent to 2 MED, 6 times, twice weekly

cytes and the functional state of these melanocytes (table II). In split epidermal preparations, there was at least a twofold increase in the population of the melanocytes. These melanocytes showed enlarged perikaryon, marked arborization of the dendritic processes, and increased tyrosinase activity. A marked increase in the number of melanin granules were seen in the horizontal sections stained with hematoxylin and eosin or diamine silver. These granules were distributed not only in the basal layers, but also in an entire suprabasal layer of the upper epidermis. UV-A plus 8-MOP treated skin showed a marked increase in the thickness of the epidermis, including the horny layer. Occasionally, there were dyskeratotic cells in the epidermis exposed to UV-B or UV-A plus 8-MOP.

Electron Microscopical Findings[2]
After a Single Exposure to either UV-A, UV-B,
or UV-A plus 8-MOP
A single exposure to UV-A or UV-B resulted in basically similar subcellular changes in the epidermal melanin unit. In skin specimens exposed to UV-A or to UV-B, there was an increase in the number of melanosomes both in the melanocytes and in the keratinocytes (table II). There was no change in the size or in the ratio of single melanosomes to single-plus-aggregated (complex) melanosomes. The number of the melanosomes present in each of the melanosome complexes appeared to be increased with UV-A (table II).

The melanocytes and keratinocytes of the skin area treated with a single exposure to UV-A plus 8-MOP contained more melanosomes than those exposed to just UV-A or to UV-B. This increase was not apparent until day 7 after exposure. There were neither any alterations in the size of melanosomes, nor in the ratio of single to complex melanosomes in the keratinocytes. The number of melanosomes in each of the melanosome complexes appeared to be increased (table II).

---

2   No electron micrographs are presented because of limitations of space and the high cost of printing.

---

for 3 weeks. UV-A plus 8-MOP = subject I received 40 mg 8-MOP orally and 2 h later was exposed to 4 J/cm² of Sylvania black light UV-A; subjects II-V received 60 mg 8-MOP orally twice weekly for 3 weeks and 2 h later exposure to UV-A from Westinghouse high intensity 400 W lamp, 5–7.5 J/cm²/day, 6 times, twice weekly for 3 weeks.

After Repeated Multiple Exposure to either UV-A (21 times),
UV-B (6 times), or UV-A plus 8-MOP (6 times)

After multiple repeated exposures to UV-A, UV-B, and UV-A plus 8-MOP, it became clear that the melanocytes respond specificially and differently to these three different stimuli. The difference was more recognizable in the synthesis, melanization, and degradation of melanosomes than in the transfer and distribution pattern of these organelles. Even though UV-B exposed melanocytes contained many well-developed Golgi apparatuses very similar to those observed in melanocytes exposed to UV-A or UV-A plus 8-MOP, the melanocytes exposed to UV-B contained less numerous and less melanized melanosomes than did melanocytes exposed to UV-A or UV-A plus 8-MOP. Melanocytes treated with UV-A plus 8-MOP had the greatest number of highly melanized melanosomes. In skin treated with UV-B or UV-A plus 8-MOP, the melanosomes in the keratinocytes often showed a large aggregation that was formed by fusion of several small melanosome complexes. Such an aggregation, however, was not seen in skin biopsies treated with UV-A.

In the melanocytes treated with UV-A, UV-B, or UV-A plus 8-MOP, the size of melanosomes appeared to be independent of the type of wavelengths of UV light (i.e. either UV-A or UV-B), although UV-A plus 8-MOP always showed the most obvious increase in the size of the melanosomes. In addition, there was a marked increase in the number of melanosomes transferred from the melanocytes to the keratinocytes. There was an apparent shift in the distribution pattern of melanosomes from the complexed or aggregated form to the single or non-aggregated form. There was also a decrease in the number of the melanosomes in each of the individual melanosome complexes. Such changes in the ratio of single melanosomes to single-plus-complexed melanosomes and in the number of melanosomes per melanosome complex were most prominently seen in the skin treated with UV-A plus 8-MOP (table II).

Discussion

The present study demonstrates that the photobiological processes after a single exposure to UV-A, UV-B, or UV-A plus 8-MOP are different from those occurring after multiple exposures, and that each type of UV irradiation caused, to a certain extent, distinct and specific cellular and subcellular changes in epidermal melanin units (i.e. in melanocytes and in

associated pool of keratinocytes). The increased melanin pigmentation after a single exposure to UV primarily reflected changes in the functional
activity of the melanocytes, whereas multiple exposures stimulated not
only functional activity, but also the numerical changes in the epidermal
melanin units. It also became clear that exposures to UV-A alone can
stimulate new melanogenesis and induce an increase in the number of melanocytes. In addition, 8-MOP in combination with UV-A can significantly enhance the functioning phase of these melanocytes and their numerical increase. UV-A was less erythemogenic and induced less intracellular
degenerative changes. UV-A therefore appeared to be more effective in
the induction of new melanogenesis than was UV-B. It is generally believed that melanogenesis (DT) can be initiated only by the ultraviolet
light of the so-called erythema spectrum (i.e. by UV-B). As early as 1962,
PATHAK et al. [5] showed that irradiation of human skin with longwave ultraviolet (UV-A) and visible light will not only stimulate IT reaction but
also new melanogenesis or DT reaction. Subsequent studies by KLIGMAN
and co-workers [6, 7] reemphasized the profound stimulation of melanin
pigmentation (DT) by UV-A. Thus, the generally held concept of the initiation of melanogenesis (DT) only by UV-B should be modified; long-
wave ultraviolet light (UV-A) must be included in the melanogenic spectrum. It is, however, still not clear whether the high efficiency of UV-A in
the induction of new melanogenesis is related to the high quantum yield
of the wavelengths or simply is due to the fact that the less energy associated with UV-A quanta (about 70–80 kcal/mol) causes less cellular degeneration than does the quanta of UV-B (about 95–100 kcal/mol). Differences in the depth of transmission and absorption of UV-A and UV-B
radiation within epidermis are also important factors in the activation of
epidermal melanocytes. In this study, it was also observed that multiple
repeated exposures to either UV-A, UV-B, or UV-A plus 8-MOP caused
increased melanin pigmentation in which the size of the newly synthesized
melanosomes and the distribution pattern of these melanosomes in the
keratinocytes were similarly altered (i.e. there was an increase in the size
as well as in the number of non-aggregated, single melanosomes in keratinocytes).

Summary

Light and electron microscopic observations on delayed tanning (DT) reactions
induced by single and repeated multiple (6–21 times) exposures to UV-A (320–400

nm), UV-B (290–320 nm), or UV-A in combination with oral 8-methoxypsoralen (8-MOP) were examined *in vivo* in human skin. A single exposure to either UV-A, UV-B, or UV-A plus 8-MOP did not reveal any change in the number of functional melanocytes, but did cause an increase in the synthesis, melanization, and transfer of melanosomes without any noticeable change in the size of melanosomes. Multiple exposures to either UV-A, UV-B or UV-A plus 8-MOP caused a marked increase in the number of the melanocytes, the number of melanosomes synthesized, the degree of melanization, and the number of melanosomes transferred to keratinocytes. Differences in the visual and macroscopic degree of melanin pigmentation induced by UV-A, UV-B, or UV-A plus 8-MOP were primarily related to differences in the rate of synthesis, melanization, and transfer of melanosomes, and not to any significant alterations in the size and distribution pattern of the melanosomes. UV-A irradiation did indeed stimulate new melanogenesis and appears to be more effective for induction of DT than is UV-B irradiation. DT stimulated by multiple exposures to UV-B, and UV-A plus 8-MOP resulted in some alterations in the size of melanosomes and in the distribution pattern of melanosomes in keratinocytes.

References

1   QUEVEDO, W. C., jr.; FITZPATRICK, T. B.; PATHAK, M. A., and JIMBOW, K.: Light and skin color; in PATHAK *et al.* Sunlight and man, pp. 194–216 (University of Tokyo Press, Tokyo 1974).
2   JIMBOW, K.; PATHAK, M. A., and FITZPATRICK, T. B.: Effect of UV on the distribution pattern of microfilaments and microtubules and on the nucleus in human melanocytes. Yale J. Biol. Med. *46:* 411–426 (1973).
3   STARICCO, R. J. and PINKUS, H.: Quantitative and qualitative data on the pigment cells of adult human epidermis. J. invest. Derm. *28:* 33–45 (1957).
4   KARNOVSKY, M. J.: Formaldehyde-glutaraldehyde fixation of high osmolarity for use in electron microscopy. J. Cell Biol. *27:* 137a (1965).
5   PATHAK, M. A.; RILEY, A. C.; FITZPATRICK, T. B., and CURWEN, W. L.: Melanin formation in human skin induced by long wave ultraviolet and visible light. Nature, Lond. *193:* 148 (1962).
6   LANGER, A. and KLIGMAN, A. M.: Tanning without sunburn with aminobenzoic acid-type sunscreen. Archs Derm. *106:* 338 (1972).
7   KAIDBEY, K. H. and KLIGMAN, A. M.: Photopigmentation with trioxsalen. Archs Derm. *109:* 674–677 (1974).

Dr. M. A. PATHAK, Department of Dermatology, Massachusetts General Hospital at Harvard Medical School, *Boston, MA 02114* (USA)

Pigment Cell, vol. 3, pp. 299–310 (Karger, Basel 1976)

The Effect of X-Irradiation on the
Dormant (Amelanotic) Melanocytes of the Hair Germ[1]

A. F. SILVER, H. B. CHASE and C. S. POTTEN

Division of Biological and Medical Sciences, Brown University, Department of Biology, Rhode Island College, Providence, R. I., and Christie Hospital, Holt Radium Institute, Manchester

Introduction

It has been known for about 50 years that radiation may produce loss of pigment of hairs [2]. More recently, CHASE [1] showed that the maximum depigmentation effect results when hair follicles are irradiated during the resting stage of the hair cycle. Follicles so treated will produce a new grey or white hair in every cycle thereafter. In 1970, POTTEN and CHASE [4] presented limited histological evidence of an absence of melanocytes in mid to late anagen follicles after irradiation during the resting stage. The precise fate of the dormant amelanotic melanocytes of the telogen hair germ after irradiation was not determined. It is our purpose in this report to elucidate that fate.

The resting (telogen) hair germ contains precursor cells to all the cell types found in the late anagen (active stage) hair bulb; sheath cells, keratinocytes, medullary cells, and melanocytes [5]. The melanocyte precursor cell may justifiably be styled a melanoblast. It is a small amelanotic cell, with a smooth rounded outline, scanty basophobic cytoplasm, and a few rudimentary dendrites [8]. It is situated low in the hair germ, maintaining contact with the basement membrane between germ and dermal papilla [8]. During telogen, the melanoblasts are dormant, in that they do not divide, or produce pigment, or synthesize nucleic acids [6]. In telogen, they are only partially differentiated, and they become fully differentiated only after being activated.

Activation occurs periodically as the hair follicles alternate between telogen and anagen (when a new hair is formed). All the cells in the hair

1   Acknowledgement of support, PHS RR-07085-08 sub. No. 22.

germ, initially after activation, proceed to synthesize RNA, then DNA and then they divide. Thus, they enter the 'cell cycle' at stage G1. During the subsequent 19 days (in the case of the dorsum of the mouse) they continue to divide and differentiate, and they create a new hair. Following anagen, the follicle goes through a brief stage (catagen) where resorption of external sheath tissue by lysosomes and macrophages occurs [3].

Activation is commonly brought about experimentally by plucking telogen (club) hairs.

The follicles of the mouse dorsum are normally in telogen between approximately 60 and 95 days of age, between the second and third spontaneous cycles of activity [7].

Material and Methods

Mice (DBA and C57 black) were irradiated at a distance of 38 cm over a period of 4 min, with a total dose of 950 r. This dose is lower than that which produces epilation for resting follicles [1]. A Picker 280 kV therapy machine was used, with HVL of 2.7 mm³. The area irradiated was dorsal skin, 9×5 mm, using a thick lead shield with the appropriate area cutout. The mice were anesthetized with Nembutal (95 mg/kg) during irradiation.

Skin samples were prepared as for EM, the technique described by SILVER et al. [8]. Thick-thin epon sections were routinely cut serially, and mounted in 10 groups of 5, on single microscope slides to facilitate serial examination.

Experimental Procedures

Three procedures were used, permitting observation of hair germs in various conditions relative to both the hair cycle and the time of X-ray. In all cases, irradiation was carried out on telogen skin.

A. In procedure 1, we studied the effect of X-rays on the melanocytes of anagen and telogen follicles, one hair cycle removed from the time of irradiation. The entire dorsum of 28 male DBA mice (aged 60–70 days) was plucked, and one side was irradiated. The animals were permitted to complete the experimentally initiated cycle, so that the new white hairs on the irradiated side could be seen. Ten of the mice were then sacrificed, 38–40 days after X-irradiation, in order to examine telogen germs. It was necessary to wait that long, since preliminary experiments showed a delay in the cycle of irradiated animals. The remaining 18 mice were then plucked again, and were sacrificed on days 1, 2, 4, 6, and 10 after the final plucking, in order to examine anagen follicles. Each side of the dorsal skin was treated separately, the unirradiated side serving as control for the X-rayed side.

B. In procedure 2, we studied the effect of X-irradiation during telogen on the

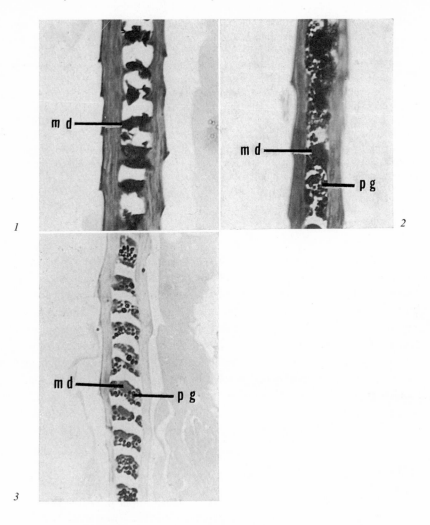

Fig. 1. White hair of DBA mouse which had been irradiated during telogen preceding the cycle which produced this hair. Abbreviations for figures 1–22: c = club hair ending; dp = dermal papilla; e = extension of dermal papilla; g = germ; ga = germ area; md = medullary cell; pg = pigment granules. Magnification as in figure 19.

Fig. 2. Control hair of DBA mouse. Magnification as in figure 19.

Fig. 3. Control hair of C57 black mouse. Magnification as in figure 19.

melanocytes of anagen follicles during the cycle immediately following X-ray. Twelve C57 black mice were plucked and irradiated on day 0, at 60–70 days of age. Two mice were sacrificed at each of the following times thereafter: 18 h, and 2, 4, 10, and 20 days. Controls consisted of 12 C57 black mice which were plucked but not irradiated; and sacrificed after the same time intervals.

C. In procedure 3, we studied specifically the extended effect of X-irradiation on the dormant melanoblasts of telogen follicles. The follicles were not activated. Twelve C57 black mice, aged 60–65 days, were irradiated, and then the hair of the exposed area was gently cut short for later identification. The animals were sacrificed at the following times after X-irradiation: 6 h, 18 h, and 2, 4, 10, and 20 days. Controls consisted of 20 C57 black mice aged 60–90 days, whose dorsal follicles were in telogen, and to whom nothing was done before sacrifice.

Results

A. In the case of the cycle once removed from the time of X-raying (procedure 1), the hairs were white to begin with. Figure 1 (cf. fig. 2 and 3) shows the irradiated hair shaft to be normally organized, except for the absence of pigment granules in the medullary cells. The telogen germs (one cycle removed from X-ray) showed no melanoblasts as compared to controls (fig. 4, 5). During the subsequently initiated cycle, follicles showed a general absence of melanoblasts in the early stages of anagen (fig. 6–9), and of melanocytes in mid to late anagen (fig. 10–13). Occasionally, there was a single abnormal melanocyte with reduced dendrites and sparse pigment in an anagen follicle which would normally have many melanocytes with elaborate dendrites and pigmentation (fig. 10, 11).

Fig. 4. Germ area of telogen DBA follicle, which had been irradiated during the preceding telogen period.

Fig. 5. Germ area of control telogen DBA follicle from the unirradiated side of same mouse as in figure 4. Arrow points to amelanotic melanocyte. Magnification as in figure 4.

Fig. 6. Germ area of DBA follicle 1 day after plucking. Follicle was irradiated during telogen preceding the cycle before this one. Magnification as in figure 4.

Fig. 7. Germ area of control DBA follicle 1 day after plucking. Arrow points to amelanotic melanocyte. Magnification as in figure 4.

Fig. 8. Lower portion of DBA follicle 4 days after plucking. Follicle was irradiated during telogen preceding the cycle before this one.

Fig. 9. Lower portion of control DBA follicle, 4 days after plucking, for the unirradiated side of same mouse as in figure 8. Arrow points to one of several amelanotic melanocytes, which alternate with the darkly staining medullary cells. Magnification as in figure 8.

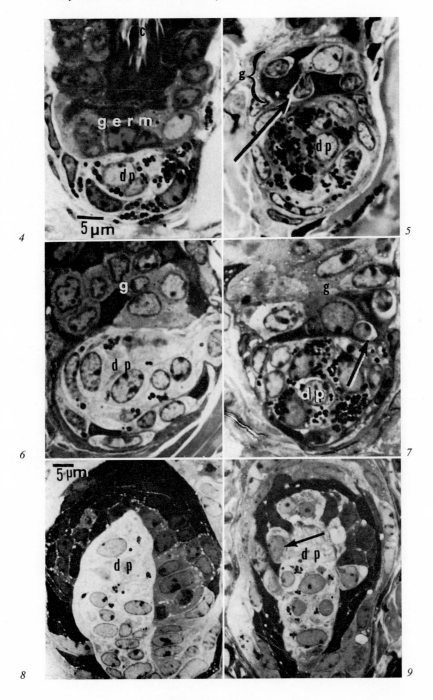

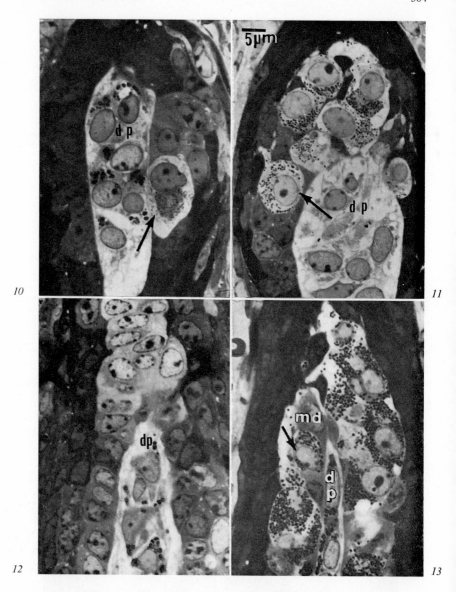

Fig. 10. Lower portion (core of anagen bulb) of DBA follicle 6 days after plucking. Follicle was irradiated during telogen preceding the cycle before this one. Arrow points to the single melanocyte present in the entire follicle. The nucleus is deformed, and dendrites are lacking. Some pigment is nevertheless beginning to be deposited. Magnification as in figure 11.

Table I. Effect of X-ray (950 r) on dormant C57 BL mouse melanoblasts. Tally of 8 telogen germs of 7 mice serially examined

Tissue type (procedure)	Tissue No.	Follicle No.	Total number of germ sections	Est. number of germ cells	Total pyknotic[a] mel'bl[b]	Total normal mel'bl[b]
Control, telogen	CT 114	slide D1 fol. 1 post.	18	48	–	3
Control, telogen	CT 62C	slide K3 fol. 2 ant.	18	36	–	1
18 h after X-ray and plucking (before mitosis)	XP 18 h a	slides H_1, H_2 fol. 1 ant.	21	54	2	–
18 h after X-ray and plucking (before mitosis)	XP 18 h a	slides H_1, H_2 fol. 2 ant.	29	60	2	–
10 days after X-ray (no plucking)	XT 10b	slide P_5 fol. 1 post.	15	28	–	2
20 days after X-ray (no plucking)	XT 20a	slide A2 fol. 1 post.	17	30	2	1
20 days after X-ray (no plucking)	XT 20b	slide L4 fol. 2 ant.	15	33	2	–
20 days after X-ray (no plucking)	XT 20d	slide A2 fol. 1 post.	17	30	2	1
			ε	319	18	

[a] Or otherwise abnormal; [b] melanoblasts.

Fig. 11. Lower portion (core of anagen bulb) of control DBA follicle, 6 days after plucking, from the unirradiated side of same mouse as in figure 10. Arrow points to one of several melanocytes, which are now producing pigment.

Fig. 12. Upper core of anagen bulb of DBA follicle, 10 days after plucking. Follicle was irradiated during telogen preceding the cycle before this one. Magnification as in figure 11.

Fig. 13. Upper core of anagen bulb of control DBA follicle, 10 days after plucking. Arrow points to one of many melanocytes, which are now filled with large melanosomes. Magnification as in figure 11.

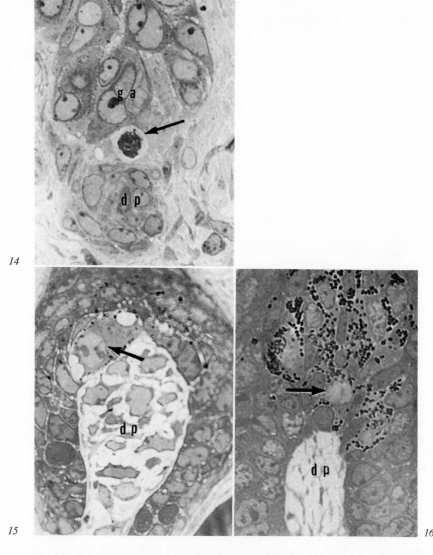

14

15

16

Fig. 14. Germ area of C57 black follicle which had been irradiated and plucked 4 days previously. The follicle is delayed morphogenetically, since the germ area should normally have grown down over the dermal papilla by 4 days after plucking, as in figures 8 and 9. Arrow points to the pyknotic nucleus of an amelanotic melanocyte. Magnification as in figure 19.

Fig. 15. Upper core of anagen bulb of C57 black follicle which had been irradiated and plucked 10 days previously. Arrow points to single melanocyte which ap-

B. In the case of the cycle directly subsequent to X-irradiation (procedure 2) many melanoblasts exhibited varying degrees of autolysis consisting of chromatin clumping, nuclear pyknosis and cell fragmentation, by 18–48 h after irradiation. Later anagen stages were often delayed, and very few normal melanocytes were present (fig. 14–16).

C. In the case of telogen melanoblasts which remained dormant after irradiation (procedure 3), radiation injury was detected 18–24 h after X-ray, and was obvious by 2 days (fig. 17, 18). As late as 20 days after irradiation, many melanoblasts of telogen germs exhibited abnormalities (fig. 19, 20).

D. Miscellaneous findings: (1) Not all the dormant melanoblasts were affected by irradiation. A small proportion appeared to be unchanged. (2) Other follicle cells were occasionally found to be pyknotic after irradiation. This was relatively rare. (3) Serial examination of telogen germs showed that the average germ of small follicles contains approximately 40 cells, of which less than 10% are melanoblasts. Table I gives the data for several C57 black hair germs, both control and irradiated. There are 2–3 melanoblasts in C57 black telogen germs, and 1–2 in the case of DBA germs. (4) Delay in the anagen schedule was seen in many irradiated follicles. (5) Anagen follicles of previously irradiated skin were, on the whole, properly organized, and produced a hair likewise relatively normal except for the lack of melanin (fig. 1, 2). (6) Catagen follicles, obtained in a few cases, showed an easily recognizable germ closely associated with the dermal papilla, in both control and experimental animals. Amelanotic melanocytes were present in the catagen germ of control follicles, but were absent in the case of irradiated follicles in catagen (fig. 21, 22).

Discussion

Less than 10% of the telogen hair germ cells are melanoblasts. If all hair germ cells were equally sensitive to X-ray, and all the cells subject to random hits, then less than 10% of the germs would produce white hairs.

---

pears to have slipped into dermal papilla, and has reduced dendrites. Very few melanosomes are present (cf. fig. 16). Magnification as in figure 19.

Fig. 16. Upper core of anagen bulb of control C57 black follicle 10 days after plucking. Arrow points to one of many dendritic melanocytes filled with melanosomes. Magnification as in figure 19.

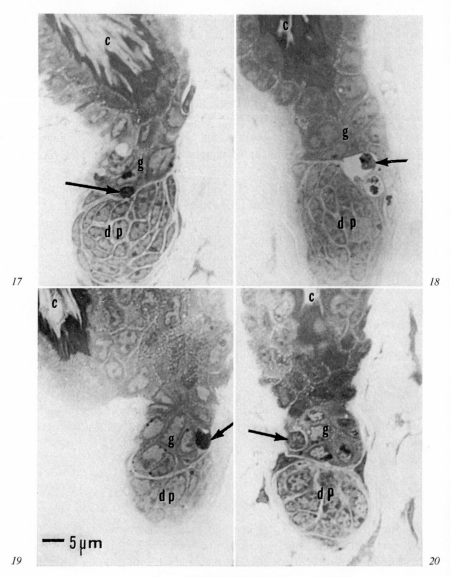

Fig. 17. Germ area of telogen C57 black follicle which had been irradiated 2 days previously. Arrow points to abnormal nucleus of amelanotic melanocyte, which has blebs. Magnification as in figure 19.

Fig. 18. Germ area of telogen C57 black follicle which had been irradiated 2 days previously (a different mouse than that of fig. 17). Arrow points to pyknotic nucleus of amelanotic melanoblast, which seems to be slipping into dermal papilla. Magnification as in figure 19.

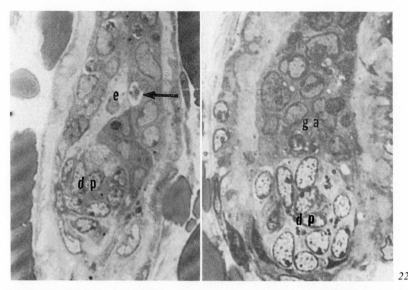

Fig. 21. Lower part of control catagen C57 black follicle, 19 days after pluck-ing. An amelanotic melanocyte (arrow) is situated adjacent to an extension (e) of the dermal papilla. Magnification as in figure 19.

Fig. 22. Lower part of catagen DBA follicle which had been irradiated 28 days previously. Delay in the cycle is evinced, as well as absence of melanocytes. Magni-fication as in figure 19.

This is not the case. CHASE [1] showed by hair counting that 95% of C57 black follicles so irradiated produce grey or white hairs.

Other cell types of the telogen hair germ are almost unaffected by this dosage of X-ray. The hair produced by irradiated follicles is relatively normal except for the absence of melanin. Thus, there seems to be no doubt that dormant melanocytes are exceptionally sensitive to X-ray.

This sensitivity has nothing to do with the general sensitivity dis-played by dividing cells, since the telogen melanoblasts are in G_0 of the cell cycle. Perhaps there is some connection between this unique sensitivi-ty to X-ray and the unique relationship of pigment cells in general to elec-tro-magnetic vibrations.

Fig. 19. Germ area of telogen C57 black follicle which had been irradiated 20 days previously. Arrow points to abnormal nucleus of amelanotic melanoblast.

Fig. 20. Germ area of control telogen C57 black follicle showing amelanotic melanocyte (arrow). Magnification as in figure 19.

Summary

It is known that a light dose of X-ray (950 r), less than the epilation dose, administered to murine telogen hair germs, produces a greyed or white hair in 95% of follicles during the next and subsequent hair cycles. Histological serial examination of epon thick-thin sections demonstrates that the dormant amelanotic melanoblasts which make up less than 10% of the hair germ cell population, and which are the progenitors of the pigmented anagen melanocytes, are unusually sensitive to X-irradiation. By 2 days after X-ray, many melanoblasts show signs of autolysis. If the irradiated telogen germs are plucked to initiate anagen, few or no pigmented melanocytes are seen in the mid – to late anagen follicles, thus accounting for the white hairs. If telogen germs are left undisturbed after irradiation, they may continue to show abnormal melanoblasts as late as 20 days after X-ray.

References

1 CHASE, H. B.: Greying of hair. I. Effects produced by single doses of X-rays on mice. J. Morph. 84: 57–80 (1949).

2 COOLIDGE, W. D.: High voltage cathode rays outside the generating tube. Science 62: 441–442 (1925).

3 PARAKKAL, P. F.: Morphogenesis of the hair follicle during catagen. Z. Zellforsch. 107: 174–186 (1970).

4 POTTEN, C. S. and CHASE, H. B.: Radiation depigmentation of mouse hair; Split dose experiments and melanocyte precursors (amelanotic melanoblasts) in the resting hair follicle. Radiat. Res. 42: 305–319 (1970).

5 SILVER, A. F. and CHASE, H. B.: DNA synthesis in the adult hair germ during dormancy (telogen) and activation (early anagen). Devl Biol. 21: 440–451 (1970).

6 SILVER, A. F. and CHASE, H. B.: Melanocyte precursor cells in the adult hair follicle: Activation and nucleic acid synthesis (abstr.). Yale J. Biol. Med. 46: 716 (1973).

7 SILVER, A. F.; CHASE, H. B., and ARSENAULT, C. T.: Early anagen initiated by plucking compared with early spontaneous anagen; in MONTAGNA and DOBSON Advances in Biology of Skin. Hair Growth, vol. 9, pp. 265–286 (Pergamon Press, Oxford 1969).

8 SILVER, A. F.; CHASE, H. B., and POTTEN, C. S.: Melanocyte precurser cells in the hair follicle germ during the dormant stage (telogen). Experientia 25: 299–301 (1969).

Dr. A. F. SILVER, Division of Biological and Medical Sciences, Brown University, Department of Biology, Rhode Island College, Providence, RI 02912 (USA)

Pigment Cell, vol. 3, pp. 311–321 (Karger, Basel 1976)

Light-Sensitive Pigment Cells of the Sea Urchin
Centrostephanus longispinus

W. Weber and M. Dambach

Zoological Institute, University of Cologne, Department of Animal Physiology, Cologne

Introduction

Physiological color change in vertebrate and invertebrate species is generally understood as a rapid reaction of the chromatophore system to various environmental and endogeneous stimuli. Hereby, the chromatic reaction is achieved by intracellular displacement (aggregation or dispersion) of pigment granules within a cell of relatively fixed outline. With respect to the extracellular regulative mechanisms two modes of action can be distinguished: (1) The indirect response to light, mediated through light receptors, which on their part trigger a nervous and/or hormonal action on the effector system. This 'background' or *secondary color response* is most widespread among fishes, amphibians, reptiles and crustaceans [3]. (2) The other system – considered to be more ancient from the evolutionary point of view – is characterized by a direct action of light on the chromatophore, which in this case acts as a stimulus-response system [4]. Known as the *primary color response* it has been shown to occur among others in larval stages of *Xenopus* [2], in isolated skin pieces of the frog *Rana esculenta* [22] and of the lizard *Anolis* [9]. It also occurs in adult forms, but may be masked by the more effective secondary response.

The phenomenon discussed in this paper is closely related to the 'primary color response' and was first observed by von Uexküll [15] and later elaborated by Kleinholz [10], Yoshida [19] and Millott [12]. It was conclusively shown that in several *diadematid sea urchins,* color change depends not on background illumination, but on the *incident light* [5, 6].

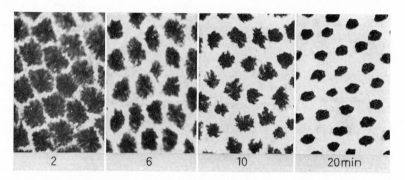

Fig. 1. Chromatophores from skin pieces after dark adaptation.

Since no further information on the morphology and physiology was available, we have focused our attention during recent years on the diadematid *Centrostephanus longispinus*, which is found primarily on the shores of the Bay of Naples.

This paper will present some new details about the structure of the pigment cells and their reaction to light on the cellular level.

Phenomenology

When stimulated with white light for about 45 min, *Centrostephanus longispinus* appears dark brown or black; the chromatophores in the integument disperse their pigment. In complete darkness, the integument of the animal turns pale within 30 min as the pigment aggregates to small dark dots measuring about 30 μm in diameter. As shown in a series of micrographs taken from skin pieces (fig. 1), a successive aggregation of the chromatophores can be observed with the onset of darkness. Under conditions of a constant weak light (e.g. 0.4–53 lx) the chromatophores are arrested in an intermediate state, and the degree of pigment dispersion is proportional to light intensity [6].

In contrast to most other cells involved in color change, *Centrostephanus* chromatophores have ameboid properties; they change shape in response to illumination or darkness [16]. The ameboid activity of the cell is facilitated by the relatively simple structure of the epithelium (fig. 2). The latter consists mainly of a unicellular layer of supporting cells, whose slender processes reach down to the basement lamella. A thin nerve plex-

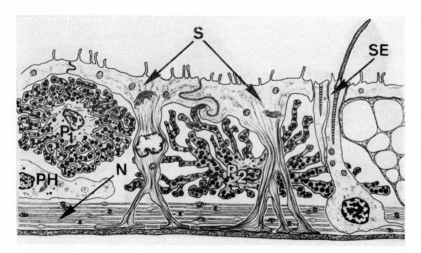

Fig. 2. Schematic drawing of the epithelium of *Centrostephanus longispinus*. S = Supporting cell; Se = sensory cell; Np = nerve plexus; Ph = phagocyte; P_1 = aggregated pigment cell; P_2 = dispersed pigment cell.

us consisting of very fine fibers spreads out in close proximity to the basement lamina. Epithelial cells intermingled with ciliated sensory cells leave an extensive intercellular space, which is occupied by pigment cells and phagocytes. Neither cell type has permanent contact with the surrounding tissue, but simply 'floats' in the intercellular fluid. Dispersion is attained by extending pigmented cell branches between the neighboring cells. The mean diameter of a fully dispersed pigment cell is about 3–4 times that of an aggregated cell.

Reaction to Cytochalasin B

One of the questions arising from the light-induced motor response of the cell concerns the ultrastructural correlates of motility. As revealed by electron microscopy, microtubules and filamentous structures are present within the chromatophore. We tested the possible role of the latter in chromatophore motility by treating with the drug Cytochalasin B (stock solution: 1 mg CB dissolved in 1 ml DMSO; final concentration: 10 μg CB/ml sea water) [7], which is known to interfere with contractile mechanisms based on cytofilaments [18].

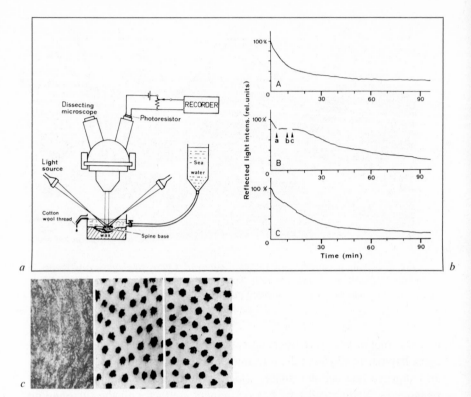

Fig. 3. Reaction to CB. (a) Diagrammatic representation of the set-up used for light stimulation and photometric recording. (b) Continuous recordings of pigment dispersion reactions elicited by illumination. (c) Chromatophore states on spine bases after dark adaptation. With CB (left); with sea water and DMSO (middle); with sea water (right). For explanations, see text.

The experimental set-up is shown in figure 3a. A dark-adapted spine base was placed in a small bowl filled with sea water, which could be replaced by sea water containing CB. For continuous recording of the light reflected from the chromatophore layer, a photoresistor was mounted on one eyepiece of a dissecting microscope and coupled to a chart recorder.

Figure 3b shows the time course of pigment dispersion in the presence and absence of CB. In A, the normal reaction curve is demonstrated. Starting with a reflected light intensity of 100% relative units, we observe the normal decrease in the intensity of the reflected light from the skin piece as it darkens. The decrease is exponential with time and reaches a plateau after 50 min. The second recording (B) – taken from

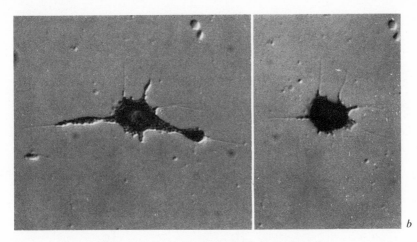

Fig. 4. Isolated pigment cell: (a) light-adapted; (b) dark-adapted.

the same skin piece after readaptation to the dark – again shows a normal decrease in reflectance for the first phase of illumination. At 'a' normal sea water was quickly replaced by sea water with CB. The flattening of the curve indicates a halt in pigment dispersion for the duration of CB treatment. After 7 min, the drug solution was washed out with sea water ('b'); pigment dispersion as measured by the intensity of the reflected light then continues ('c'). Curve C demonstrates a nearly complete recovery of the reaction.

Inhibition of pigment concentration by CB can also be shown: 3 spine bases were exposed to light until the chromatophores were fully dispersed. One piece was then exposed to CB plus DMSO in sea water, the second with DMSO in sea water and the control in sea water alone. After 10 min more of light, all three objects were brought into darkness for 40 min in order to induce pigment concentration. As demonstrated in figure 3c, CB completely arrested the chromatophores in the dispersed state, whereas the chromatophores of DMSO specimens showed the same degree of pigment concentration as the untreated sea water control.

Reaction of Isolated Pigment Cells

Within the cellular structure of the epithelium, dispersion and aggregation of the pigment might theoretically be influenced by humoral fac-

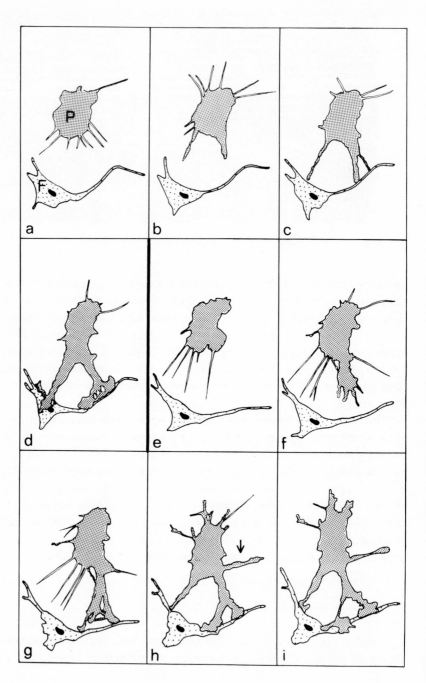

tors emerging from the underlying nerve plexus or from the intercellular fluid. In order to test their endogeneous properties, pigment cells were isolated, transferred into fresh sea water, and observed microscopically under different conditions of illumination.

Figure 4a shows an isolated pigment cell in the light-adapted state. From the vicinity of the cell body, pigmented cell branches, which change into extremely thin filopodia, radiate centrifugally. They give the cell an irregular stellate appearance. Subjected to darkness for 20 min (fig. 4b), the cell has retracted almost all of its pigment branches. The remaining filopodia will also be drawn in, if darkness continues.

As interpretation of cell motility cannot be based only on a series of static pictures gained from light and electron microscopy, time-lapse cine-matography – taken at 1-sec intervals – was performed on isolated pig-ment cells during light adaptation after a previous dark phase. Figure 5 shows tracings of projected frames from a movie of an isolated pigment cell and a fibroblast. 20 sec after the onset of illumination a number of unpigmented filopodia, measuring less than $0.5 \mu m$ in diameter, can be seen extending from the pigmented cell body (a). The formation of these protuberances proceeds very rapidly within a few seconds, as if under considerable pressure. Under continued illumination (b), the filopodia elongate slowly and simultaneously a centrifugal immigration of pigment granules into the filopodia takes place. The evaluation of consecutive frames shows that the pigment migration is discontinuous, in the sense that single pigment granules travelling in a centrifugal direction may re-verse and go centripetally for a few seconds. With continued illumination, the pigment-filled processes increase in length and diameter. After they have established contact with the fibroblast (c), they spread out further on the substratum (d). Figure 5e shows the same pigment cell illuminated for 20 sec after a previous dark adaptation. It has rounded up during the dark phase and again, after the outgrowth of filopodia, the cell flattens by a centrifugal migration of pigmented processes (f). Finally, the mass movement comes to a halt after the cell branches have anchored at the fi-broblast. Between figures 5g and h the whole cell body has been drawn in

---

Fig. 5. Tracings of projected frames from 16-mm movie of isolated pigment cell (P) and fibroblast (F): (a) 20 sec after onset of illumination; (b) 5 min, 50 sec; (c) 7 min, 50 sec; (d) 18 min, 50 sec; (e) 20 sec after onset of illumination (after pre-vious dark adaptation for 6 min); (f) 3 min, 30 sec; (g) 6 min; (h) 14 min; (i) 19 min (see text).

the direction of the arrow. Either under a coverglass or in a Petri dish, the cell can be repeatedly induced to change shape by altering illumination.

Discussion

In recent literature, the phenomenon of the 'primary color response' has been described in a number of invertebrate and vertebrate species. In these examples however, pigment movement takes place within cells of fixed shape. The results of the present experiments demonstrate a 'primary response' of pigment cells, which are exceptional both in their *intrinsic photosensitivity* and in their *motility*. As hormonal and nervous influences can be ruled out, the isolated unicellular system provides a fascinating model for studying the basic sensory mechanisms and transformation of intracellular excitation into a motor response [17]. The problems involved are complex and only partially understood.

Looking for a functional interpretation of this specific color-change mechanism, one should keep in mind that the pigment cells lie just above the supraepithelial nerve plexus, which is a part of the light-sensitive ecto-neural nervous system [21]. Therefore, the pigmentary system may act as a *protective screen*, keeping basic nervous activity on a constant level by light-induced graded chromatophore responses [6].

It is tempting to suggest that the naphthoquinone pigment, which has been shown to be widely distributed in *Diadema antillarum* [13], may be involved in photoreception. This pigment shows an absorption maximum at 463 nm, which is very close to the maximum sensitivity of the chromatophores at 470 nm [20]. However, given the probable mechanism of sensory transduction in other photoreceptors, we would favor the speculative idea of a photopigment (carotenoid?) bound to the plasmalemma, which on illumination triggers a photomechanical transduction process by means of permeability changes.

The ameboid property of the cell raises the basic question of the location of the contractile apparatus necessary for movement, the nature of which is still explained by the controversial theories of hydraulic pressure flow [11] and the front zone contraction [1]. It seems difficult to explain the motility of our chromatophores on the basis of one of these theories alone. As in all motile systems, cytoplasmic filaments constitute the structural correlates for motility in these pigment cells. The reversible inhibition of aggregation as well as dispersion by the drug CB strongly supports this view [7]. It is conceivable that a pressure gradient exerted by concentration of a filamentous network within the center of the cell causes a centrifugal cytoplasmic flow in dispersing chromatophores. As revealed by time-lapse cinematography, the direction of pigment granule movement is not continuous, but is often interrupted and even reversed. It resembles a 'shuttling' motion, which has also been observed in fish chromatophores [8, 14]. For the reverse reaction, pigment aggregation and retraction of cell processes, one might expect a contraction of a filament system, which inserts at the cell membrane. Special attention should also be given to the filopodia, which are extruded from the cell body immediately after illumination begins. They are comparable in size with microspikes found in cultured nerve cells. From the functional point of view, one gains the impression that, once they have contacted a neighboring cell, they serve as 'anchors' for centrifugal pigment movement. It is evident from our cinematographic observation, that from these adhesion points a force is exerted, which pulls the cell in a definite direction. Therefore, the motility of the chromatophore might possibly be attained by the interplay of an *intercellular push-pull mechanism*.

In this report, only some of the relevant problems could be discussed. Numerous physiological and structural questions, such as spectral sensitivity, sites of photoreception, and the effector system of motility, open a wide field for further research on this intriguing little object.

Summary

The chromatophores of the diadematid sea urchin *Centrostephanus longispinus* have ameboid properties and show a 'primary color response'. On illumination, a successive extension of the pigmented cell processes takes place. Darkness leads to a retraction of the cell branches. The drug Cytochalasin B reversibly inhibits dispersion and aggregation. Pigment cells isolated from the epithelium display light sensitivity in the same manner as in normal tissue. Functional aspects of this stimulus-response system are discussed.

Acknowledgments

These studies were supported by Deutsche Forschungsgemeinschaft (Grant: We 527/2 and 527/3).

We thank Miss M. E. GROSMANN and Mrs. A. DAMBACH for their skillful technical assistance. We are also indebted to Prof. Dr. P. SCHROEDER for correction of the English manuscript.

References

1   ALLEN. R. D.: A new theory of ameboid movement and protoplasmic streaming. Expl Cell Res., suppl. *8:* 17–31 (1961).

2   BAGNARA, J. T.: Control of melanophores in amphibians; in DELLA PORTA and MÜHLBOCK Structure and control of the melanocyte. 6th Int. Pigment Cell Conf., pp. 16–28 (Springer, Berlin 1966).

3   BAGNARA, J. T. and HADLEY, M. E.: Chromatophores and color change. The comparative physiology of animal pigmentation (Prentice-Hall, New Jersey 1973).

4   BURGERS, A. C. J.: Biological aspects of pigment cell research; in DELLA PORTA and MÜHLBOCK Structure and control of the melanocyte. 6th Int. Pigment Cell Conf. (Springer, Berlin 1966).

5   DAMBACH, M.: Die Reaktion der Chromatophoren des Seeigels *Centrostephanus longispinus* auf Licht. Z. vergl. Physiol. *64:* 400–406 (1969).

6   DAMBACH, M. und JOCHUM, F.: Zum Verlauf der Pigmentausbreitung beim Farbwechsel des Seeigels *Centrostephanus longispinus Peters.* Z. vergl. Physiol. *59:* 403–412 (1968).

7   DAMBACH, M. and WEBER, W.: Inhibition of pigment movement by cytochalasin B in the chromatophores of the sea urchin *Centrostephanus longispinus.* Comp. Biochem. Physiol. *50A:* 49–52 (1975).

8   GREEN, L.: Mechanism of movements of granules in melanocytes of *Fundulus heteroclitus.* Proc. natn. Acad. Sci. USA *59:* 1179–1186 (1968).

9   HADLEY, C. E.: Color changes in excised and intact reptilian skin. J. exp. Zool. *58:* 321–331 (1931).

10 KLEINHOLZ, J. H.: Color changes in echinoderms. Publ. Staz. zool. Napoli *17:* 53–57 (1938).

11 MAST, S. O.: Structure, movement, locomotion and stimulation in Amoeba. Z. Morph. *41:* 347–425 (1926).

12 MILLOT, N.: The sensitivity to light, reactions to shading, pigmentation and color changes of the sea urchin, *Diadema antillarum Philippi.* Biol. Bull. mar. biol. Lab. Woods Hole *99:* 329–330 (1950).

13 MILLOT, N. and YOSHIDA, M.: The spectral sensitivity of the echinoid *Diadema antillarum Philippi.* J. exp. Biol. *34:* 394–401 (1957).

14 SCHLIWA, M. and BEREITER-HAHN, J.: Pigment movements in fish melanophores. Morphological and physiological studies. III. The effects of colchicine and vinblastine. Z. Zellforsch. *147:* 127–148 (1973).

15 UEXKÜLL, J. VON: Vergleichende sinnesphysiologische Untersuchungen. III. Der Schatten als Reiz für *Centrostephanus longispinus.* Z. Biol. *34:* 319–339 (1896).

16 WEBER, W. und DAMBACH, M.: Amoeboid bewegliche Pigmentzellen im Epithel des Seeigels *Centrostephanus longispinus.* Ein neuartiger Farbwechselmechanismus. Z. Zellforsch. *133:* 87–102 (1972).

17 WEBER, W. and DAMBACH, M.: Light-sensitivity of isolated pigment cells of the sea urchin *Centrostephanus longispinus.* Cell. Tiss. Res. *148:* 437–440 (1974).

18 WESSELS, N. K.; SPOONER, B. S.; ASH, J. F.; BRADLEY, M. M. O.; LUDUENA, M.

A.; TAYLOR, E. L.; WRENN, J. T., and YAMADA, K. M.: Microfilaments in cellular and developmental processes. Science, Wash. *171:* 135–143 (1971).

19   YOSHIDA, M.: On the response of the chromatophore of the sea urchin, *Diadema setosum* (Leske). J. exp. Biol. *33:* 119–123 (1956).

20   YOSHIDA, M.: Spectral sensitivity of chromatophores in *Diadema setosum* (Leske). J. exp. Biol. *34:* 222–225 (1957).

21   YOSHIDA, M. and MILLOTT, N.: Light-sensitive nerve in an echinoid. Experientia *15:* 13–14 (1959).

22   ZETTNER, A.: Über die Lichtreaktion der Froschhautchromatophoren. Z. Biol. *108:* 210–216 (1956).

Prof. Dr. W. WEBER, Zoological Institute, Department of Animal Physiology, University of Cologne, Weyertal 119, *D–5 Cologne 41* (FRG)

Pigment Cell, vol. 3, pp. 322–335 (Karger, Basel 1976)

Adrenoreceptors of Teleost Melanophores

Barrie C. Finnin, Olga Dudinski and Barry L. Reed

Victorian College of Pharmacy, Parkville, Vic.

In the introduction to a monograph on molecular pharmacology, DE JONGH [2] has suggested that: 'To most modern pharmacologists the receptor is like a beautiful but remote lady. He has written her many a letter and quite often she has answered the letters. From these answers the pharmacologist has built himself an image of this fair lady. He cannot, however, truly claim ever to have seen her, although one day he may do so.'

This paper concerns some of the letters the authors have written this lady, together with an interpretation of her various replies.

Drug receptors are defined by DE JONGH as 'molecules of the organism which are the point of attack of drug molecules'. A great many workers have looked at the effects of drugs on the melanophores of teleost fishes, but very few have sought to characterize the properties of the receptor types of this diverse and highly developed pigment cell.

In previous investigations, the melanophores of the freshwater angelfish *Pterophyllum eimekei* have been shown to be under adrenergic control, and to possess alpha-adrenoreceptors which mediate melanosome aggregation (paling) and beta-adrenoreceptors which mediate melanosome dispersal (darkening) [3, 4, 7–9]. Evidence for the existence of beta-adrenoreceptors was based on the observation that the beta-adrenoreceptor agonists isoprenaline (isoproterenol), orciprenaline and isoxuprine produced pigment dispersal in angelfish melanophores maintained in a state of partial pigment aggregation either by nerve stimulation at low pulse rates or by the injection of melatonin [7, 8]. This report was the first indication of the existence of beta-adrenoreceptors on teleost melanophores [6]. The present paper extends these observations to include the results of experiments with a range of beta-adrenoreceptor agonist and antagonist drugs delivered to melanophores *in vivo* by a subcutaneous injection technique.

In addition, dose response curves for single fish have been determined for epinephrine and norepinephrine, using an exposed melanophore preparation, and the relationship between melanophore response and the concentration of alpha-adrenoreceptor agonist has been investigated.

Materials and Methods

All experiments reported in this paper were performed with wild-type freshwater angelfish *Pterophyllum eimekei,* Ahl, the characteristics of which have been described previously [3]. Melanophore responses were detected and measured photometrically by the transmitted light technique of Finnin and Reed [3]. This technique involves the measurement and continuous recording of light transmitted through pigmented fins or pigmented areas of the body of living spinal-sectioned fishes. The fish were spinal-sectioned in the cervical region and were kept completely immobilized under water on the stage of an inverted microscope. Fluctuations in the amount of light passing through the fish (which directly indicate changes in melanosome dispersion) were recorded continuously on a chart recorder. The melanophores of spinal-sectioned fishes are free from the control of central pigment-aggregating impulses and normally remain in a state of maximal pigment dispersion until stimulated either via sympathetic nerves or by drugs. Stimulation of nerves to melanophores was by square wave pulses delivered to electrodes inserted into the spinal cord immediately posterior to the point of section. The melanophores of the fish could be maintained in any desired state of partial pigment aggregation by the selection of suitable parameters of stimulation [3].

Drugs were administered either by local subcutaneous (s.c.) injection or by direct application to exposed melanophores. Subcutaneous injections were delivered into an area immediately adjacent to the area of melanophores under study. All s.c. injections were given with 5-μl syringes fitted with fixed 32 gauge needles. The dose volume in all cases was 1 μl and the injection vehicle had the following composition: NaCl 7.5 g, KCl 0.19 g, CaCl$_2$ · 2H$_2$O 0.2 g, water to 1 litre.

Drugs injected s.c. act locally on the melanophores of only one side of the fish; the melanophores of the other side are still in the light path, however, and tend to mask the drug-induced responses obtained because they do not receive the drug administered. The sensitivity of the preparation, therefore, could be increased greatly by the removal from the other side of the fish of those scales and melanophores that would otherwise be in the light path. This modification of the original technique was adopted in all experiments where drugs were given by s.c. injection.

In other experiments drugs were administered by direct application to exposed fin melanophores (the 'stripped fin' technique). To achieve this, all structures covering the area of melanophores to be studied were stripped from the fin so as to expose the melanophores to the environment in which the fish were maintained. The fish were kept in an isotonic buffer of the following composition during all stripped fin experiments: NaCl 6.0 g, KCl 0.19 g, $CaCl_2 . 2H_2O$ 0.2 g, Tris(hydroxymethyl) aminomethane 1.92 g, citric acid 1.05 g, water to 1 litre. Melanophores maintained in this solution showed normal responses to drugs and to stimulation of the spinal cord for the duration of all experiments. Melanophore responses were measured for melanophores of the lower surface of the fin only, as the melanophores of the upper surface were removed during the stripping process. Drugs to be administered to the stripped fin preparation were dissolved in the buffer solution in which the fish was immersed. The solution was removed completely with each change of drug, and drug-containing solutions were alternated with drug-free buffer solution to allow the fish to return to a steady baseline prior to subsequent drug exposure. Epithelial cells were found to grow over the exposed melanophores during the course of several hours, and these cells routinely were removed by gentle suction each time the buffer solution was replaced. A constant level device was used to ensure that the dish was filled to the same level each time so that the light path through the solution was of constant length. Full details of this revised technique will be published elsewhere. A minimum of 5 and a maximum of 25 fish were given each dose of each drug or drug combination tested.

Results and Discussion

Each of the beta-adrenoreceptor agonist drugs investigated (isoproterenol, trimetoquinol, orciprenaline, salbutamol and soterenol) was found to produce melanosome dispersal (darkening) within the melanophores of the angelfish.

A tracing of a typical experiment is shown in figure 1. Initially, the fish were subjected to a period of stimulation (square wave pulses 5 V, 20 Hz, 1 msec duration for 20 sec, repeated every 5 min) until the paling response elicited by stimulation became constant. The fish then were stimulated continuously at a low pulse rate (within the range 0.75–2 Hz) so as to maintain the melanophores of the fish in an intermediate state of melanosome aggregation (a stimulation plateau). All drugs given in this series of experiments were administered by s.c. injection to fish maintained on a stimulation plateau. A number of fish showed a drop in the level of the stimulation plateau following s.c. injection of the vehicle (this phenomenon is well demonstrated in fig. 1). This injection artefact was allowed for by injecting test fish with vehicle alone on two occasions prior to the administration of drugs (as shown in fig. 1) and by injecting an equal number of control fish with vehicle alone on 3 occasions. The drop in plateau level (darkening) produced by the injection of beta-agonist was

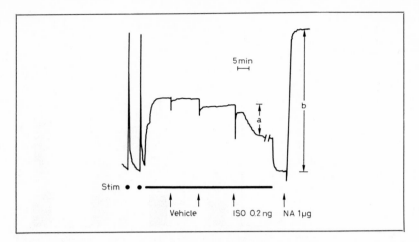

Fig. 1. A trace from a typical experiment showing the effect of a beta-adreno-receptor agonist on melanophores. Fish were stimulated (Stim) at 20 Hz for 20 sec where indicated ●, followed by continuous stimulation at 1.5 Hz ━━━. Fish were injected twice with vehicle alone, with isoproternol (ISO), and with a large dose of norepinephrine (NA), where indicated by the arrows. The darkening response induced by isoproterenol is shown by distance 'a', and the maximal fading response to norepinephrine by distance 'b'.

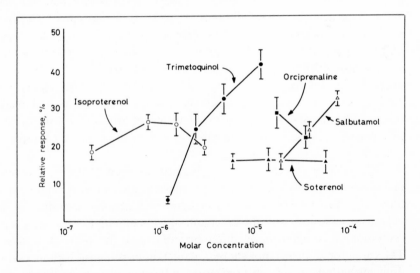

Fig. 2. Relative percent response of angelfish melanophores versus molar concentration (log scale) for 5 beta-agonists. The standard error of the mean for each point is shown (the relative percent response for controls was 6.1±2.2).

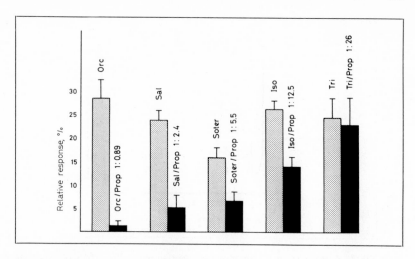

Fig. 3. Blockade by propranolol (Prop) of the response of angelfish melanophores to the beta-agonists orciprenaline (Orc), salbutamol (Sal), soterenol (Soter),
isoproterenol (Iso) and trimetoquinol (Tri). The standard error of the mean is indicated in each case together with the molar ratio of agonist to antagonist used.

taken as the difference between the plateau level before and after the
injection of drug (shown as distance 'a' in fig. 1). Results were expressed
as a 'relative percent response' by expressing the drop in plateau level
('a') as a percentage of a 'maximal fading response' produced by a large
dose of norepinephrine given at the end of each experiment (distance 'b'
in fig. 1), i.e. relative percent response = $(a/b) \times 100$. The relative percent response for each of the beta-agonists investigated was compared
statistically with that of the controls by means of Student's t-test (the relative percent response for controls was 6.1 with a standard error of
± 2.2).

The relative percent response obtained for each of the beta-agonists
investigated compared with the molar concentration of drug administered
(dose volume constant) is shown in figure 2. Each concentration of the
beta-agonists tested, with the exception of trimetoquinol in its lowest concentration, was significantly different from controls ($p < 0.05$, 2-sided).
The curve for isoproterenol shows a reduction in response with increasing
drug concentration; this phenomenon can be explained by an action of isoproterenol on alpha-adrenoreceptors at high doses as observed by Reed
and Finnin [8]. Trimetoquinol and salbutamol both showed an increase

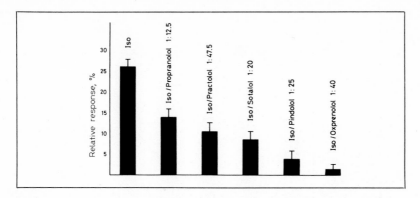

Fig. 4. Blockade of the response of angelfish melanophores to isoproterenol (Iso) produced by 5 beta-adrenoreceptor-blocking drugs. The standard error of the mean is indicated in each case together with the molar ratio of agonist to antagonist used.

in response with increasing concentration, while soterenol and orciprenaline showed non-significant changes in response with increasing concentration in the concentration range investigated.

The capacity of the beta-antagonist drug propranolol to block the melanosome-dispersing action of the beta-agonist drugs investigated was studied by injecting propranolol together with each of the beta-agonists. The results obtained are shown in figure 3. The doses of the beta-agonists were chosen to give approximately the same response (a relative percent response of approximately 25), with the exception of soterenol which could not produce this degree of agonist activity (refer fig. 2).

The molar ratio of propranolol to agonist was selected on the basis of preliminary experiments and was increased until a significant blockade of response was produced. Propranolol produced a significant blockade of response of each of the beta-agonists studied (with the exception of trimetoquinol) in the ratios shown in figure 3. It was not possible to block the response produced by trimetoquinol with propranolol, even in the ratio of 1:26. Control fish maintained on a stimulation plateau showed no significant response to the administration of propranolol alone within the dose range used in these experiments. (Higher doses of propranolol than these produced a rise in the level of the stimulation plateau, presumably because propranolol blocked the intrinsic beta activity of the neurotransmitter at these dose levels.)

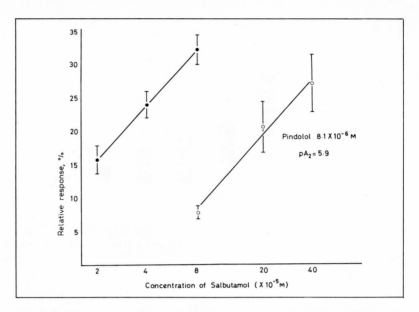

Fig. 5. Relative percent response of angelfish melanophores versus molar concentration of salbutamol (log scale), with (O), and without (●) the beta-antagonist pindolol. Linear regression lines are shown together with the standard error of the mean for each point. The pA₂ value calculated from the displacement of the lines is 5.9.

The beta-adrenoreceptor antagonist drugs propranolol, practolol, sotalol, pindolol, and oxprenolol were tested for their ability to block the melanosome-dispersing response of a fixed dose of isoproterenol (which produced a relative percent response of approximately 25). The results obtained together with the molar ratios used are shown in figure 4. The molar ratios of antagonist to isoproterenol were selected on an arbitrary basis to produce a statistically significant block, no attempt was made to compare the potencies of these compounds. Each of the beta-antagonists tested was capable of producing a highly significant blockade of the beta-agonist activity of isoproterenol ($p < 0.001$, 1-sided).

The effect of the beta-adrenoreceptor antagonist pindolol on the dose response relationship obtained for salbutamol is shown in figure 5. The linear regression lines calculated for the two sets of points are shown, together with the standard error of the mean for each point. The slopes of the two lines do not differ significantly (27.2 for salbutamol alone and

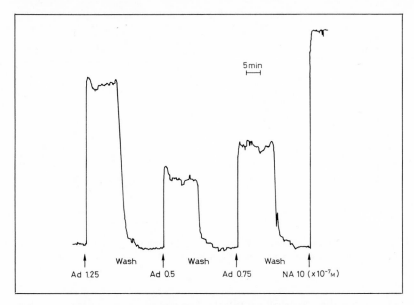

Fig. 6. A tracing of the response shown by the melanophores of an angelfish stripped fin preparation to 3 different concentrations of epinephrine (Ad). The melanophores were exposed to each concentration of epinephrine for about 10 min after which the solution was replaced with buffer alone (wash). A maximal fading response produced by a large dose of norepinephrine (NA) is shown on the right of the trace.

27.9 for salbutamol with pindolol), and the linear regression coefficients for the two lines are 1 and 0.99, respectively. The observation that pindolol causes a parallel displacement of the dose response line for salbutamol indicates that pindolol is acting as a competitive antagonist. For a competitive antagonist, it can be shown that:

$$D'/D = 1 + GK_G,$$

where D' is the concentration of agonist needed to produce the same response in the presence of an antagonist (concentration G) as was produced by the agonist alone at a concentration of D. K_G is the affinity constant for the competitive antagonist. The K_G for pindolol on the angelfish melanophore calculated from the data presented in figure 5 is 7.6×10^5. A scale for comparing the potency of antagonists (pA values) has been devised by SCHILD [10]. The $pA\chi$ value is defined as the negative logarithm (base 10) of the molar concentration of an antagonistic drug which

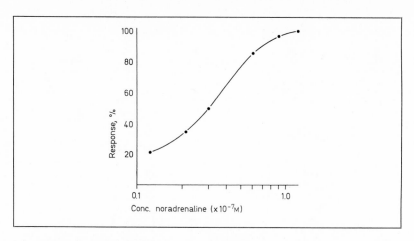

Fig. 7. Percent response of angelfish melanophores versus molar concentration of norepinephrine (noradrenaline) (log scale).

will reduce the effect of a multiple dose (χ) of an active drug to that of a single dose. For example, if the concentration of the antagonist is such that twice the original dose is required to produce the same effect as the original dose given alone, then the pA_2 value is the negative logarithm of this concentration of antagonist. In theory, $pA_2 = \log K_G$ for a competitive antagonist. Since K_G for pindolol on the angelfish melanophore is 7.6×10^5, the $pA_2 = 5.9$. Antagonists with high pA_2 values (e.g. a value of 10) have a high specificity for antagonism, while low pA_2 values (e.g. 4) usually indicate a non-specific antagonism. Before any conclusions can be drawn on the nature of the antagonism in this case, it will be necessary to determine the pA_2 values for pindolol and other antagonists against various agonists in different concentrations. For true competitive antagonism, the pA_2 value will be independent of agonist concentration, and for agonists which act on the same receptor the pA_2 value will be independent of the agonist used. Further, if the antagonism is competitive it can be shown that $pA_2 - pA_{10} = 0.95$; experimental determination of this figure, therefore, would confirm the competitive nature of the antagonism.

The beta-adrenoreceptors of mammals have been classified into 2 subgroups according to the responses of different organs to various beta-adrenoreceptor agonists [5]. The beta-adrenoreceptors of heart and intestinal smooth muscle are of the β^1 type, while those of the smooth mus-

Table I. Comparison of the beta-adrenoreceptors of the angelfish melanophore with some mammalian beta-receptors

	Potency ratios		
	guinea pig heart force	guinea pig trachea	angelfish melanophore
Isoproterenol	1	1	1
Trimetoquinol	>10,000	2	2.5
Orciprenaline	63	144	20
Salbutamol	2,500	5	40
Soterenol	>10,000	5	>20
Range	1–10,000	1–144	1–40

cle of the trachea, for example, are of the β^2 type. More recently, doubt has been thrown on the validity of this classification because of its inflexibility, although there is little doubt that any particular tissue behaves more like some tissues than others in response to a given beta-adrenoreceptor stimulant (see review by BRITTAIN *et al.* [1]). The relative potencies of 5 beta-adrenoreceptor agonists on guinea pig heart force, guinea pig trachea and the angelfish melanophore are shown in table I. (The figures for the guinea pig are taken from BRITTAIN *et al.* [1]). The potency ratios for the angelfish melanophore were determined by expressing the molar concentration of agonist necessary to produce a 25% relative response as a fraction of the molar concentration of isoproterenol necessary to produce the same response. A value of >20 was recorded for soterenol since it did not produce a 25% relative response at any of the concentrations tested. The values recorded in table I indicate that the angelfish melanophore is more like guinea pig trachea than guinea pig heart force in its response to these beta-adrenoreceptor agonists. If the classification of LANDS *et al.* [5] is valid, therefore, the angelfish melanophore appears to possess beta-adrenoreceptors of the β^2 type.

When angelfish melanophores are exposed to solutions containing epinephrine or norepinephrine, using the stripped fin preparation, they respond with melanosome aggregation. For any particular concentration, the melanophores rapidly adopt a corresponding degree of aggregation which is maintained for as long as the melanophores are exposed to the solution. When the drug is washed from the melanophores, they rapidly assume their normal resting state of maximal melanosome dispersal. A tracing of response heights to various concentrations of epinephrine for

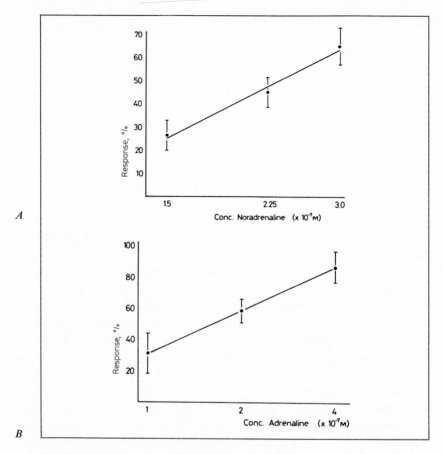

Fig. 8. A Percent response of angelfish melanophores versus molar concentration of norepinephrine (noradrenaline) (log scale) determined for a single fish. The linear regression lines and the 95% confidence limits for each point are shown. *B* Percent response of angelfish melanophores versus molar concentration of epinephrine (adrenaline) (log scale) determined for a single fish. The linear regression lines and the 95% confidence limits for each point are shown.

angelfish melanophores of a stripped fin preparation is shown in figure 6. A maximal reference response produced by a high concentration of norepinephrine is shown on the right of the trace. The melanophores were exposed to the epinephrine-containing solutions for 10 min in each case and were allowed approximately 10 min to return to their resting state between doses. Figure 7 shows a dose/response curve for norepinephrine

Table II. Mean results from linear regression analysis

	Slope[1]	Inter-cept[1]	Concentration ($\times 10^{-7}$ M) for 50% response		r[1]
			mean	range	
Norepinephrine	107 ± 23	93 ± 46	0.61	0.18–2.35	0.99 ± 0.01
Epinephrine	90 ± 20	60 ± 20	0.98	0.41 ± 1.88	0.995 ± 0.005

r = Linear regression correlation coefficient.
1 $\pm 95\%$ confidence limits.

where the percent response of melanophores is plotted versus the molar concentration of norepinephrine (log scale). Percent response in this case refers to the change in absorption of light caused by a particular concentration of drug expressed as a percentage of the maximum possible change in absorption (the response of a very large dose of norepinephrine). There appears to be a sigmoid log dose/response relationship displayed in figure 7, but there are insufficient points in the central portion of the curve to confirm the expected linearity of this region. A similar dose/response relationship was found for epinephrine. To investigate this further, angelfish melanophores in a stripped fin preparation were exposed to 3 different concentrations of catecholamines each on 3 occasions (the order of exposure being based on a latin square arrangement). Concentrations were chosen to produce a response within the range 20–80%. Typical results for experiments designed in this way shown in figure 8. The percent response versus log concentration curve for norepinephrine is shown in figure 8A and the curve for epinephrine in figure 8B. Linear regression lines are shown in each case together with the 95% confidence limits about each point. The results from 6 experiments on each catecholamine are summarized in table II. The average slopes of the linear regression lines for epinephrine and norepinephrine do not differ significantly; any difference in slope that is present, however, makes a comparison of potency between the 2 catecholamines more difficult. As evidenced by the wide 95% confidence limits, the slopes of individual lines for either catecholamine varied widely. Thus, comparisons of potency of agonists and antagonists should be made only on the basis of comparisons performed with the same melanophores (which would be expected to yield lines with the same slope for the two agonists, provided they both act on the same receptors). This is necessary also because individual fish vary widely in sensitivity. The intercepts shown in table II, together with their 95% confidence limits, serve as a rough indication of relative potency; a better indication of potency is obtained from the concentration required to produce a 50% response. The wide range of values obtained for the 2 catecholamines precludes the determination of an exact potency ratio in this study, the potency ratio of norepinephrine to epinephrine, however, appears to be of the order of 1:1.5. The correlation coefficients for the linear regression lines are close to 1 (table II) and have narrow 95% confidence limits which indicates that the points for each line fit a straight line well.

Summary

Experiments with 5 beta-adrenoreceptor agonists and 5 beta-adrenoreceptor blocking drugs on an *in vivo* melanophore preparation have confirmed the existence of beta-adrenoreceptors on the melanophores of the freshwater angelfish *Pterophyllum eimekei*. These beta-adrenoreceptors mediate melanosome dispersal (darkening) in the angelfish and have some of the characteristics of the β^2-adrenoreceptors proposed for higher animals.

Dose/response curves determined for single fish for the alpha-adrenoreceptor agonists epinephrine and norepinephrine show that the melanosome aggregation (paling) induced by these agents is proportional to the logarithm of the concentration exposed to the melanophores.

Acknowledgements

Gratitude is expressed to Dr. RONALD R. NOVALES for his generous assistance in the presentation of this paper.

This investigation was carried out during the tenure of grants from the Australian Research Grants Committee and the Pharmaceutical Society of Victoria, Australia.

References

1   BRITTAIN, R. T.; JACK, D., and RITCHIE, A. C.: Recent β-adrenoreceptor stimulants. Adv. Drug Res. 5: 197–253 (1970).
2   JONGH, D. K. DE: Some introductory remarks on the conception of receptors; in ARIËNS Molecular pharmacology, vol. 1, pp. xiii–xvi (Academic Press, New York 1964).

3 FINNIN, B. C. and REED, B. L.: The continuous recording of melanophore responses in teleost fishes. Life Sci. *9:* 321–333 (1970).

4 FINNIN, B. C. and REED, B. L.: The action of reserpine on teleost melanophores. Eur. J. Pharmacol. *22:* 239–248 (1973).

5 LANDS, A. M.; LUDUENA, F. P., and BUZZO, H. J.: Differentiation of receptors responsive to isoproterenol. Life Sci. *6:* 2241–2249 (1967).

6 NOVALES, R. R.: Discussion. Endocrine regulation of pigmentation. Am. Zool. *13:* 895–897 (1973).

7 REED, B. L. and FINNIN, B. C.: Adrenergic innervation of melanophores in a teleost fish. Proc. 7th Int. Pigment Cell Conf., Washington 1969 (abstr.). J. invest. Derm. *54:* 95–96 (1970).

8 REED, B. L. and FINNIN, B. C.: Adrenergic innervation of melanophores in a teleost fish; in RILEY Pigmentation: its genesis and biologic control, pp. 285–294 (Appleton Century Crofts, New York 1972).

9 REED, B. L. and FINNIN, B. C.: Fish as test animals in pharmacology. Aust. J. Pharm. Sci. *NS3:* 23–25 (1974).

10 SCHILD, H. O.: pA, a new scale for the measurement of drug antagonism. Br. J. Pharmacol. *2:* 189–206 (1947).

Dr. BARRIE C. FINNIN, Victorian College of Pharmacy, 381 Royal Parade, *Parkville, Vic. 3052* (Australia)

Pigment Cell, vol. 3, pp. 336–344 (Karger, Basel 1976)

Beta Adrenoceptors, Cyclic AMP and Melanosome Dispersion in Guppy Melanophores[1]

Ryozo Fujii and Yoko Miyashita[2]

Department of Biology, Sapporo Medical College, Sapporo

Introduction

It is well established that melanophores of fish are primarily controlled by adrenergic melanosome-aggregating nerves [6]. Further, recent studies have shown that the cellular receptors concerned are of alpha-adrenergic nature [5]. It is also known that in many fish species a pituitary principle, possibly a melanophore-stimulating hormone, takes part in dispersing melanosomes, resulting in the gradual darkening of the integument [1]. However, the rapid darkening reactions seen among living animals are not explained by the hormonal mechanism alone.

Using *in vitro* preparations from a popular tropical fish, we have attempted here to characterize the cellular receptors involved in dispersing melanophore inclusions, and have further tried to couple the events at the receptor level with the intracellular mechanical ones. Details of first part of this work appear elsewhere [7].

Material and Methods

Adult female guppies *(Lebistes reticulatus)* were used as the experimental material. Procedures, apparatuses and drugs employed for pharmacological studies on split tail-fin preparations were fundamentally the same as described elsewhere [5]. The drugs were freshly prepared in the physiological solution which had the fol-

1   This work was supported by Grants Nos. 754165 and 854176 from the Ministry of Education of Japan.
2   We thank Mr. H. Tadano for his skilled help in electron microscopy.

lowing composition (mM): NaCl, 128; KCl, 2.7; CaCl$_2$, 1.8; glucose, 5.6; HEPES-NaOH buffer, 5.0 (pH 7.2).

In some experiments, the preparations were irrigated with nucleotide solutions, which were also made up with the physiological saline. The nucleotides used included adenosine 5′-monophosphate (5′-AMP, Nutritional Biochemicals, Cleveland), adenosine 3′-monophosphate (3′-AMP, Nutritional Biochemicals), adenosine 2′-monophosphate (2′-AMP, Sigma Chemical, St. Louis), adenosine 5′-diphosphate, sodium (ADP, P-L Biochemicals, Milwaukee), adenosine 5′-triphosphate, disodium (ATP, Sigma Chemical), guanosine 5′-triphosphate, sodium (GTP, Sigma Chemical), uridine 5′-monophosphate, disodium (UMP, Kohjin, Tokyo), cytidine 5′-monophosphate, disodium (CMP, Kohjin), adenosine 3′,5′-cyclic monophosphate, sodium (cyclic AMP, Sigma Chemical), dibutyryl-adenosine 3′,5′-cyclic monophosphate (P-L Biochemicals) and guanosine 3′,5′-cyclic monophosphate, sodium (cyclic GMP, Kohjin). Their stock solutions were neutralized beforehand with NaOH, when necessary. Other drugs employed were theophylline (Tokyo Chemical Ind., Tokyo) and caffeine (Wako Pure Chemical Ind., Osaka). These methylxanthines were also dissolved in the saline.

For the iontophoretic microinjection of a nucleotide into the melanophore, an inverted microscope was employed in combination with a micromanipulator. The nucleotides tested comprized cyclic AMP, 5′-AMP, ATP and cyclic GMP. Micropipettes containing one of these solutions were prepared according to the method of TSIEN [12] with the slight modifications that 1.0-M solutions were used for adenine nucleotides, and 0.1-M solutions for cyclic GMP, because of its poor solubility. By means of an electronic stimulator (Nihon Kohden, MSE-3), the hyperpolarizing current was applied through a micropipette as 1-sec rectangular pulses at 0.5 Hz. For monitoring the current intensity, a dual beam oscilloscope (Nihon Kohden, VC-7) was put to use. A melanophore was impaled vertically around the center of the cell from the dermal side of a split fin preparation. When the injection was attempted into an aggregated melanophore, the bathing medium had been changed from a normal to an isotonic K-rich saline, in which all Na ions were replaced with K ions.

By using conventional methods, tail-fin pieces were processed for fine structural observations of melanophores. Ultrathin sections were stained with uranyl acetate and lead citrate, and observed in a JEM-100B electron microscope.

Results and Discussion

As expected, nervous stimulation, catecholamines and some related monoamines induced the pigment aggregation in melanophores of the present material. That these effects were mediated through alpha-adrenoceptors has recently been shown in one of our foregoing papers [5]. Whenever one works on fish melanophores, on the other hand, it has been rather difficult to examine an agent as to whether it is melanin-dis-

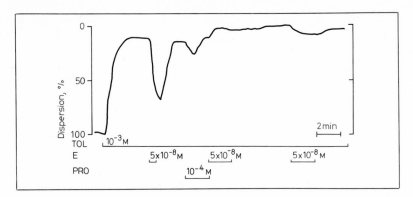

Fig. 1. Typical photoelectric recording of the melanophore response of the guppy, *Lebistes reticulatus,* showing the melanosome-dispersing action of weak epinephrine (E) solution, and the effect of propranolol (PRO) on the former. A 10^{-3}-M tolazoline (TOL) solution was employed to induce melanin aggregation.

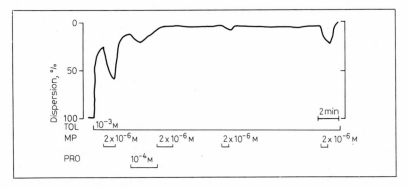

Fig. 2. Typical recording showing the melanosome-dispersing action of a synthetic beta stimulant, metaproterenol (MP), and the effect of propranolol (PRO) on the former. TOL = Tolazoline.

persing or not, since the cells in isolated preparations normally assume dispersed state in physiological solutions. By making use of split fin preparations of guppies, we could mostly overcome these difficulties. In moderately strong solutions (e.g. 10^{-3} M) of tolazoline, an alpha-adrenergic-blocking agent, the melanophore pigment becomes aggregated to a high degree. This may be due to the sympathomimetic action possessed by the blocking agent itself. During this phase, various agents could be examined for their possible dispersing effects.

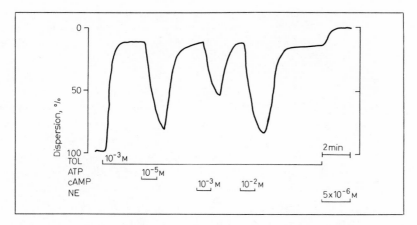

Fig. 3. Typical recording showing the effect of ATP and cyclic AMP (cAMP) on melanophores. TOL = Tolazoline.

First, substances currently suspected or proved to be neurotransmitters in variety of synapses were examined for their effects on aggregated melanophores. They included acetylcholine, 5-hydroxytryptamine, dopamine, histamine, gamma-amino butyric acid, glycine, glutamic acid and aspartic acid, and were all shown to be ineffective in dispersing melanosomes.

Catecholamines and some related sympathomimetic amines were then put to the same procedure. Such substances included norepinephrine, epinephrine, phenylephrine, isoproterenol, methoxyphenamine, and protokylol. In response to their strong solutions, a further aggregation of pigment was usually observed beyond the level attained by the coexistence of tolazoline. We were rather amazed to find that their weaker solutions did have a reverse action; the dispersion of melanosomes. In the left part of figure 1, such a response to epinephrine was demonstrated, which is known to have either an alpha or beta effect on adrenergically innervated tissues. Other beta agonists tested were metaproterenol and isoxsuprine. They were without the melanin-aggregating effect, and exhibited a very strong action to disperse melanosomes over a wide range of concentration (fig. 2). These monoamine-induced dispersion responses were quite reproducible, and were easily antagonized by propranolol (fig. 1 and 2) or by dichloroisoproterenol, both of them being beta-adrenergic-blocking agents. These results favor the view that, as in some amphibians and reptiles [2], beta-adrenoceptors are present

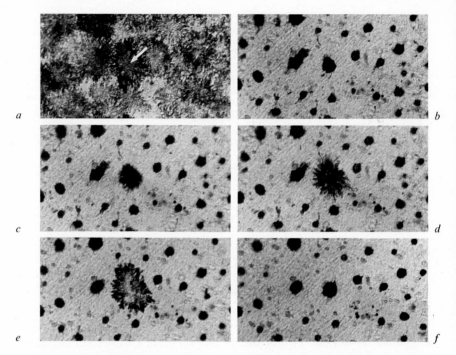

Fig. 4. Serial photomicrographs of web skin of a split fin preparation, showing the effect of iontophoretic injection of cyclic AMP into a melanophore seen in the center of each print. (a) Initial dispersed state of melanophores in the physiological saline. White arrow indicates the site of micropipette impalement. (b) Aggregated state induced under the influence of K-rich saline for 4 min. Iontophoretic current was just turned on. (c) 15 sec afterwards. (d) 1 min afterwards. The current was turned off at the same time. (e) 4 min afterwards, when the maximal degree of pigment dispersion was attained in the injected cell. Melanosomes were so dispersed that the cell body became mostly devoid of them. (f) 23 min after shutting the current off. Melanosomes were again aggregated. × 135.

in the melanophore, and take part in the darkening response of this fish species. The only pertinent paper published thus far was by REED and FINNIN [9] who, working on angelfish melanophores *in vivo*, observed a transient melanin dispersion in response to isoproterenol injected intraperitoneally.

The functional endogenous beta-stimulating amine may be epinephrine, and adrenal chromaffin cells are naturally thought to be its source. However, our preliminary observations using a histochemical fluores-

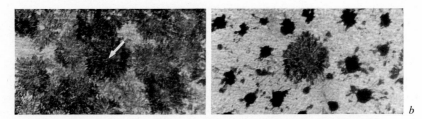

a   *b*

Fig. 5. Photomicrographs of web skin of a split preparation, showing the effect of cyclic AMP into a dispersed melanophore and that on the response to K ions. (a) After a 1-min application of the pulses into the melanophore seen in the center. In the physiological saline. White arrow indicates the site of the pipette penetration. (b) 3 min after changing the medium to K-rich saline. Melanosomes in the injected cell remained fully dispersed, while those in other cells became aggregated. × 135.

cence technique suggest that the peripheral chromaffin cell system might be another candidate, storing the amine.

It has been shown in a variety of cells and tissues, that adenyl cyclase is stimulated by catecholamines and that the receptors of beta-adrenergic type may be involved in this process [10]. On the other hand, it has become probable that an increase or decrease in the intracellular cyclic AMP levels produces dispersion or aggregation of melanosomes, respectively, within amphibian and reptile melanophores [2]. In some cases, the sequence is thought to be beta receptor-mediated. Since NOVALES and FUJII [8] on killifish, and SCHLIWA and BEREITER-HAHN [11] on angelfish, showed that cyclic AMP added to the bathing media accelerated melanin dispersion, the participation of this nucleotide seems to be the case also in fishes. Using a number of nucleotides, we have studied this on the material which is now known to have beta adrenoceptors.

It was found that both cyclic AMP and its dibutyryl derivative dispersed melanosomes to a greater or less degree, and a case in which cyclic AMP was very effective is exemplified in figure 3. Methylxanthines were also potent pigment-dispersing agents. The tested nucleotides which contain other bases than adenine were all ineffective in dispersing the pigment. Contrary to our expectation, adenine nucleotides other than cyclic monophosphate strongly dispersed melanosomes, even when very weak solutions, such as 10^{-5} M, were applied. In figure 3, the marked dispersing effect of ATP is exhibited. Up to the present, we do not know the mechanism by which those nucleotides act to drive the cellular inclu-

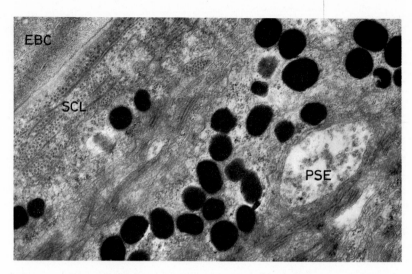

Fig. 6. Electron micrograph of the dermis of tail fin. Note a number of microtubules in cross sections or in profiles in the cytoplasm of melanophore processes. EBC = Epidermal basal cell; PSE = presynaptic element; SCL = subepidermal collagenous layer. × 18,500.

sions. One explanation might be that one of those substances tried or a related substance acts on the pigment cells as a chemical mediator released from so-called 'purinergic' nerves, as recently suggested by BURNSTOCK [3] in a few autonomically innervated effector cells. These circumstances in a certain way created a necessity for a more direct approach to the problem concerning the validity of the second messenger hypothesis in pigment cells.

Trials were thus made to inject cyclic AMP or some other nucleotides iontophoretically into the melanophores. In most experiments, including those exhibited in figures 4 and 5, the current through the micropipette was adjusted to be about 10^{-10} A. Adopting 0.3 as the transport number for cyclic AMP iontophoresis [12], therefore, the quantity of the nucleotide ejected through the pipette was roughly estimated to be 3×10^{-16} mol per sec [4]. On the other hand, the total volume of an average-sized guppy melanophore was calculated to be about 5×10^{-12} liter. Thus, the increase in the intracellular concentration of the nucleotide may be about 6×10^{-5} M per 1-sec pulse. Even when we take account of the continuing destruction by phosphodiesterase or leakage through injured membranes, therefore, sufficient amounts of the nucleotide may have been supplied during the pulse application.

As shown in figure 4, the cyclic AMP injection brought about a rapid and reversible dispersion of pigment within the aggregated melanophore. Such a dispersion was not observed, when 5′-AMP, ATP or cyclic GMP was applied by iontophoresis. Figure 5a typically demonstrates that cyclic AMP injected did not produce the aggregation of melanosomes. The other nucleotides tested were also found ineffective in aggregating the pigment. In addition, we observed that injected cyclic AMP counteracted the action of K ions, which were potently pigment-aggregating in untreated cells (fig. 5b).

In view of the above results, it may be concluded here that the second messenger theory for cyclic AMP is applicable to the fish melanophores, and that beta-adrenoceptors of the cell play a role at least partly in accelerating centrifugal movement of melanosomes. Working on glutaraldehyde-fixed fin pieces, we could find a number of microtubules in the melanophores of the present material (fig. 6). Although quite a few workers are in agreement with the opinion that these tubular elements may be involved in transferring pigment granules in melanophores [11], the link between the cyclic AMP changes and the movement remains still a matter of speculation. For understanding this, further studies are deservedly needed.

Summary

Using split fin preparations of the guppy, *Lebistes reticulatus,* regulatory mechanisms of pigment dispersion in melanophores were studied. Weak solutions of adrenergic monoamines, especially of beta stimulants, were found to disperse melanosomes. Such an effect was easily antagonized by beta-adrenergic-blocking agents. Cyclic AMP and other adenine nucleotides added to the medium induced the pigment dispersion. However, intracellular iontophoresis of some nucleotides revealed that only cyclic AMP was effective. It was concluded that beta-adrenoceptors mediate the melanosome dispersion by increasing cyclic AMP levels in the pigment cells.

References

1   ABBOTT, F. S.: Endocrine regulation of pigmentation in fish. Am. Zoologist *13:* 885–894 (1973).

2   BAGNARA, J. T. and HADLEY, M. E.: Chromatophores and color change (Prentice-Hall, Englewood Cliffs 1973).
2   BURNSTOCK, G.: Purinergic nerves. Pharmacol. Rev. *24:* 509–581 (1972).
4   CURTIS, D. R.: Microelectrophoresis; in NASTUK Physical techniques in biological research, vol. 5, pp. 144–190 (Academic Press, New York 1964).
5   FUJII, R. and MIYASHITA, Y.: Receptor mechanisms in fish chromatophores. I. Alpha nature of adrenoceptors mediating melanosome aggregation in guppy melanophores. Comp. Biochem. Physiol. *51C:* 171–178 (1975).
6   FUJII, R. and NOVALES, R. R.: Nervous control of melanosome movements in vertebrate melanophores; in RILEY Pigmentation: its genesis and biologic control, pp. 315–326 (Appleton, New York 1972).
7   MIYASHITA, Y. and FUJII, R.: Receptor mechanisms in fish chromatophores. II. Evidence for beta adrenoceptors mediating melanosome dispersion in guppy melanophores. Comp. Biochem. Physiol. *51C:* 178–187 (1975).
8   NOVALES, R. R. and FUJII, R.: A melanin-dispersing effect of cyclic adenosine monophosphate on *Fundulus* melanophores. J. cell. Physiol. *75:* 133–136 (1970).
9   REED, B. L. and FINNIN, B. C.: Adrenergic innervation of melanophores in teleost fish; in RILEY Pigmentation: its genesis and biologic control, pp. 285–294 (Appleton, New York 1972).
10   ROBISON, G. A.; BUTCHER, R. W., and SUTHERLAND, E. W.: Cyclic AMP (Academic Press, New York 1971).
11   SCHLIWA, M. and BEREITER-HAHN, J.: Pigment movements in fish melanophores. Morphological and physiological studies. IV. The effect of cyclic adenosine monophosphate on normal and vinblastine-treated melanophores. Cell Tissue Res. *151:* 423–432 (1974).
12   TSIEN, R. W.: Adrenaline-like effects of intracellular iontophoresis of cyclic AMP in cardiac Purkinje fibres. Nature new Biol. *245:* 120–122 (1973).

Dr. RYOZO FUJII, Department of Biology, Sapporo Medical College, *Sapporo 060* (Japan)

Pigment Cell, vol. 3, pp. 345–356 (Karger, Basel 1976)

The Effects of Laser Irradiation on Fish Chromatophores

Joyce W. Hawkes

Oregon Regional Primate Research Center, Beaverton, Oreg.

Introduction

The laser produces a coherent beam of highly monochromatic light which can be focused to a spot as small as 0.1 μm, and in this dimension is used as a microsurgical knife in cell biology [1–3]. On a macroscopic surgical scale, the precision with which the intense beam can be focused and the selective absorption of light by melanin in the pigment epithelium of the eye are the bases of photocoagulation therapy [13] in, for example, repairing a detached retina. When an unfocused beam is pulsed at a tissue, whatever molecules absorb the particular wavelength become potential sites of injury [16]. Fish skin has numerous melanophores underneath the epidermis and at several depths in the dermis [9, 10], which contain melanin granules that absorb light over a wide spectrum in the visible range. The unfocused ruby laser beam, at an energy density which does not damage the nonabsorbing tissue, would be expected to cause various effects in these layered melanophores. This paper reports the ultrastructural effects of an unfocused laser pulse on melanophores (black) and associated chromatophores (yellow) and iridophores (iridescent) of coho salmon skin.

Methods

Yearling coho salmon, *Oncorhynchus kisutch,* were obtained through the courtesy of the National Marine Fisheries Service, Portland, Oregon, and maintained in laboratory aquaria at 15° C. In preparation for laser irradiation, the fish were anestheized in MS-222 (ethyl-*m*-aminobenzoate methanesulfonate) and placed in a container full of water with a clear quartz window on one side. The laser beam passed first through the quartz window and then through 4 cm of water to the fish skin. The salmon received a 30-nsec pulse of 6,943 Å light from a Q-switched ruby laser at an energy density of about 1 J/cm² at the exit pupil of the laser. A circle of skin just below the dorsal fin and 0.5 cm in diameter was the target for all experiments. In addition, some fish were branded on the head, which lacks scales. For comparison, one experiment was performed on green swordtails, *Xiphophorus helleri,* with a 10- to 20-msec pulse of 6,943 Å light.

Pieces of irradiated and nonirradiated salmon skin were excised and processed for electron microscopy 5 min; 5, 26, and 50 h; and 14, 20, 41, and 82 days after treatment. The fixative contained 0.75% glutaraldehyde, 3% formalin, 1% acrolein in 0.1 M sodium cacodylate buffer with 0.02% $CaCl_2 \cdot 2H_2O$, 0.02 M s-collidine and 5.5% sucrose. Initial fixation was followed by a buffer wash and postfixation in 1% osmium tetroxide [9]. Tissues were dehydrated, embedded in Spurr medium [17], and sectioned with either a glass or a diamond knife. Thin sections for electron microscopy were triple stained with lead citrate, uranyl acetate, and lead citrate and were examined with a Philips EM-300. For light microscopy, sections were cut 1 μm thick and stained with toluidine blue.

Results

A nanosecond laser pulse caused a momentary blanching of the salmon skin, followed by a gradual darkening that resulted in a black area corresponding precisely to the irradiated area. The skin remained dark for 6–8 months, gradually lightened to brown, and eventually regained its normal color. A millisecond pulse laser caused a bubble of gaseous material to appear under the epidermis within 5 min and to remain for about a day. At its largest diameter, the bubble was 2.5 mm across and slowly decreased until it was no longer distinguishable. The skin darkened locally, but regained its normal color within a month. Since the long-term effects of the nanosecond pulse laser were more complex than those of the millisecond pulse laser, this report is limited to the former.

Fig. 1. Light micrograph of coho salmon skin 5 min after laser irradiation. All the melanophores (M) in the field are vesiculated, but the drosopterin-containing xanthophore (arrow) shows no overt damage. E = Epidermis; S = scale. × 500.

Fig. 2. Electron micrograph of coho salmon skin 5 min after irradiation. The epidermal cells, as in figure 1, appear normal. The melanophores that receive the most direct impact of the light have empty areas (M), but the underlying melanophore that was presumably shaded from the laser pulse appears normal. The closely associated iridophore is severely damaged (I). E = Epidermis; D = dermis. × 4,300.

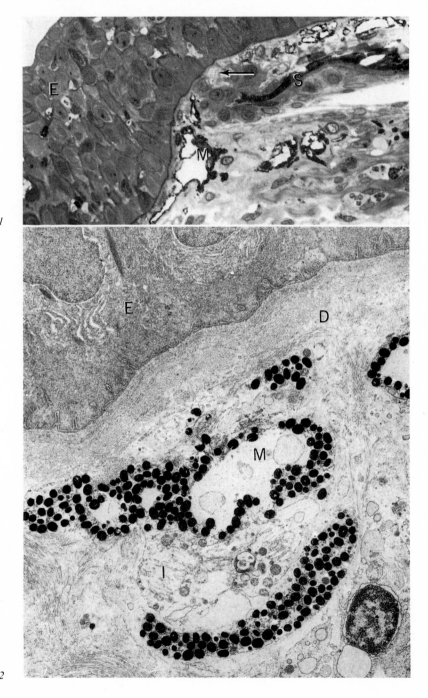

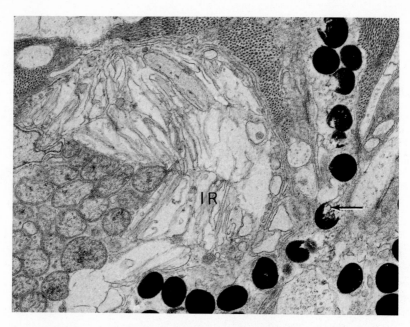

Fig. 3. Electron micrograph of iridophores (IR) at the edge of the irradiated zone 26 h after treatment. The membranes around the crystalline platelets are disrupted. Melanosomes in the adjacent melanophore show typical laser induced damage (arrow). × 15,000.

No overt irradiation damage, neither generalized loss of cells nor apparent necrosis, can be observed in the epidermis (fig. 1). Judging from the number of metaphase figures, mitosis increases slightly in the basal layer of cells by 20 days after irradiation, and the basal lamina is about three times thicker than in normal animals.

The effects in the dermis, a complex, multilayered structure in salmon [9], ranged from severe in the most superficial melanophores to none in, for example, the fibroblasts. The deep green of the dorsal skin is produced by three dermal cells which together form a 'chromatophore unit' [10]. Each of these cells contributes a different quality to the skin color and each responds differently to the laser. The yellow xanthophores, which contain vesicles of drosopterins and carotenoids, are not directly damaged by ruby laser pulses (fig. 1, 4). In some areas, however, where the melanophores were so extensively damaged that the dermis had scattered vacuous areas, there is some question about whether the xan-

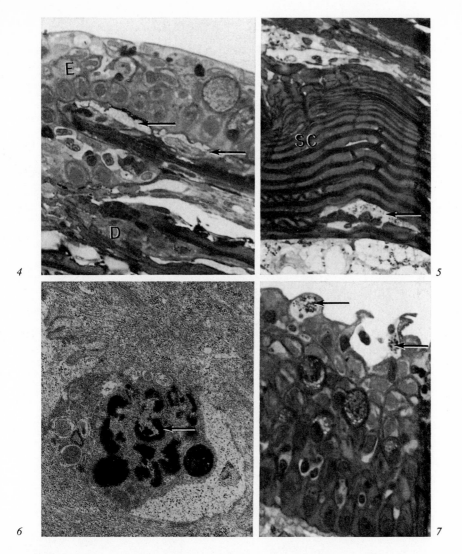

Fig. 4. Light micrograph of laser pulsed coho skin 20 days post-treatment. The nonpigmented components of the epidermis (E) and dermis (D) still appear normal. Xanthophores (arrows) also look the same as in untreated skin. × 580.

Fig. 5. 20 days after irradiation. Cells with melanosomes (arrow) have invaded the deep parts of the dermis, the stratum compactum (SC), from the underlying pigmented layer where melanophores were disrupted. × 620.

Fig. 6. Electron micrograph of the contents of the pigment-containing cells shown in figure 7. Note the broken fragments of melanosomes (arrow). × 19,000.

Fig. 7. Light micrograph of coho salmon skin 41 days after laser irradiation. Phagocytic cells containing damaged melanosomes are sloughing at the surface of the epidermis (arrows). × 620.

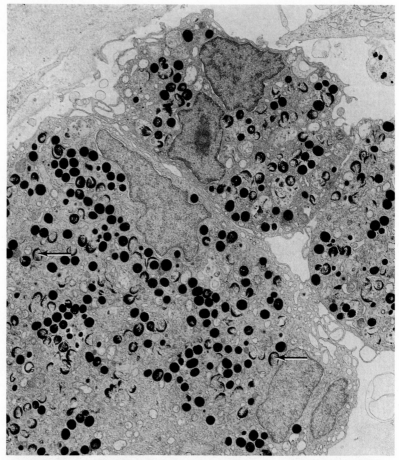

8

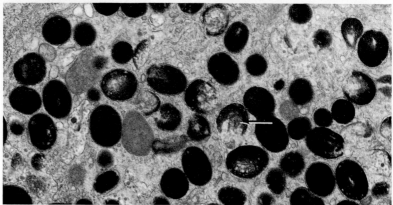

9

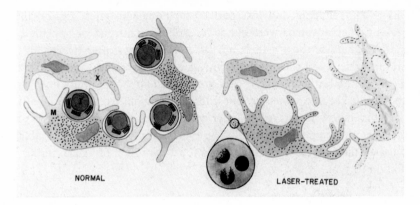

Fig. 10. Summary diagram comparing the untreated and treated chromato-phore unit. See Conclusions section for explanation.

thophores incurred any secondary damage. In the severely damaged zones, vesicles that could be fragments of pterinosomes from the xan-thophores can be seen. However, in regions of moderate damage, the xan-thophores appeared healthy and remained so for the duration of the study.

The extremely sensitive iridophores, on the other hand, disappeared from the treated area between 26 and 50 h and were not replaced (fig. 2, 3). By 20 days, the edge of the irradiated area glittered with a rim of iri-dophores which seem more numerous than in normal skin, but did not move into the irradiated zone.

The melanophores responded variously. The most striking reaction, and the one that produced the darkened skin tone, was the inability of all the melanophores to aggregate melanosomes. When a solution of 0.1% KCl was applied to both irradiated and nonirradiated skin, the melano-somes in the normal melanophores aggregated to the cell center and caused the skin tone to become light. However, no lightening occurred in the irradiated area. Beyond this generalized reaction, the melanophore re-sponse ranged from total disruption to very mild damage. In the most se-vere cases, the melanophores died, the cell membrane broke up, and the cell fragments were picked up by phagocytic cells (fig. 5) and sloughed off at the surface (fig. 6, 7). Other melanophores became vesiculated, as an

Fig. 8. Electron micrograph of melanocytes in salmon skin 20 days after laser irradiation. There are numerous damaged melanosomes (arrows). × 4,700.

Fig. 9. Disrupted melanosomes (arrow) 72 days after irradiation. × 8,500.

immediate reaction, and lost part of their melanosomes (fig. 2); the remaining melanosomes were either fractionally damaged or appeared normal. The fate of these cells is not clear; by 20 days after treatment, there are no vesiculated cells in the skin (fig. 8), but whether they recovered or died cannot be ascertained. Still other melanophores were not harmed enough to become vesicular, but a loss of material from portions of some of the melanosomes gave the latter a crescent shape (fig. 8) whereas most melanosomes appeared normal. These melanophores remained viable and retained their damaged melanosomes for a minimum of 72 days after irradiation (fig. 9).

Discussion

The initial response of fish skin to nanosecond pulses of the ruby laser appears to depend on the selective absorption of light by one group of cells, the melanophores. The absorbing substance is melanin, which is associated with proteins and is contained in vesicles, 0.5 μm in diameter, the melanosomes. The selective destruction of these melanosomes is a highly localized effect which sometimes occurs without the death of the melanophores. This means that the nucleic acids, enzymatic systems, and structural proteins of the cell have not incurred enough damage to be destroyed and that ,therefore, heat energy does not travel far from the melanosomes. The fact that thermal effects from Q-switched laser pulses are highly localized in other cell systems is substantiated by theoretical considerations [11, 16, 20]. However, the nanosecond time pulse of the Q-switched laser produces biological effects in retinal tissue that are not fully explained by thermal considerations [8], and the disruption that ensues from mechanical forces is an important source of pathologic changes [15]. Acoustic shock waves, Brillouin scattering, free radical formation, and harmonic generation have been postulated as injury-producing agents [12]. Direct evidence for such effects, however, is scanty.

Melanin treated with millisecond laser pulses or heated to 350 °C [12] showed no changes in electron density; but after a picosecond pulse, some of the melanosomes of the rhesus eye lost electron density (melanin?) and resembled typical mammalian premelanosomes [8]. In the retina of rabbits, nanosecond pulses did not cause fragmentation in the melanosomes [15]. In the fish, nanosecond pulses produced both fragmentation and internal damage which appeared as electron-transparent areas in otherwise whole melanosomes. The brevity of the Q-switched and mode-locked lasers effect immediate and local heating so that the absorbing loci, but not the surrounding tissue, are hot. Expansion of material within the melanosomes could fragment it. Judging from currently available information, there are two plausible explanations for the rupture of melanosomes in fish skin. One is that the water in the melanosome is heated locally and, when it expands, blows the melanosome into fragments. The other hypothesis is that the melanin itself is broken down. To break the carbon-carbon bond would require about 3.5 eV, whereas one 6,943-Å photon has an energy of only 1.80 eV. Therefore, a two-photon capture mechanism must be postulated to supply the required energy. Further work with an *in vitro* system is being done to test both hypotheses which are not mutually exclusive.

An additional question arises: Is the lability of melanin in the path of a ruby laser pulse due to some unique property of fish melanin? This is probably not the case, because fish melanin is formed by the same enzymatic pathways as other vertebrate melanins [4, 5]; how premelanosomes are formed, however, is not entirely resolved. Premelanosomes, which have the typical periodicity characteristic of mammalian premelanosomes, have been found in the eyes of *Fundulus heteroclitus* [18]; but premelanosomes are rarely observed in fish. In xanthic goldfish, however, small electron-dense vesicles coalesce and form larger and larger aggregates until the typical and final melanosome is completed [19]. After laser treatment, a vesicular substructure is quite evident in salmon melanosomes. Furthermore, this effect is basically similar to the change in appearance of melanosomes in rhesus melanocytes to typical mammalian premelanosomes after a short laser pulse [7].

The survival of the xanthophores is predictable since they would not be expected to absorb the red wavelength. The extreme sensitivity of the iridophores, however, seems unusual. Unlike the iridophores located in the ventral aspects of the body, these cells, situated in the dorsal part of the skin, do not reflect a silvery sheen. Instead, their iridescence appears in various shades of green. To some extent, this tone is expected to be mediated by overlying yellow xanthophores, so the true reflected color is probably in the blue region. What happens to the red wavelengths? If red light were absorbed, the temperature could increase enough to kill the cell: hypoxanthine, one of the crystalline components of iridophores [14], decomposes at 150 °C and the cell volume is 1/3 to 1/2 filled with the long, thin crystalline platelets [10]. In other fish iridophores, the nonreflected light is transmitted rather than absorbed. Whatever the mechanism that destroys the iridophores, they may serve as a biological thermometer in a system where direct temperature measurements are unfeasible simply because, as yet, there is no thermocouple that responds in the nanosecond time range.

Conclusions

The local darkening of fish skin which results from mild doses of ruby laser light (6,943 Å) is due, not to damage to the epidermis, but to the effect on the chromatophores in the underlying dermis. Color in the normal coho salmon, *Oncorhynchus kisutch,* is produced by a dermal chromatophore unit made up of three cell types – xanthophores (yellow), iridophores (iridescent), and melanophores (black) – each of which responds differently to the laser (fig. 10). The xanthophores (X) are least affected by laser irradiation and look normal, whereas the iridophores (I) are extremely sensitive and disappear from the treated area. The melanophores (M) have a wide range of responses, the most striking of which is the loss of ability to aggregate their melanosomes, which produces the darkened skin tone. Some melanophores die and are removed by macrophages which slough off at the epidermal surface. Some become vesiculated with partial loss of melanosomes; the remaining melanosomes are either fractionally damaged or appear normal. In other melanophores, no vesiculation occurs, but there is a loss of material from some of their melanosomes which then have a crescent shape. These melanophores remain viable, retaining their damaged melanosomes for a minimum of 82 days after irradiation.

Acknowledgments

This work is Publication No. 803 of the Oregon Regional Primate Research Center supported in part by Public Health Service, National Institutes of Health Grants RR 00163 of the Animal Resources Branch, Division of Research Resources, and AM 08445 of the National Institute of Arthritis and Metabolic Diseases.

The author wishes to thank Dr. K. R. FARRELL and Mr. T. BELL, Washington State University, for the initial observation that the ruby laser turns fish skin dark and Dr. FARRELL for the use of the ruby laser. In addition, I have enjoyed discussing the theoretical aspects of the paper with Dr. G. MASSEY, Oregon Graduate Center for Physics and Chemistry, and Dr. J. FELLMAN, University of Oregon Health Sciences Center.

DEBORAH ANN LACY provided excellent technical assistance.

References

1 BERNS, M. W.: Recent progress with laser microbeams. Int. Rev. Cytol. *39:* 383–411 (1974).

2 BERNS, M. W.: Directed chromosome loss by laser microirradiation. Science *186:* 700–705 (1974).

3 BERNS, M. W. and SALET, C.: Laser microbeams for partial cell irradiation. Int. Rev. Cytol. *33:* 131–156 (1972).

4 CHAVIN, W.: Fundamental aspects of morphological melanin color changes in vertebrate skin. Am. Zoologist *9:* 505–520 (1969).

5 CHAVIN, W.; KIM, K., and TCHEN, T. T.: Endocrine control of pigmentation. Ann. N.Y. Acad. Sci. *100:* 678–685 (1963).

6 DENTON, E. J. and LAND, M. F.: Mechanism of reflection in silvery layers of fish and cephalopods. Proc. R. Soc. Lond. *178:* 43–61 (1971).

7 HAM, W. T., jr.; MUELLER, H. A.; GOLDMAN, A. I.; NEWNAM, G. E.; HOLLAND, L. M., and KUWABARA, T.: Ocular hazard from picosecond pulses of Nd:YAG laser radiation. Science *185:* 362–363 (1974).

8 HAM, W. T., jr.; WILLIAMS, R. C.; MUELLER, H. A.; GUERRY, D., III; CLARKE, A. M., and GEERAETS, W. J.: Effects of laser radiation on the mammalian eye. Trans. N.Y. Acad. Sci. *28:* 517–526 (1966).

9 HAWKES, J. W.: The structure of fish skin. I. General organization. Cell Tissue Res. *149:* 147–158 (1974).

10 HAWKES, J. W.: The structure of fish skin. II. Chromatophore unit. Cell Tissue Res. *149:* 159–172 (1974).

11 HAYES, J. R. and WOLBARSHT, M. L.: Thermal model for retinal damage induced by pulsed lasers. Aerosp. Med. *39:* 474–480 (1968).

12 HAYES, J. R. and WOLBARSHT, M. L.: Models in pathology – mechanisms of action of laser energy with biological tissue; in WOLBARSHT Laser applications in medicine and biology, vol. 1 (Plenum Press, New York 1971).

13 HOCHHEIMER, B. F.: Lasers in ophthalmology; in WOLBARSHT Laser applications in medicine and biology, vol. 2 (Plenum Press, New York 1974).

14 MARKERT, J. R. and VANSTONE, W. E.: Pigments in the belly skin of coho salmon *(Oncorhnychus kisutch)*. J. Fish Res. Board Can. *23:* 1095–1098 (1966).

15 MARSHALL, J.: Thermal and mechanical mechanisms in laser damage to the retina. Investve Ophthal. *9:* 97–115 (1970).

16 MORENO, G.; SALET, C., and VINZENS, F.: Ultrastructure of mitochondria after laser microirradiation (French). J. Microscopie *16:* 269–278 (1973).

17 SPURR, A. R.: A low viscosity epoxy resin embedding medium for electron microscopy. J. Ultrastruct. Res. *26:* 31–43 (1969).

18 SZABO, G.: Melanin pigmentation. Dis. nerv. Syst., suppl. *29:* 58–62 (1968).

19 TURNER, W. A., TAYLOR, J. D., and TCHEN, T. T.: Melanosome formation in the goldfish: the role of multivesicular bodies. J. Ultrastruct. Res. *51:* 16–31 (1975).
20 VASSILIADIS, A.: Ocular damage from laser radiation; in WOLBARSHT Laser applications in medicine and biology, vol. 1 (Plenum Press, New York 1971).

Dr. JOYCE W. HAWKES, Oregon Regional Primate Research Center, 505 N.W. 185th Ave., *Beaverton, OR 97005* (USA)

Pigment Cell, vol. 3, pp. 357–366 (Karger, Basel 1976)

The Epidermal Melanocytes of the Mongolian Gerbil

Their Postnatal Development and Response to Carcinogens[1]

WALTER C. QUEVEDO, jr., CHARLES J. McDONALD, JACOB DYCKMAN, THERESA C. BIENIEKI, ROBERT D. FLEISCHMANN and THOMAS J. HOLSTEIN

Division of Biological and Medical Sciences, Brown University, Providence, and Department of Biology, Roger Williams College, Bristol, R.I.

Introduction

The Mongolian gerbil *(Meriones unguiculatus)* offers unique opportunities for inquiries into the action of chemical and physical agents on the cutaneous melanocyte system. In earlier publications, it was established that topical applications of 7,12-dimethylbenz(*a*)anthracene (DMBA) elicit a striking increase in melanogenically active melanocytes in both the dermis and the normally non-pigmented interfollicular epidermis of the adult hairy (dorsal) trunk skin [8, 16]. Although croton oil shares with DMBA the ability to produce a marked hyperpigmentation of the dermis, it fails to stimulate increased pigmentation of the epidermis [16]. The source of the increased numbers of melanogenic melanocytes in treated skin remains to be established. In the dermis, it may involve the activation and proliferation of previously amelanotic melanocytes and/or the proliferation of melanotic melanocytes which normally form scattered perifollicular and interfollicular dermal networks. In the epidermis, it may derive from the stimulation-proliferation of melanocytes which become melanogenically inactive during the first month of life, or from the migration of melanocytes from hair follicles and/or the dermis [8, 13, 15, 18]. A similar explanation may hold for the sporadic occurrence of numerous melanocytes within DMBA-induced papillomas and squamous cell carcinomas [8]. The present study was undertaken to examine further by light and electron microscopy the structure of normal and carcinogen-treated gerbil skin to determine whether any distinction can be made between the

1 Supported by PHS Research Grant CA-06097 from the National Cancer Institute.

various hypotheses advanced in explanation of the chemically induced cutaneous hyperpigmentation.

Materials and Methods

Age-dependent changes in the melanocyte populations of interfollicular epidermis of the mid-dorsal trunk were examined in a total of 16 gerbils ranging from 1 to 180 days of age. Skin specimens from which the hypodermis was removed by scraping, or epidermal sheets split from the underlying dermis following treatment with 2N NaBr, were incubated in dopa-reagent and prepared as whole mounts employing methods fully described elsewhere [14, 17]. The numbers of melanocytes were estimated per mm² over the surface area of the skin in plane projection. In each specimen, the calculations were based on actual counts of melanocytes within an area of 1.11 mm².

A group of 5- to 6-month-old male and female gerbils was treated once weekly with 1 ml of 0.1% DMBA in acetone released from a calibrated syringe on the shaved dorsum of each animal. In each case, two or three animals were killed one week after receiving 1, 3, 5, 7, or 9 applications. Two additional animals received 12 weekly treatments with 1 ml of 0.1% DMBA in acetone and sacrificed approximately one month after the last application. Standard histological procedures were followed in preparing paraffin sections and epidermal sheets from representative skin specimens. Representative specimens of DMBA-treated (3 and 12 applications) and normal skin were also prepared for electron microscopy. They were fixed in paraformaldehyde-glutaraldehyde, post-fixed in osmium tetroxide and embedded either in Spurr low-viscosity epoxy resin or epon-araldite. Sections were made on a Sorval Porter-Blum MT2-B Ultramicrotome, stained with uranyl acetate and lead citrate, and examined in a Zeiss EM9S-2 electron microscope.

Results

In excess of 400/mm² on the first day of life, the number of dopa-reactive epidermal melanocytes in the interfollicular epidermis of the mid-dorsal trunk skin rapidly declined during the first two weeks until only a few were still present by 180 days of age (fig. 1). It was not possible to determine the fate of the melanocytes at the light microscope level.

Examination of adult skin with the electron microscope revealed an epidermis consisting of several layers of viable keratinocytes capped by a well-developed cornified layer (fig. 2). The non-keratinocytes of the normal epidermis fell into three classes: Langerhans cells, Merkel cells, and indeterminate cells. Indeterminate cells lacked the desmosomes and tonofilaments characteristic of keratinocytes but possessed no unique orga-

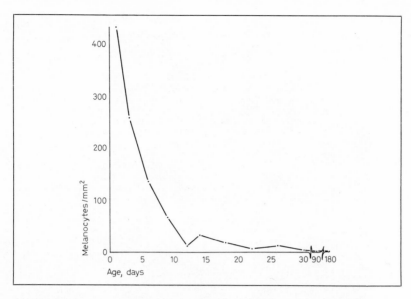

Fig. 1. Age-dependent changes in populations of dopa-reactive epidermal melanocytes. At 90 and 180 days, the points represent averages for 4 and 2 animals, respectively. All others are based on one animal.

nelles which would permit their further identification. Langerhans cells and indeterminate cells were found both in the suprabasal and basal layers. The small number of Merkel cells detected were in the basal layer evidently proximal to hair follicles. The non-keratinocytes of the basal layer were usually substantially separated from the basal lamina by a thin extension of the cytoplasm from flanking keratinocytes. Although observed by light microscopy, no epidermal melanocytes were found in the non-treated epidermis of adult gerbils examined by electron microscopy.

In DMBA-treated skin, melanocytes first appeared in the external root sheaths of hair follicles and in the adjacent epidermis. Later, they formed dense populations throughout the epidermis. Following three weekly applications of DMBA, numerous melanocytes containing melanosomes in various stages of formation were observed in the interfollicular epidermis (fig. 3).

The cytoplasm of keratinocytes contained mature melanosomes deployed either as single entities or grouped two or more within membrane-limited vesicles forming melanosome complexes. Consistent with their status as non-keratinocytes, the epidermal melanocytes were usually

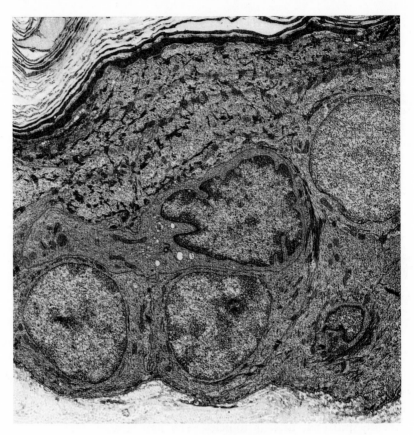

Fig. 2. Survey of normal epidermis in the gerbil. Note the well-keratinized epidermis and dendritic Langerhans cell above the basal layer. × 5,580.

Fig. 3. Epidermal melanocyte in gerbil skin following three applications of DMBA. Note the keratinocyte cytoplasm extending beneath much of the basal surface of the melanocyte. × 5,580.

Fig. 4. Epidermal melanocyte in gerbil skin following three applications of DMBA. The cell appears somewhat shrunken and possesses an electron-dense cytoplasm. × 5,580.

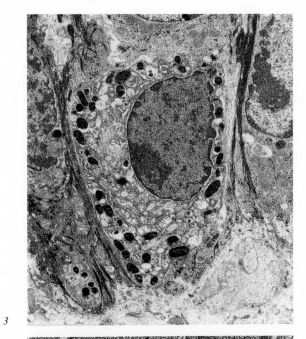

3

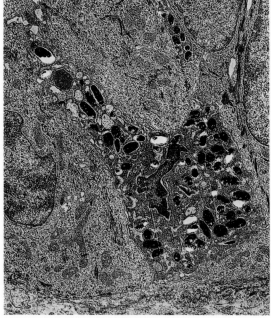

4

'cushioned' by keratinocyte cytoplasm extending beneath a substantial portion of their proximal surfaces. In some cases, the more mature melanosomes appeared to be distributed mainly in the peripheral cytoplasm of the melanocytes. Occasional melanocytes, apparently dislodged from the basal layer, were found at high levels in the epidermis among the ascending keratinocytes. There were indications that some melanocytes were damaged and perhaps destroyed by DMBA treatment. A somewhat shrunken, possibly necrotic, melanocyte with an electron-dense cytoplasm was found in the basal layer of DMBA-treated epidermis (fig. 4). In addition, along with large numbers of melanosomes, phagosomes containing debris possibly of melanocyte origin were found in occasional keratinocytes (fig. 5).

In the hyperpigmented dermis of DMBA-treated skin, dermal melanocytes in some cases contained only fully melanized (stage IV) melanosomes; in others, melanosomes at stages I–IV of development [5]. In addition, melanosomes were found in dermal macrophages where they were arranged in groups of two or more within membrane-limited lysosomal structures.

Raised blue nevus-like perifollicular tumors were found in DMBA-treated skin [16]. They were composed of cells containing numerous round to elliptical melanosomes (fig. 6). There was the suggestion that the round granules consisted of small electron-dense spherical bodies. Occasionally, aggregates of filaments were present within possible stage I–II melanosomes. In some cells, several melanosomes formed complexes within membrane-limited bodies which also contained myelin-like structures.

Discussion

The source of epidermal melanocytes in the DMBA-treated epidermis of gerbils remains to be established. Although it is possible that indeterminate cells are in reality amelanotic melanocytes, no definite precur-

---

Fig. 5. Numerous melanosomes within a keratinocyte of skin treated three times with DMBA. In addition, note phagosomes containing non-pigmentary debris possibly of melanocyte origin. × 14,570.

Fig. 6. DMBA-induced blue nevus-like tumor. Note the numerous round to elliptical melanosomes distributed in the tumor cells adjacent to a hair follicle. × 5,580.

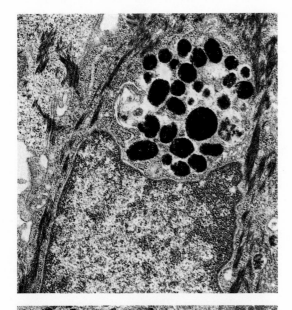

5

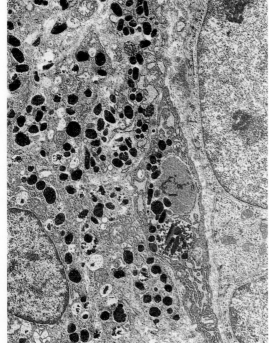

6

sor melanocytes were observed in non-treated skin. The initial appearance of active melanocytes near hair follicles following application of DMBA is consistent with either the migration of melanocytes from hair follicles or more effective penetration of carcinogen into the skin at the pilosebaceous canal leading to early melanocyte activation. It is possible that careful tracing of the age-dependent loss of epidermal melanocytes in neonatal gerbils by electron microscopy may resolve the question of the affinities of indeterminate cells. At present, there is a strong possibility that they are related to Langerhans cells [3].

In addition to possessing the ability to elicit melanogenesis within melanocytes, DMBA also appears to be capable of damaging melanocytes possibly resulting in their death and degradation. This effect of DMBA on melanocytes has also been reported by KLAUS [6] for guinea pig melanocytes treated in cell culture. Damaged epidermal melanocytes may be removed by detachment from the basal layer followed by their ascent along with keratinocytes [1]. Less definite is their removal by the phagocytic activity of neighboring keratinocytes [20]. The DMBA-induced high rate of melanogenesis may lead to the accumulation of cytotoxic melanin precursors resulting in damage to melanocytes [7].

The source of the increased numbers of active dermal melanocytes in the skin of gerbils treated with DMBA or croton oil also is not clear. It is possible that they originate from the proliferation of the small population of dermal melanocytes normally present in the dermis as interfollicular and perifollicular networks and/or the activation and proliferation of normally non-pigmented dermal melanocytes [16]. In general histology, the melanotic tumors induced by DMBA appear most comparable to the DMBA-induced, blue nevus-like tumors in Syrian hamsters and may have a similar origin, possibly from dermal melanocytes or neural elements associated with hair follicles [9–12]. The pathway of melanosome formation within the blue nevus-like tumors may differ from that detected in the DMBA-activated dermal and epidermal melanocytes of treated skin [4].

Coupled with our previous studies, it is clear that DMBA possesses a marked ability to elicit the appearance of both epidermal and dermal melanocytes. Significantly, croton oil activates only dermal melanocytes [8, 16]. In view of the failure of croton oil to elicit the appearance of epidermal melanocytes, it seems evident that simple epidermal hyperplasia in itself is not sufficient to account for the changes in populations of active epidermal melanocytes. Pigmented mice treated with croton oil exhibit essentially identical pigmentary responses to those found in the gerbil [19]. The hyperpigmentation is essentially restricted to the dermis. However, methylcholanthrene leads to the appearance of numerous epidermal and dermal melanocytes in pigmented mice [19]. These findings are of particular interest in that our preliminary observations indicate that croton oil acts as a 'promoter' for papilloma induction in the gerbil, a property already well-documented for the mouse [2].

Summary

Light microscope examination of the dorsal hairy (trunk) skin of Mongolian gerbils reveals that dopa-positive melanocytes are numerous in the interfollicular epidermis at birth, but decline sharply during the first month. Electron microscope observations on the interfollicular epidermis of adult gerbils demonstrates that Langerhans cells and indeterminate cells are the dominant non-keratinocytes.

Topical application of DMBA once weekly for 9 weeks results in a striking increase in melanogenically active epidermal melanocytes. The epidermis becomes heavily melanized and there is the suggestion that some melanocytes become damaged and either dislodged from the basal layer or phagocytized by adjacent keratinocytes. There is a marked increase in dermal melanocytes and macrophages in DMBA-treated skin. Dermal blue nevus-like tumors elicited by DMBA contain cells laden with round to elliptical melanosomes. In overall response to chemical carcinogens there appears to be a striking similarity between mice and gerbils.

References

1 BARLA-SZABÓ, L.: Ejection of melanocytes and melanin from fetuses and new-born mammalian animals. Acta morph. hung. 18: 213–225 (1970).

2 BAIRD, W. M. and BOUTWELL, R. K.: Tumor-promoting activity of phorbol and four diesters of phorbol in mouse skin. Cancer Res. 31: 1074–1079 (1971).

3 BREATHNACH, A. S.; SILVERS, W. K.; SMITH, J., and HEYNER, S.: Langerhans cells in mouse skin experimentally deprived of its neural crest component. J. invest. Derm. 50: 147–160 (1968).

4 EPSTEIN, J. H.; EPSTEIN, W. L., and NAKAI, T.: Production of melanomas from DMBA-induced 'blue nevi' in hairless mice with ultraviolet light. J. natn. Cancer Inst. 38: 19–30 (1967).

5 FITZPATRICK, T. B.; QUEVEDO, W. C., jr.; SZABÓ, G., and SEIJI, M.: Melanocyte system. Biology of the melanin pigmentary system; in FITZPATRICK, ARNDT, CLARK, EISEN, VAN SCOTT and VAUGHAN Dermatology in general medicine, chap. 5, pp. 117–146 (McGraw-Hill, New York 1971).

6 KLAUS, S. N.: Effects of DMBA on melanocytes in culture. Dermatologica *148:* 104–107 (1974).

7 LERNER, A. B.: On the etiology of vitiligo and gray hair. Am. J. Med. *51:* 141–147 (1971).

8 MCDONALD, C. J.; QUEVEDO, W. C., jr.; BIENIEKI, T. C., and FAUSTO, N.: Role of melanocytes in responses of the skin of Mongolian gerbils to chemical carcinogens. J. invest. Derm. *54:* 92–93 (1970).

9 NAKAI, T.: The induction and ultrastructural study of amelanotic dermal melanocytoma in the Syrian albino hamster. Lab. Invest. *12:* 554–562 (1963).

10 NAKAI, T. and RAPPAPORT, H.: A study of the histogenesis of experimental melanotic tumors resembling cellular blue nevi. The evidence in support of their neurogenic origin. Am. J. Path. *43:* 175–199 (1963).

11 QUEVEDO, W. C., jr.; CAIRNS, J. M., and SMITH, J. A.: The effects of croton oil and 7,12-dimethylbenz(*a*)anthracene (DMBA) on melanocytes in hamsters. Am. Zoologist *1:* 381 (1961).

12 QUEVEDO, W. C., jr.: The role of melanocytes in skin carcinogenesis. Natn. Cancer Inst. Monogr. *10:* 561–575 (1963).

13 QUEVEDO, W. C., jr.; YOULE, M. C.; ROVEE, D. T., and BIENIEKI, T. C.: The developmental fate of melanocytes in murine skin; in DELLA PORTA and MÜHLBOCK Symp. Structure and Control of the Melanocyte, pp. 228–241 (Springer, Berlin 1966).

14 QUEVEDO, W. C., jr.; BIENIEKI, T. C.; MCMORRIS, F. A., and HEPINSTALL, M. J.: Environmental and genetic influences on radiation-induced tanning of murine skin; in MONTAGNA and HU Adv. Biol. Skin, vol. 8, pp. 361–377 (Pergamon Press, Oxford 1967).

15 QUEVEDO, W. C., jr. and SMITH, J.: Electron microscope observations on the postnatal 'loss' of interfollicular epidermal melanocytes in mice. J. Cell Biol. *39:* 108a (1968).

16 QUEVEDO, W. C., jr.; BIENIEKI, T. C.; FAUSTO, N., and MAGALINI, S. I.: Induction of pigmentary changes in the skin of the Mongolian gerbil by chemical carcinogens. Experientia *24:* 585–586 (1968).

17 QUEVEDO, W. C., jr.; SZABÓ, G., and VIRKS, J.: Influence of age and UV on the populations of dopa-positive melanocytes in human skin. J. invest. Derm. *52:* 287–290 (1969).

18 QUEVEDO, W. C., jr.: Genetic control of melanin metabolism within the melanin unit of mammalian epidermis. J. invest. Derm. *60:* 407–417 (1973).

19 ROHRBACH, R.: Die Stimulierung Dopaoxydase-positiver Melanocyten während der Carcinogenese der Haut. Virchow's Arch. Abt. B Zellpath. *3:* 219–228 (1969).

20 WEISS, L. W. and ZELICKSON, A. S.: Dendritic cells in developing mammalian epidermis. J. invest. Derm. *58:* 171 (1972).

Dr. WALTER C. QUEVEDO, jr., Division of Biological and Medical Sciences, Brown University, *Providence, RI 02912* (USA)

Pigment Cell, vol. 3, pp. 367–377 (Karger, Basel 1976)

Some Animal Models of
Human Hypomelanotic Disorders

K. Jimbow, W. C. Quevedo, jr., T. B. Fitzpatrick and H. Sugano

Department of Dermatology, Harvard Medical School and Massachusetts General Hospital, Boston, Mass., and Division of Biological and Medical Sciences, Brown University, Providence, R.I.

Introduction

Hypomelanosis[1], i.e. a decrease in normal melanin pigmentation, is a prominent clinical feature of a number of cutaneous disorders in man. Careful examination of a variety of pigmentary disorders has revealed differences not only in the clinical expression of hypomelanosis, but also in the underlying cellular events of which it is the ultimate expression. The present paper discusses new findings in several human pigmentary disorders that illustrate the diversity of mechanisms accounting for hypomelanosis. Some of these entities occur in animals and reasonably approximate the specific human pigmentary diseases. In such cases, the animal models to be reported provide the opportunity for clarification of the etiology of the comparable human condition.

Melanin pigmentation in man, as viewed macroscopically, reflects primarily microscopic variations in the function of the epidermal melanin unit [1]. An epidermal melanin unit consists of a melanocyte and the pool of keratinocytes with which it is associated. Melanocytes synthesize melanosomes that are acquired and transported by keratinocytes. Four major biological processes of the 'melanosome pathway' have been recog-

---

1   The terms hypomelanosis, amelanosis and depigmentation are not synonymous. 'Amelanosis' denotes a total lack of melanin. 'Depigmentation' literally means a loss of melanin that had previously existed in the melanocytes, as exemplified by the reversible circumscribed white macules that occur at the site where hydroquinone has been applied and by the irreversible circumscribed white macules that occur at the site where monobenzyl ether of hydroquinone has been applied.

nized: melanosome synthesis, melanization, transfer, and degradation. Variations in the function of epidermal melanin units are expressed in the racial differences in skin color: skin color can be differentiated by the differences in the size, rate of synthesis, and degree of melanization of melanosomes, the rate of their transfer from melanocytes to keratinocytes, and the mode of their degradation in keratinocytes [2]. This report will demonstrate that human hypomelanotic disorders that occur clinically as congenital and circumscribed can be characterized by defects in this 'melanosome pathway'.

Alteration in Synthesis or Structure of Melanosomes

1. Piebaldism
a) Macroscopic and Light and Electron Microscopic Characterization of Hypomelanosis of Piebaldism in Man
Piebaldism (PB) is characterized by hypomelanosis affecting the hair and skin in a pattern distinctive both for its distribution and for the islands of pigmentation (fig. 1a).

BREATHNACH *et al.* [3] reported that the hypomelanotic skin occurring in PB contained melanocytes that synthesize a few partially melanized melanosomes and peculiar round granules. COMINGS and ODLAND [4], however, reported an absence of melanocytes and melanosomes in such hypomelanotic lesions. In our study, none of the four subjects showed at the light microscope level the presence of dopa-positive melanocytes in the hypomelanotic lesions of skin and hair. The electron microscope revealed a total absence of functioning melanocytes, except in one case in which only one melanocyte was found in the hypomelanotic lesion of the upper thigh. This melanocyte showed abnormal, unmelanized melanosomes that were spherical in overall shape and contained a granular interior. There were no melanized melanosomes. A characteristic finding in our study was an island of the hypermelanosis located usually in the center of the hypomelanotic skin (fig. 1a). This island contained melanocytes that were normal in population density and synthesized both normal (ellipsoidal and lamellar) and abnormal (spherical and granular) melanosomes (fig. 1b, c). These melanosomes showed various degrees of melanization. These melanosomes, when transferred to keratinocytes, underwent a marked degradation within the phagosomes and often fused with each other in the lower epidermis (fig. 1b).

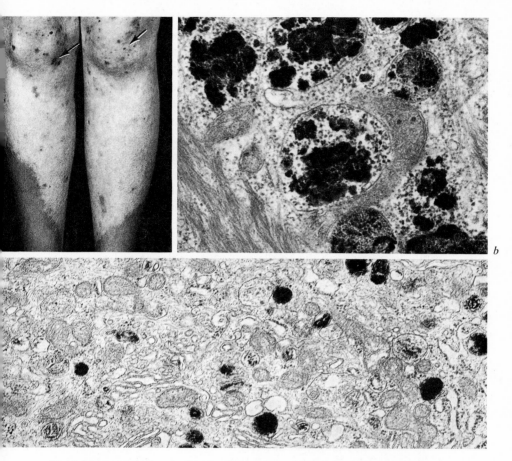

Fig. 1. Macroscopical and microscopical aspects of Piebaldism (PB). (a) Arrows indicate the islands of hypermelanosis in the center of hypomelanosis. (b) Abnormal degradation and fusion of melanosome complexes in the keratinocytes of hyper-melanotic skin. $\times$ 12,000. (c) Formation of abnormal melanosomes (i.e. spherical and granular) in the melanocytes of hypermelanotic lesion. $\times$ 10,000.

b) Comparative Characterization of Hypomelanosis of Piebaldism in Man with Animal Models

In a comprehensive study of the comparative developmental genetics of 'white-spotting' in mice, MAYER [5–8] established that specific genes influence pigment patterns by either *type 1* action at the neural-crest level, resulting in the production of cells having either no or limited ability to differentiate into melanocytes; *type 2* action at the tissue environment level, where they establish a climate hostile to or inadequate for melanoblast survival and differentiation: or *type 3*, a combination of actions at the neural-crest and tissue-environmental levels.

The survival and differentiation of melanocytes is obviously determined by the genotype of the melanoblast, which sets the minimal environmental requirements necessary for differentiation, and by the adequacy of the local tissue environment, which often changes significantly throughout embryonic and postnatal development. The animal studies may indicate that the absence of melanocytes in the hypomelanotic lesions in man is due to a similar cause. The presence of a few melanocytes in the hypomelanotic lesions of the extremities supports the view that melanoblasts in PB subjects invade all regions, with the possible exception of the white-forelock region; their failure to differentiate in some regions would then be due to the hostile environments during embryonic periods. The melanocytes that survive in the hyper- and hypomelanotic regions are not entirely normal and synthesize abnormal melanosomes with an ultrastructure similar to that of Harding-Passey mouse melanoma melanosomes. No comparable findings have been reported for the ultrastructure of melanocytes in white-spotted mice.

2. Tuberous Sclerosis
a) Macroscopic and Light and Electron Microscopic Characterization of Hypomelanosis of Tuberous Sclerosis in Man

The white macules in tuberous sclerosis (TS) occur anywhere on the body and are readily detectable, even in the fairest skin, with Wood's light (fig. 2a) [9]. They are irregularly scattered and isolated and, rarely, may follow a dermatomal distribution. A special feature of the white macules is their shape, which may be either oval or like a thumbprint or lance-ovate, the shape of the leaflet of the mountain-ash tree. In a small number of patients, the hypomelanosis may occur on the hair and skin of the scalp.

Light microscopy of split-dopa preparation of normal and hypomelanotic skin revealed no obvious difference in the population of functioning melanocytes. Within the melanocytes of the hypomelanosis, however, the perikaryon was smaller and the dendrites were less developed than those in the normal control skin of the same subject. The electron microscope showed that these melanocytes contained organelles involved in melanogenesis that were smaller in size and fewer in number than those in

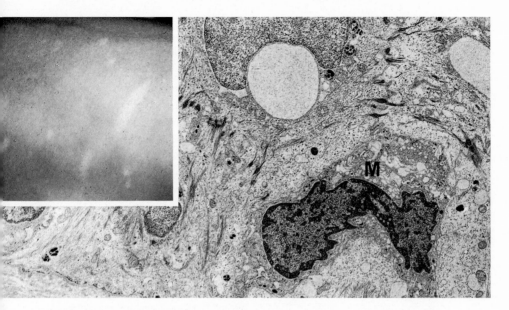

Fig. 2. Macroscopical and microscopical aspects of TS. (a) A Wood's light view of hypomelanotic lesions in a Negroid subject. (b) An electron microscopical view of hypomelanotic skin in the Negroid subject of *a*. Only a few melanosomes are seen in the melanocyte (M). Note that the melanosomes transferred to keratinocytes are all in an aggregated form, whereas in a control specimen of the same subject, the melanosomes in keratinocytes are larger in size and singly distributed. × 8,600.

the melanocytes of normal control tissues. Also, there was a reduction in the number and size of the melanosomes within the melanocytes of the hypomelanotic skin and hair. This reduction in the synthesis and size of melanosomes resulted in a decrease in population densities of melanosomes transferred to keratinocytes of the hypomelanotic skin and hair. Interestingly, most of the melanosomes transferred into keratinocytes were arranged in complexes in all the specimens examined. This aggregation of melanosomes was observed even in the hypomelanotic skin of a Negroid (fig. 2b) and in the hypomelanotic hair of a dark-haired Caucasoid, whereas in the control sites of these subjects, the melanosomes were mostly nonaggregated and singly distributed. There was no abnormal degradation of melanosomes in keratinocytes, nor was there any abnormal fusion of melanosome complexes in keratinocytes.

b) Comparative Characterization of
Hypomelanosis of Tuberous Sclerosis in Man with Animal Model

It is not yet known whether the hypomelanotic skin of TS in man results from gene action within the melanocytes or at the tissue environment. It is also not certain whether there is an animal model corresponding to human TS. In the skin of PET/mr mice, however, there are 'miniature' melanocytes that are, like the melanocytes in human TS, generally
weak in dopa reaction and smaller in overall size than typical melanocytes
[10]. These 'miniature' melanocytes did not respond to the UV irradiation
and nitrogen-mustard application that caused an increase in the number
and size of typical melanocytes of the same mice. Although the hypomelanotic skin of TS shows clinically a weak tanning reaction to UV irradiation, the question of whether the melanocytes in this hypomelanotic region will, like those in normal skin, show an increase in population, size
of perikaryon, and activity of dopa oxidase after irradiation is under
investigation.

Alteration in Melanization of Melanosomes

1. Albinism

Witkop *et al.* [11] have investigated and reviewed the several types
of albinism known to occur in man. Recently, we found a new type of albinism in which the color of the hair and skin are not totally diluted, but
the iris is translucent, which is the distinctive feature of this trend. There
is no change in visual acuity, including nystagmus, as invariably occurs in
recessive oculocutaneous albinism [12]. The propositus was a 5-year-old
boy who had, since birth, marked skin intolerance to sunlight, characterized by easy sun burning. He had blond hair, pale-blue irises and very fair
skin that tanned only slightly. Biopsy specimens of the child's exposed
skin were indistinguishable, by both light and electron microscopy, from
specimens of fair Caucasoid skin. There was a normal population of dopa-positive melanocytes with a few partially melanized melanosomes. Incubation of epilated hair bulb in tyrosine solution indicated the presence
of active tyrosinase in the follicular melanocytes. Fair skin, blond hair,
decreased tolerance of the skin to sunlight, pale-blue irises, which were
translucent and normal visual acuity without nystagmus were present in
the father, paternal uncle, and paternal grandmother, indicating a Men-
delian dominant trait for the moderate dilution of the skin and hair color.

Other members of the family, including a paternal aunt and paternal grandfather, had dark brown hair, dark skin, brown eyes, and a marked ability to tan. This heritable syndrome, which we call 'dominant oculocutaneous hypomelanosis' [12], provides an example of linkage between eye, skin, and hair color in which there are none of the serious visual defects present in the recessive oculocutaneous albinism. The possible adaptive advantage of the diluted eye color in this syndrome in a particular environmental setting remains to be determined. There does not appear to be any clear animal model for the 'dominant oculocutaneous hypomelanosis' of man.

Alteration in Transfer and Degradation of Melanosomes

1. Nevus Depigmentosus
a) Macroscopic and Light and Electron Microscopic Characterization of Nevus Depigmentosus in Man

The clinical aspects of the three patterns of hypomelanosis occurring in ND have been described in detail [13]. Briefly, these patterns are: (1) isolated, circular or rectangular, anywhere on the body but especially on the trunk; (2) typically dermatomal; (3) atypically dermatomal, with either a bizarre, sharply angulated streaking of hypomelanosis (fig. 3a), or a distribution of hypomelanosis in a whirl formation [14].

Light microscopy showed a normal population of dopa-positive melanocytes in the hypomelanotic lesions. These melanocytes, however, revealed 'stubby' dendrites, which might indicate some kind of abnormality either in the transfer and degradation of melanosomes, or in the symbiosis between melanocytes and keratinocytes. Electron microscopy revealed that the melanosomes in melanocytes are occasionally aggregated in the membrane-limited vacuoles of autophagosomes (fig. 3b). Usually, these autophagosomes contained small aggregates of 4-10 melanosomes; rarely, however, the aggregates were huge, consisting of at least 45 melanosomes. Within the vacuoles, the melanosomes often showed a partial degradation, and were associated with a myelin pattern and fine electron-dense grains (fig. 3c). In the keratinocytes, the number of melanosomes was decreased, and those transferred melanosomes showed either nonaggregated or aggregated patterns, following the genetic background of the subjects [2].

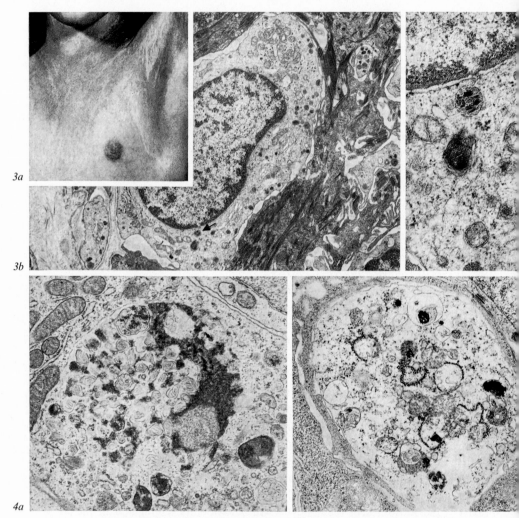

Fig. 3. Macroscopical and microscopical view of ND. (a) An atypical, dermatomal pattern of hypomelanosis. (b) An electron microscopical view of the melanocyte in the hypomelanotic skin. Note that the melanosomes in this melanocyte are
more numerous than those of TS lesion (fig. 2b). An arrow indicates the abnormal
aggregation of melanosomes in the melanocyte. × 4,900. (c) A high power view of
the melanosome aggregation within the melanocyte. Note that each melanosome is
partially degraded within a membrane-limited vacuole. × 23,500.

Fig. 4. Hypomelanosis in White Leghorn chicken feather. (a) Abnormal aggregation and degradation of melanosomes within the melanocyte. 11-day-old embryo.
× 17,000. (b) A degradation of the whole melanocyte at day 16 of embryonic
growth. × 8,000.

b) Comparative Characterization of Hypomelanosis of
Nevus Depigmentosus in Man with Animal Model

Our previous study [15] of the hypomelanosis in White Leghorn chicken feathers indicated that similar melanosome aggregation might be the cause of the hypomelanosis associated with the ND that occurs in man. In White Leghorns, these intramelanocytic aggregates of melanosomes were present in the acid-phosphatase-positive autophagic vacuoles and were presumed to be subjected to lysosomal degradation within the melanocytes before they were transferred into the epithelial cells (fig. 4a, b). It is not certain whether the intramelanocytic aggregation of the melanosomes is the cause of hypomelanosis in ND. It is remarkable, however, that melanosomes in melanocytes are more numerous in ND than in other forms of congenital circumscribed hypomelanosis, i.e. TS and PB, in which the transfer and degradation processes are not impaired, and that the number of melanosomes in the keratinocytes are decreased in ND as well as in TS. It is therefore suggested that the transfer and degradation of melanosomes are impaired in ND, perhaps through this mechanism of intramelanocytic aggregation of melanosomes.

Perspectives

The epidermal melanin unit (EMU) concept stresses that the basic mechanism for melanin pigmentation in mammals is multicellular in design, consisting of a melanocyte and an associated population of keratinocytes. It suggests that the 'melanosome pathway' of synthesis, melanization, transfer, and degradation is regulated at levels of biological organization that transcend the properties of the individual cells. The EMU represents but one expression of complex cellular interactions which are initiated during embryonic development and maintained throughout life. A variety of evidence indicates that, in adult mammals, the tissue environment may act to specify melanocyte performance. The abnormal melanosomes associated with melanocytes in hypermelanotic and hypomelanotic skin of PB subjects suggest that this is the case in man. The available animal models for human hypomelanosis may permit experimental analysis of the extent to which the observed changes in melanocytes of the hypomelanotic skin in ND and TS result from events that are intrinsic to melanocytes or are initiated at some more elevated level in the hierarchy of organization of the EMU.

Summary

Decrease or absence of melanin pigmentation in mammalian skin may involve changes in one or more of four major biological processes of melanin metabolism: the formation, melanization, transfer, and degradation of melanosomes. In broad outline, the cellular and subcellular processes operative in a number of different kinds of hypomelanosis in man have been characterized by light and electron microscopy. In some cases, there exist experimental animals which express in approximate or identical form the same manifestations.

Piebaldism in man exhibits features which based on experimental analysis in white-spotted mice might be explained by a failure of melanoblasts to invade certain areas of the embryonic skin, their failure to differentiate in certain skin regions owing to a hostile local environment, or a combination of the two factors. New ultrastructural findings suggest an important role of the local tissue environment in human piebaldism. Although melanocyte populations appear to be normal, an absence of melanin deposition within melanosomes as a result of the intrinsic genetic programming of melanocytes is found in tyrosinase negative oculocutaneous albinism in man and mice. It is not known whether the hypomelanosis of tuberous sclerosis in man results from gene action within melanocytes or through the cells of their tissue environment. A defect in melanosome transfer occurs in the feather follicle melanocytes of White Leghorn chicken embryos. As a consequence, melanosomes are retained by melanocytes and accumulated and degraded within autophagic vesicles; this event may be central to the observed programmed death of the melanocytes. The hypomelanosis of Chédiak-Higashi syndrome and nevus depigmentosus shows some of the features of melanocyte morphogenesis within White Leghorn chicken embryos. The condition in man results from complex changes in the structure and function of melanocytes.

References

1 Fitzpatrick, T. B. und Breathnach, A. S.: Das epidermale Melanin-Einheit-System. Derm. Wschr. *147:* 481 (1963).

2 Szabo, G.; Gerald, A. G.; Pathak, M. A., and Fitzpatrick, T. B.: Racial differences in the fate of melanosomes in human epidermis. Nature, Lond. *222:* 1081 (1969).

3 Breathnach, A. S.; Fitzpatrick, T. B., and Wyllie, L. M. A.: Electron microscopy of melanocytes in human piebaldism. J. invest. Derm. *45:* 28 (1965).

4 Comings, D. E. and Odland, G. F.: Partial albinism. J. Am. med. Ass. *195:* 519 (1966).

5 Mayer, T. C.: Temporal skin factors influencing the development of melanoblasts in piebald skin. J. exp. Zool. *166:* 397 (1967).

6 Mayer, T. C.: A comparison of pigment cell development in albino, steel, and dominant-spotting mutant mouse embryos. Devl Biol. *23:* 297 (1970).

7 Mayer, T. C. and Maltby, E. L.: An experimental investigation of pattern de-

velopment in lethal spotting and belted mouse embryos. Devl Biol. *9:* 269 (1964).

8   MAYER, T. C. and GREEN, M. C.: An experimental analysis of the pigment defect caused by mutations at the W and S1 foci in mice. Devl Biol. *18:* 62 (1968).

9   FITZPATRICK, T. B.; SZABO, G.; HORI, Y.; SIMONE, A. A., and REED, W. B.: White leaf-shaped macules: earliest visible sign of tuberous sclerosis. Archs Derm. *98:* 1 (1968).

10 REAMS, W. M. and HOWARD, V. M.: Refractoriness of miniature melanocytes to ultraviolet light (abstr.). J. invest. Derm. *60:* 106 (1973).

11 WITKOP, C. J.; HILL, C. W.; DESNICH, S.; THIES, J. K.; THORN, H. U.; JENKINS, M., and WHITE, J. G.: Ophthalmologic, biochemical, platelet, and ultrastructural defects in the various types of oculocutaneous albinism. J. invest. Derm. *60:* 443 (1973).

12 FITZPATRICK, T. B.; JIMBOW, K., and DONALDSON, D. D.: Dominant oculo-cutaneous albinism (abstr.). Br. J. Derm. *91:* 23 (1974).

13 JIMBOW, K.; FITZPATRICK, T. B.; SZABO, G., and HORI, Y.: Congenital circumscribed hypomelanosis: a characterization based on electron microscopic study of tuberous sclerosis, nevus depigmentosus, and piebaldism. J. invest. Derm. *64:* 50 (1975).

14 MONTGOMERY, D. W.: The cause of the streaks in naevus linearis. J. Cut. Genito-Uri. Dis. *9:* 455 (1910).

15 JIMBOW, K.; SZABO, G., and FITZPATRICK, T. B.: Ultrastructural investigation of autophagocytosis of melanosomes as programmed death of melanocytes in White Leghorn feathers: a study of morphologic events leading to hypomelanosis. Devl Biol. *36:* 8 (1974).

KOWICHI JIMBOW, MD, PhD, Department of Dermatology, Sapporo Medical College, Minami 1, *Nishi 16, Sapporo* (Japan)

Pigment Cell, vol. 3, pp. 378–383 (Karger, Basel 1976)

The Role of Melanin in Human Neurological Disorders[1]

PETER PROCTOR

Department of Physics, M. D. Anderson Hospital, Houston, Tex.

Our interest in the melanins began indirectly with investigations into the etiology of the Lesch-Nyhan syndrome (juvenile hyperuricemia). This inborn error of metabolism is characterized by a greatly increased rate of purine synthesis and of increased systemic levels of the chief purine meta-bolite, uric acid [13]. The Lesch-Nyhan syndrome is accompanied by a number of interesting neurological abnormalities; these are self-mutila-tion, hyperactivity, choreoathetosis, and psychotic behavior (e.g. our at-tention was first drawn to this disorder because of a hyperuricemic patient who had originally been misdiagnosed as a schizophrenic).

In the course of these investigations, both the ability of the purines to catalyze oxidations and the electron-donor properties of the purines were observed [18]. It was also brought to our attention that the phenothiazine tranquillizers (e.g. chlorpromazine) may also be strong electron donors. Most significantly, one of the side-effects of long-term phenothiazine treatment is choreoathetoid tardive dyskinesia; another is very striking hyperpigmentation [9], which is where melanin enters the picture [4].

A role for brain melanin in extrapyramidal diseases [4] and schizo-phrenia [9] has been suggested. Prompted by the apparent partial overlap of both symptoms and electronic structure between the Lesch-Nyhan syn-drome and phenothiazine side-effects, we attempted to determine if such symptomology represented a general case for charge-transfer agents in man. We first determined from literature sources all of the known cir-cumstances resulting in the chronic presence of charge-transfer agents in man [18].

1 Supported by a grant from the Retina Research Foundation, Houston, Tex. and by PHS Grant CA05099.

Table I. Charge-transfer agent associated disorders

Syndrome	C-T agent	Psychosis	Dyskinesia	Pigmentary abnormality
Juvenile hyperuricemia	purines	+	+	?
Dopa treatment	dopa	+	+	+ ?
Phenothiazine treatment	chlorpromazine	?	+	increased
Alcaptonuria	homogentisic acid	?	+	increased
Homocystinuria	homocysteine	+	?	decreased
Hyperthyroidism	thyroid hormones	+	+	increased
Iodism	iodide	+	?	increased
Bromism	bromide	+	+	increased
Wilson's disease	copper	+	+	increased
Manganese poisoning	Mn^{++}	+	+	?
Hemochromatosis[1]	iron	+	?	increased

References in PROCTOR [18].
Dyskinesia includes Parkinsonism, tremor, choreoathetosis, ataxia, etc.
1 deafness common

Table I lists syndromes, the charge-transfer agents associated with them, and some of their symptoms. A very striking trend emerges from table I: it appears as though two or more of three symptoms – psychosis, dyskinesia, and pigmentary abnormalities – are common to disorders involving the chronic presence of charge-transfer agents. Deafness is also present, but only occasionally. The presence of pigmentary abnormalities is particularly significant, since certain brain nuclei (e.g. the substantia nigra and the locus ceruleus) concerned with fine motor control and the regulation of sensory imput are heavily melanized. It has been suggested that this melanin is nothing more than an end product of tyrosine or catecholamine metabolism, but perhaps not.

For example, while the effects of charge-transfer agents can be explained in other fashions [18], the association of pigmentary abnormalities with neurological symptoms holds even where there is no evidence for the presence of a charge-transfer agent. A list of such disorders is given in table II. Of great interest is the common association of deafness with

Table II. Association of pigmentary abnormalities with neurological disorders

Syndrome	Psychosis	Dyskinesia	Pigmentary abnormality	Deafness
WAARDENBURG [22]	?	?	piebald	+
TELLFER et al. [21]			piebald	
JEUNE et al. [12]	?	+	pigmented spots	+
Usher's syndrome [10]	+	+	retinitis pigmentosa	+
HAMMERSCHLAG [11]	?	+	piebald	+
CROSS et al. [5]	?	+	hypopigmented	?
Varitint-Walder mouse [2]	+[1]	+	piebald	+

1 Behavioral effects analogous to those of amphetamine in mice (i.e. analogous to amphetamine psychosis in man).

many of these disorders. LINDQUIST [14] presented evidence for a role for inner ear melanin in the etiology of deafness. It may be of significance that deafness has also been reported in hyperuricemia [20] and in paranoid schizophrenia [3]. This list is also relevant to the common association of retinitis pigmentosa and other pigmentary retinopathies 10, 14 with deafness and/or ataxia.

From these clinical observations, it seems reasonable to hypothesize that melanin may play some active role in non-illuminated pigmented tissues such as the midbrain and the inner ear. What this role might be is open to question. Melanin is an electron acceptor and so forms charge-transfer complexes with electron donors such as those we have considered. Perhaps melanin acts as a kind of trap for free radicals or excited state species [17] generated in metabolic processes (for a review of the evidence for such species see CILENTO [1]). Of particular relevance are the activated forms of oxygen (singlet oxygen, superoxide anion radical or hydroxyl radical) used by leukocytes as bacteriocidal agents [15].

Another possibility is that melanin acts as an inhibitor of nervous depolarization [7]. The ability of melanin to act as a bistable switch at physiological potentials is of interest in this regard [16]. Power must be expended to switch melanin to the *on* (highly conductive) state and to keep it there. Potentials much greater than those required to switch melanin ($\sim$300 V/cm) are available near a depolarizing axon, and neuromelanin may be concentrated at the axon hillock. Perhaps the power required to switch these particles *on* means that membrane depolarization would be inhibited in the vicinity of neuromelanin particles in brain, ear, or retinal cells.

On the other hand, perhaps it is simply a question of abnormalities in melanin metabolism somehow affecting the development of the nervous system and of neural connections, as in the case of the Siamese cat [6]. Likewise, it is possible that the pigmentary abnormalities in table II merely reflect some neural crest defect or some defect in (say) trace metal or tyrosine transport or metabolism which happens to be also expressed as a pigmentary abnormality. A good example of the plethora of possibilities is provided by the Lesch-Nyhan syndrome, in which excess purine production can result in the presence of potentially melanin-binding charge-transfer agents such as the purines, the production of activated forms of oxygen such as peroxide, superoxide anion, hydroxyl radical, or singlet oxygen by uric acid or xanthine oxidase (see particularly FRIED *et al.* [8]), or the inhibition of some cerebral cyclic nucleotide phosphodiesterase by purines – all of which could affect melanized brain structure either directly or indirectly.

In summary, it seems likely that melanin plays some active role in such melanized structures as the midbrain and the inner ear, and that, at least in certain special cases, it may also have a role in the etiology of symptoms involving these structures. In the case of the midbrain, these symptoms are psychosis and dyskinesia, and in the case of the inner ear, deafness. Final definition of the role of melanin in such disorders must necessarily await the elucidation of the role of melanin in non-illuminated structures and in the retina.

In any event, the analysis presented here has some immediate clinical implications. For example, we become interested in the melanins because of the Lesch-Nyhan syndrome, but there is still no direct evidence that skin melanin metabolism is altered in this disease (although a 'greenish yellow' skin pigmentation is commonly reported). This possibility could be examined easily. Similarly, the other blanks in tables I and II suggest other unreported symptoms which might exist in some of the listed disorders.

Finally, as reported elsewhere in this symposium by my colleagues Dr. McGINNESS and Dr. CORRY, the possible role of melanin as a potentiator of cell death in drug-induced and senile deafness [14] has implications in the treatment of melanoma by the use of ultrasound and in the etiology of such diseases as Parkinsonism [19] and various retinopathies [14] in which there is an apparent specific killing of melanized tissues.

Summary

In certain human disorders, pigmentary abnormalities accompany one or more of three neurological signs – psychosis, dyskinesia, or deafness. In many cases, such signs are also associated with the chronic presence of charge-transfer agents. A few of the possible roles of melanin in the etiology of such symptoms are reviewed.

References

1 CILENTO, G.: Excited electronic states in dark biological processes. Q. Rev. Biophys. 6: 485–501 (1964).

2 COOLS, A. R.: Neurochemical correlates of the Waltzing-Shaker syndrome of the Varitint-Wadler mouse. Psychopharmacologia 24: 384–396 (1972).

3 COOPER, A. F.; CURRY, A. R.; KAY, D. W. K.; GARSIDE, R. F., and ROTH, M.: Hearing loss in paranoid and affective psychoses of the elderly. Lancet ii: 851–854 (1974).

4 COTZIAS, G. C.; PAPAVASILIOU, P. S.; WOERT, M. H. VAN, and SAKAMOTO, A.: Melanogenesis and extrapyramidal diseases. Fed. Proc. Fed. Am. Socs exp. Biol. 23: 713–717 (1964).

5 CROSS, H. E.; MCKUSICK, V. A., and BREEN, W.: A new oculocerebral syndrome with hypopigmentation. J. Pediat. 70: 3 (1967).

6 GUILLERY, R. W.; CASAGRANDE, V. A., and OBERDORFER, M. D.: Congenitally abnormal vision in Siamese cats. Nature, Lond. 252: 193–199 (1974).

7 FORREST, F. M.: Evolutionary origin of extrapyramidal disorders in drug-treated mental patients, its significance, and the role of neuromelanin; in FORREST, CARR and USDIN The phenothiazines and structurally related drugs (Raven press, Hewlett 1974).

8 FRIED, R.; FRIED, L. W., and BABIN, D. R.: Biological role of xanthine oxidase and tetrazolium-reductase inhibitor. Eur. J. Biochem. 33: 439–445 (1973).

9 GREINOR, A. C.: Schizophrenia and the pineal gland. Can. Psychiat. Ass. J. 15: 433–447 (1970).

10 HALGREN, B.: Retinitis pigmentosa combined with congenital deafness, cerebellar ataxia, and mental abnormality in a proportion of cases. Acta psychiat. scand. 34: suppl. 138, p. 1 (1959).

11 HAMMERSCHLAG, J.: Zur Kenntnis der hereditar-degenerativen Taubstummheit. VI. Über einen mutmasslichen Zusammenhang zwischen 'hereditarie Taubheit' und 'hereditarer Ataxie'. Z. Ohrenheilk. 56: 126–138 (1908).

12 JEUNE, A., et al.: Syndrome familial associant ataxie, surdite, et oligophrenie sclerose myocardique d'évolution fatale chez l'un des enfants. Pédiatrie, Lyon 18 (1963).

13 LESCH, M. and NYHAN, W. L.: A familial disorder of uric acid metabolism and central nervous system function. Am. J. Med. *37:* 561 (1964).

14 LINDQUIST, N. G.: Accumulation of drugs on melanin. Acta radiol. suppl. *325:* 1–92 (1973).

15 MAUGH, T. H.: Singlet oxygen: a unique microbicidal agent in cells. Science *182:* 44–45 (1973).

16 MCGINNESS, J.; CORRY, P., and PROCTOR, P.: Amorphous semiconductor switching in melanins. Science *183:* 853–855 (1974).

17 MCGINNESS, J. and PROCTOR, P.: The importance of the fact that melanin is black. J. theor. Biol. *39:* 677–678 (1973).

18 PROCTOR, P.: Electron-transfer factors in psychosis and dyskinesia. Physiol. Chem. Physics *4:* 349–360 (1972).

19 PROCTOR, P.; MCGINNESS, J., and CORRY, P.: A hypothesis on the preferential destruction of melanized tissues. J. theor. Biol. *48:* 19–23 (1974).

20 ROSENBERG, A.; BERGSTROM, L.; TROOST, B., and BARTHOLOMEW, B.: Hyperuricemia and neurologic deficits. New Engl. J. Med. *282:* 992–997 (1970).

21 TELLFER, M.; SUGAR, M.; JAEGER, E., and MULCAHY: Dominant piebald trait (white forelock and leucoderma) with neurological impairment. Am. J. hum. Genet. *23:* 383–389 (1971).

22 WAARDENBERG, P. J.: A new syndrome combining developmental anomalies of eyelids, eyebrows and nose root with congenital deafness. Am. J. hum. Genet. *3:* 195 (1951).

Note added in proof

An excellent review of the anatomy of neuromelanin is BAZELON *et al.,* Neurology, *17:* 512 (1967). Likewise, LAFERRIERE *et al.,* Ann. Otol. *83:* 685 (1974), have reviewed the anatomy of inner ear melanin.

Particularly worthy of note is the fact that in both retinitis pigmentosa and in the inner ear there is a tendency for melanized cells to proliferate along the vasculature, perhaps to perform a similar function. This function might be related to protecting the vasculature against sound induced free radicals which could cause hypercoagulability by generating prostaglandin-like products. Both the retina and the ear are very sensitive to hypercoagulability syndromes.

Prof. P. PROCTOR, Department of Ophthalmology, Baylor College of Medicine, *Houston, TX 77030* (USA)

Pigment Cell, vol. 3, pp. 384–392 (Karger, Basel 1976)

Degradation of Melanosomes *in vitro* and *in vivo*

Nobuya Saito and Makoto Seiji

Department of Dermatology, Tohoku Unversity, School of Medicine, Sendai

Recent electron microscopic observations have shown that melanosomes present in compound form could be disintegrated in the melanocytes [17], dermal melanophages [6], and keratinocytes [4]. Lysosomal enzyme activities were also exhibited in individual melanosomes as well as in melanosome complexes [16], and now melanosome complexes are thought to be a kind of lysosome [10].

Lysosomes are present in the epidermal cells. Biochemical studies on degradation of melanosomes by lysosomes, isolated from mouse epidermis, were carried out and revealed that melanosomes could be degraded by lysosomes at the protein moiety but not at the melanin moiety [12]. In this paper, studies on degradation of melanosomes *in vitro* by human epidermal lysosomes, and the fate of melanosomes injected into guinea pig skin are reported.

Materials and Methods

Preparation of lysosomes: The human skin samples were taken from amputated extremities obtained at the time of surgery. The age of the patients had a wide range, and both sexes were represented. The epidermis was obtained by the (slightly modified) stretch separation method discribed by Rosett *et al.* [11]. The skin was separated from the underlying tissues and stored in ice. The skin was clamped in a vise moistened with ice water, and then stretched as tightly as possible, almost to the point of tearing. The epidermis was scraped with a scalpel blade, and the scrapings were immediately placed in chilled beaker containing 0.25 M sucrose solution. All subsequent operations were performed at 0–4 °C. The epidermis was homogenized in 0.25 M sucrose (1:10 w/v) with a conical glass homogenizer [13] for 1.5 min at top speed. The homogenate thus obtained was filtered through gauze, then separated by differential centrifugation into three fractions, consisting of the precipitate of the first centrifugation at 700 g for 10 min, and the precipitate and the supernatant of the second centrifugation at 12,000 g for 15 min. Lysosomal enzyme activities of these isolated fractions were determined.

Enzyme assay: Acid phosphatase was estimated by the methods described by KIND and KING [5]. Cathepsin was determined by SHAMBERGER's [18] modification of Anson's method.

Preparation of radioactive melanosomes: The first group of male Swiss mice with Harding-Passey melanoma (1–2 cm in diameter) was given intraperitoneal injection of 10 μCi/10 g body weight of ^{14}C-amino acid mixture [protein hydrolysate-C 14 (U) 57 mCi/mM, The Radiochemical Centre, Amersham] in 0.05 ml of distilled water. A second group of mice was given 10 μCi/10 g body weight of ^{14}C-sodium acetate (Sodium acetate-2-^{14}C, 48.0 mCi/mM, Daiichi Pure Chemicals Co. Ltd, Tokyo). The third group received ^{14}C-dopa of 5 μCi/10 g body weight [L-3(3,4-dihydroxyphenyl)alanine-3-^{14}C; 9.7 mCi/mM, The Radiochemical Centre, Amersham] in 0.05 ml of distilled water in the same way. 12 h after the injections, the animals were killed. The melanomas were removed and immediately homogenized in 0.25 M ice cold sucrose. Melanosomes were prepared by the method of SEIJI et al. [14].

Digestion of the labeled melanosomes by lysosomes in vitro: The labeled melanosomes to be digested were suspended in 0.25 M sucrose solution. 0.3 ml of each suspension was mixed with 0.3 ml of 0.1 M sodium acetate and acetic acid buffer, pH 5.0 and incubated at 37 °C for 5 min. Then 0.4 ml of lysosomes suspension was added to the reaction mixtures. Incubation was carried out for 0, 15, 30, and 60 min with continuous shaking. The amounts of cell particles used in the individual experiments are indicated in figures 1–5. At the end of each incubation, the reaction mixture was centrifuged at 12,000 g for 15 min. Then an aliquot of the supernatant obtained was transfered to vials containing 10 ml of scintillating solution (methanol, 150 ml; toluene, 350 ml; dioxane, 250 ml; POPOP, 0.5 g; PPO, 5 g; naphthalene, 25 g), and the radioactivity was measured in liquid scintillation spectrometer (Aloka, LSD-601).

Degradation of labeled melanosomes in vivo: The back hair of male albino guinea pigs weighing about 400 g was shaved with electric clippers. Then the guinea pigs received intracutaneous injections of the labeled melanosomes suspended in 0.25 M sucrose solution. For one series of the experiment, five to six animals were used. 0.1 ml of labeled melanosomes were divided into five parts and each 0.02 ml of melanosomes were injected into five sites. The skin specimens were taken with a 6-mm punch at the end of two weeks, one week, four days, two days, one day and immediately after the injection. The specimens were transferred to vials and incubated with 0.3 ml of Soluene (Soluene-100, Packard Instrument Co. Inc.) at 60 °C, overnight. 10 ml of scintillating solution, as described above, was added and the radioactivities were determined.

The effect of corticosteroid on the degradation of melanosomes in vivo: 1.0 ml of melanosome suspension labeled at the protein component was mixed with 0.1 ml of corticosteroid (triamcinolone acetonide 40 mg/ml). The mixed solution was injected into guinea pig skin. Degradation of labeled melanosomes was determined as described above.

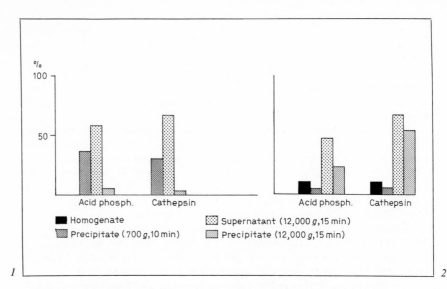

Fig. 1. Distribution of enzyme activities of the human epidermis. Most of the enzyme activities are present in the supernatant of the centrifugation at 12,000 g for 15 min. In the lysosomal fraction (the precipitate obtained after centrifugation at 12,000 g for 15 min), only a small amount of enzyme activities were detected.

Fig. 2. Specific activities of each fraction, which are expressed as relative values against that of the homogenate. In both supernatant and precipitate obtained after centrifugation at 12,000 g for 15 min, a high level of enzyme activity was found.

Results

Human epidermal lysosome: Figure 1 shows the distribution of lysosomal enzyme activity of each fraction. Most of the enzyme activities were present in the supernatant obtained after the second centrifugation at 12,000 g. The specific activities of each fraction are shown in figure 2. Higher activities were found to be present in the supernatant and precipitate obtained after centrifugation at 12,000 g. In the human epidermis, the lysosomal enzymes (acid phosphatase and cathepsin) were found to exist mainly in the soluble fraction thus prepared. In this experiment, therefore, the supernatant obtained after centrifugation at 12,000 g for 15 min, in an acetate buffer of pH 5.0, was used as the lysosomal fraction for the following digestion experiment.

Digestion of ^{14}C-amino acid-labeled melanosomes by human epider-

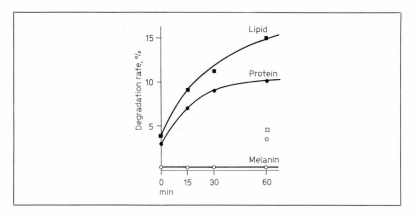

Fig. 3. Time courses of degradation of melanosomes labeled with ^{14}C-amino acids, ^{14}C-sodium acetate and ^{14}C-dopa by the action of human epidermal lysosomes. The control was incubated in the absence of added lysosome. O = ^{14}C-amino acid-labeled melanosome alone; □ = ^{14}C-sodium acetate-labeled melanosome alone. 0.3 ml of ^{14}C-amino acid-labeled melanosome suspension (1.7 mg protein, 3,140 cpm/mg protein), ^{14}C-sodium acetate-labeled melanosome (1.9 mg protein, 1,540 cpm/mg protein) and ^{14}C-dopa-labeled melanosome suspension (1.1 mg protein, 2,150 cpm/mg protein) were incubated separately with 0.4 ml of epidermal lysosomal preparation (2.1 mg protein, 748 μg phenol/60 min/mg protein) in a 0.1-M acetic acid buffer, pH 5.0 at 37 °C. After incubation for the indicated period of time, the mixture was centrifuged at 12,000 g for 15 min, and the radioactivity of the supernatant was determined. The amount of radioactivity liberated in the supernatant was expressed as a percentage of the total radioactivity used.

mal lysosomes *in vitro*: The radioactivity of the melanosomes isolated from Harding-Passey mouse melanoma injected with the ^{14}C-amino acid mixture was 3,140 cpm/mg protein. The degradation rate was expressed as a percentage of the total radioactivity of melanosomes used. As shown in figure 3, the lysosomal enzymes caused progressive solubilization of the protein component of melanosomes. At the end of 60 min, about 10% of the total radioactivity had become soluble. At zero time of incubation, the labeled melanosomes were degraded about 3%. Melanosomes incubated without the lysosomal preparation for the same period of time also showed about 4% solubility.

Degradation of lipid moiety of melanosomes by human lysosomes *in vitro*: The radioactivity of melanosomes labeled with ^{14}C-sodium acetate was 1,540 cpm/mg protein. The time course of digestion is shown in fig-

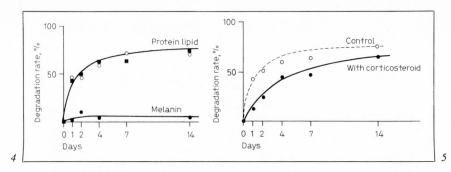

Fig. 4. Time course of degradation of melanosomes injected into guinea pig skin. Skin specimens were obtained with a 6-mm punch at indicated times and the radioactivity remaining in the injected sites was determined. Degradation rates of protein moiety (■), lipid moiety (O), and melanin moiety (●) are shown. The degradation rates of protein and lipid moiety was almost within the same range.

Fig. 5. The effect of corticosteroid on the degradation of melanosomes *in vivo.* Melanosomes labeled with ^{14}C-amino acids were mixed with corticosteroid (40 mg/ml triamcinolone acetonide, 1:10 v/v) (●). The control group received labeled melanosomes without corticosteroid (O).

ure 3. Progressive degradation was noticed. The degradation rate at the end of 60 min, zero time and without lysosomes were 25, 3.5 and 5%, respectively. It appeared that in melanosomes the lipid component was more fragile than the protein component.

Resistance of melanin moiety of melanosomes to degradation by human lysosomes *in vitro:* The radioactivity of the melanosomes labeled with ^{14}C-dopa was 2,150 cpm/mg protein. Figure 3 reveals that the melanosomes had not undergone any significant change, even at the end of 60 min. Melanin appears to be very resistant to lysosomal digestion *in vitro.*

Degradation of melanosomes *in vivo:* The degradation was expressed as a disappearence of radioactivity from the injected site. The rate was expressed as a percentage of the radioactivities injected. As shown in figure 4, the protein and lipid moiety of melanosomes were degraded and disappeared progressively with time from the injected site. The degradation rates of protein and lipid were in almost the same range. One day after injection, the degradation rate of protein and lipid of melanosomes reached about 45%. The final degradation rates of both components were about 75%. On the contrary, even at the end of two weeks after injection, no changes were noticed in the radioactivities of the melanin moiety. *In vivo* as well as *in vitro,* the protein and lipid moiety of melanosomes could be degraded, but the melanin moiety was not.

The effects of corticosteroid on the degradation of melanosomes *in vivo:* The time course of degradation of melanosomes mixed with corticosteroid is shown in figure 5, thus showing that corticosteroid decreased the degradation rate of the protein component of the melanosomes; the shorter the time after injection, the more effective the action of corticosteroid. After one day, the degradation of protein moiety was prevented about 45% by corticosteroid and at the end of two weeks, about 20%.

Discussion

The presence of lysosomes has been demonstrated in the epidermal cells of human and animal skin with electron microscopic [20], histochemical [3] and biochemical [12] methods. It is generally believed that lysosomes are localized in light mitochondrial fractions [1]. But most of the lysosomal enzyme activities of the human epidermis were found to be localized in the supernatant obtained after centrifugation at 12,000 g for 15 min. We have obtained exactly the same results with rat epidermis [12] and similar results have been reported elsewhere [19]. It is thought that the force required to sufficiently homogenize the epidermis is stronger than that needed for other tissues; thus, the lysosomes of the epidermis may be broken up during preparation [2, 12]. The glass conical homogenizer was used to homogenize the epidermis, since it was not possible to obtain a good human epidermal homogenate with the teflon homogenizer.

Morphological figures showing disintegration of melanosomes have been demonstrated in aged melanoma melanocytes [17], melanophages in the dermis [6] and in the keratinocytes [4], and the lysosomal enzyme activity was found to be present in individual melanosomes as well as compound melanosomes [16]. It is thought that lysosomes are closely related to the degradation mechanisms [7] and melanosome complexes, in which disintegration of melanosomes are seen, are lysosomes themselves [10]. Biochemical studies *in vitro* on the degradation of melanosomes by mouse liver lysosomes [9] and by rat epidermal lysosomes [12] have been carried out. In these studies, we came to the conclusion that in degradation the site attacked first would be the protein part which constitutes the skeleton of the melanosome. Experimental results showed that melanosomes were degraded at the protein and lipid moieties by lysosomal enzymes. It is assumed that in the melanoma tissues, injected ^{14}C-amino acids and ^{14}C-sodium acetate are incorporated into protein and lipid moiety of melanosomes, respectively. The ^{14}C-dopa injected into mice with melanomas is known to incorporate specifically into the newly synthesized melanin of melanosomes [15]. As shown in figure 3, the protein and lipid moiety of melanosomes were progressively degraded; on the other hand, the melanin moiety was resistant and not digested at all. In experiments *in vivo*, it is assumed that the decrease in radioactivity at the site injected is due to the degradation and disappearance of the protein moiety of melanosomes. *In vivo*, as well as *in vitro*, the degradation was observed only in the protein and lipid moiety but not in the melanin moiety.

Melanosomes consist of the outer membrane and inner membranous matrix, on which the deposition of melanin takes place. The membrane of melanosomes presumably consists of protein and lipid. Therefore, it appears that in the degradation of melanosomes, *in vitro* and *in vivo*, the initial change produced may be the disintegration of the membranous component of melanosomes; on the contrary, melanin *per se* is very tough and scarcely ever destroyed by lysosomal enzymes.

It has been said that the majority of melanosomes injected into the dermis of the hamster are phagocytized by macrophages in less than 24 h and melanosome complexes were formed [8]. At present, the melanosome complex is believed to be some kind of lysosome [10], and it is well-known that corticosteroids have a stabilizing action on lysosomes. The corticosteroid, when injected with melanosomes, showed an inhibitory effect on the degradation of melanosomes *in vivo*. These findings will be one more piece of evidence to support the hypothesis that the degradation of melanosomes *in vivo* is carried out by lysosomes.

Summary

The degradation of melanosomes by epidermal lysosomes was studied *in vitro*. The majority of the lysosomal enzymes activities were localized in the supernatant obtained after centrifugation at 12,000 g for 15 min. The protein, lipid and melanin moieties of mouse melanoma melanosomes were labeled with [14]C. Digestion of these labeled melanosomes was carried out with lysosomes of human epidermis. The progressive degradation of the protein and lipid moiety of the melanosomes was observed; but there was no significant degradation of the melanin moiety. Labeled melanosomes were injected intracutaneously into the back of guinea pigs. Radioactivity of protein and lipid moiety disappeared progressively from the injection site. But at the end of two weeks, almost all radioactivity of the melanin moiety remained at the site where the melanin-labeled melanosomes were injected. It is assumed, therefore, that melanosomes can be degraded by lysosomes at the protein and lipid moieties, but not at the melanin moiety, *in vitro* as well as *in vivo*.

References

1   DUVE, C. DE; PRESSMAN, B. C.; GIANETTO, R.; WATTIAUX, R., and APPELMANS, F.: Tissue fractionation studies. 6. Intracellular distribution patterns of enzymes in rat-liver tissue. Biochem. J. *60:* 604–617 (1955).
2   DICKEN, C. H. and BECKER, R. H.: Biochemical evidence for the presence of lysosomes in the epidermis. J. invest. Derm. *47:* 426–431 (1966).
3   HALL, J. H.; SMITH, J. G., jr., and BURNETT, S. C.: The lysosome in contact dermatitis. A histochemical study. J. invest. Derm. *49:* 590–594 (1967).
4   HORI, Y.; TODA, K.; PATHAK, M. A.; CLARK, W. H., jr., and FITZPATRICK, T. B.: A fine-structure study of the human epidermal melanosome complex and its acid phosphatase activity. J. Ultrastruct. Res. *25:* 109–120 (1968).
5   KIND, P. R. N. and KING, E. J.: Estimation of plasma phosphatase by determination of hydrolysed phenol with aminoantipyrine. J. clin. Path. *7:* 322–326 (1954).
6   MISHIMA, Y.: Cellular and subcellular activities in the ontogeny of nevocytic and melanocytic melanomas; in MONTAGNA and HU Adv. Biol. Skin, vol. 8 (Pergamon Press, Oxford 1966).
7   MISHIMA, Y. and ITO, R.: Electron microscopy of microfocal necrosis in malignant melanomas. Cancer, Philad. *24:* 185–193 (1969).
8   MISHIMA, Y.: Lysosomes and skin disease. Taisha, Tokyo *9:* 274–287 (1972).
9   OHTAKI, N. and SEIJI, M.: Degradation of melanosomes by lysosomes. J. invest. Derm. *57:* 1–5 (1971).
10   OLSON, R. L.; NORDQIST, J., and EVERETT, M. A.: The role of epidermal lysosomes in melanin physiology. Br. J. Derm. *83:* 189–199 (1970).
11   ROSETT, T.; FOGG, J. B., and CLARK, J. L.: Studies in the biochemistry of skin. III. Substrate utilization by cell-free extracts of adult rat epidermis. J. invest. Derm. *41:* 385–390 (1963).
12   SAITO, N. and SEIJI, M.: Epidermal lysosome and the degradation of melanosomes. Acta derm-vener., Stockh., suppl. *73:* 69–74 (1973).
13   SANTOIANNI, P. and ROTHMAN, S.: Deoxyribonucleic acid microdetermination in human epidermis. J. invest. Derm. *40:* 317–323 (1963).
14   SEIJI, M.; SHIMAO, K.; BIRBECK, M. S. C., and FITZPATRICK, T. B.: Subcellular localization of melanin biosynthesis. Ann. N. Y. Acad. Sci. *100:* 493–533 (1963).
15   SEIJI, M. and IWASHITA, S.: Intracellular localization of tyrosinase and site of melanin formation in melanocyte. J. invest. Derm. *45:* 305–314 (1965).
16   SEIJI, M. and KIKUCHI, A.: Acid phosphatase activity in melanosomes. J. invest. Derm. *52:* 212–216 (1969).

17 SEIJI, M. and OHTAKI, N.: Lysosomes in mouse melanoma. J. invest. Derm. *56:* 436–440 (1971).
18 SHAMBERGER, R. J.: Lysosomal enzyme changes in growing and regressing mammary tumours. Biochem. J. *111:* 375–383 (1969).
19 SMITH, J. G., jr.; YARDLEY, H. J.; ROSSETT, T., and MOORE, M. J.: Lysosomal enzymes in rat epidermis. J. clin. Invest. *45:* 1074 (1966).
20 WOLFF, K. and SCHREINER, E.: Epidermal lysosomes. Archs Derm. *101:* 276–286 (1970).

Prof. N. SAITO, Department of Dermatology, Tohoku University, School of Medicine, *Sendai 980* (Japan)

Pigment Cell, vol. 3, pp. 393–405 (Karger, Basel 1976)

Melanocyte-Keratinocyte Interaction in Pigment Transfer[1]

M. Seiji, K. Toda, K. Okazaki, M. Uzuka, F. Morikawa and M. Sugiyama

Department of Dermatology, Tohoku University School of Medicine, Sendai; Department of Dermatology, Tokyo Teishin Hospital, Tokyo; Shiseido Laboratories, Yokohama, and Yone Production, Tokyo

Introduction

In mammals, the so-called 'epidermal melanin unit' is functioning to maintain the normal skin and hair color [3, 13] and the melanin transfer step constitutes one of the four steps: melanin formation in melanocyte, melanosome transfer, dispersion of melanosomes in the keratinocyte, turnover of keratinocytes and degradation of melanosomes. The transfer mechanisms have been studied with light and electron microscope on epidermis [17, 19] hair [9, 11] and cell culture system [1, 2, 5, 6, 8, 10, 16]. It is now generally assumed that the transfer of melansomes occurs directly from cell to cell and a portion of the melanosome accumulated dendrite of melanocyte is phagocytized by the keratinocyte [1, 2, 4, 6, 8, 10], then melanosomes thus transferred disperse within the cytoplasm of the keratinocyte [5, 15, 19, 20].

The light and electron microscopic studies were carried out in order to clarify the exact sequences of melanosome transfer which takes place between melanocyte and keratinocyte in cell culture and hair follicle. The cells were observed with the time-lapse cinematography and scanning and transmission electron microscopes. Some of the results obtained are reported in this paper.

1   This work was partly supported by research grants from the Ministry of Education, Japan.

Materials and Methods

1) Epidermal cell culture: Thiersch grafts of the black guinea pig ear were incubated in the 1% trypsin solution at 37 °C for 30 min, the dermis was separated manually, then the epidermis sheets were squeezed, shaken and pulled about with forceps. The resulting cell suspension was centrifuged at 1,000 rpm for 5 min. The sediment was resuspended in the culture medium and cultured in the Rose-chamber or Falcon plastic Petri dishes at 37 °C for several days, and the culture medium was changed every other day. The culture medium used was Eagle's minimum essential medium supplemented with 20% fetal bovine serum.

2) Hair follicle tissue culture: The hair follicles were isolated manually from the newborn C57 mouse skin and cultured in Rose chamber containing Eagle's minimum essential medium supplemented with 20% fetal bovine serum.

3) Observations: The cell behaviors were recorded with time-lapse cinematography with both a phase contrast and a usual transmission light microscope; they were used as occasion demanded during the observation. For the electron microscopic observation, the cells were fixed at appropriate time during the analysis of time-lapse sequences in 2.5% glutaraldehyde and 2% osmium tetroxide solution in 0.06 M veronal acetate buffer, pH 7.2, containing 4.5% sucrose for 20 min at 4 °C. Then they were subjected to the transmission and scanning electron microscopic observations following the routine dehydration, embedding, cutting and staining procedures, and/or dehydration and coating procedures, respectively.

Results

Epidermal Cell Culture System

1) Light microscopic observations: By the end of one week, the cultures became well established and melanocytes and keratinocytes were numerous. The keratinocytes were flattened and formed sheets, the melanocytes had multiple dendrites and a large number were associated with keratinocytes. Melanosome donation was seen from the melanocytes to the keratinocytes. It appeared to begin with the contact of the actively ruffling keratinocyte membrane and the tip of the branching process of melanocyte. The tip of the dendrite containing many melanosomes seemingly penetrated into the keratinocyte, then the tip of dendrite appeared to be constricted and formed a small pouch (fig. 1). The constriction, however, was almost but not completed, the pouch was still connected with a fine string to the stem of the dendrite. 3 h later, the pouch appeared to be cut off completely from the dendrite. Then the pouch, phagocytized in the cytoplasm of the keratinocyte, gradually moved toward the perinuclear area where it tended to disperse singly or

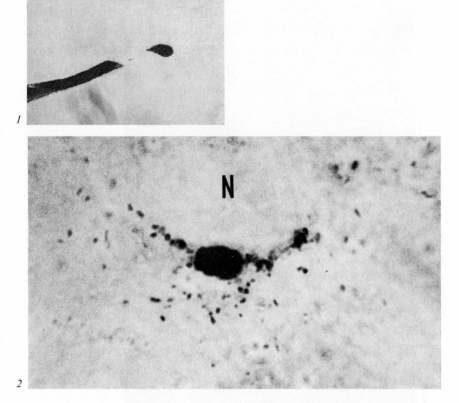

Fig. 1 and 2. Showing melanosome transfer processes taking place between cultured melanocyte and epidermal cell. A usual transmission light microscope was used. A melanocyte dendrite was constricted and about cut off by the keratinocyte (fig. 1). Melanosomes were dispersing from the cluster of melanosomes (fig. 2).

as a group of few melanosomes (fig. 2). Melanosomes were transferred from the melanocyte to the keratinocyte as a cluster enclosed with the cytoplasmic membrane of the dendritic process of melanocyte.

2) Scanning electron microscopic observation: Figure 3 shows one of the typical views of epidermal cell culture obtained from newborn guinea pig skin. One melanocyte with two long slender dendrites and a short one was in contact with two keratinocytes. The tip of the dendrite seen on the left was introduced in the cytoplasm of the keratinocyte, and seemed to be at the constricted stage. The cytoplasm of the melanocyte

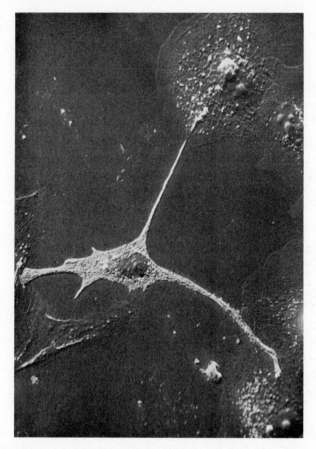

Fig. 3. A scanning electron microscopic picture of epidermal cell culture obtained from the guinea pig skin. A melanocyte was in contact with keratinocytes with its slender long two dendrites. ×600.

was found to be filled with uniform small particles. The margin of the cytoplasm of keratinocyte was clearly seen so that the relationship between the dendrite of melanocyte and the keratinocyte cytoplasm could be defined more precisely.

3) Transmission electron microscopic observations: Various steps of melanosome transfer from the melanocyte to the keratinocyte are observed in more details in the vertical sections of the cultured cells. Figure 4 shows that a tip of the dendrite of melanocyte was penetrated into the keratinocyte and enfolded with the cytoplasmic membrane and with

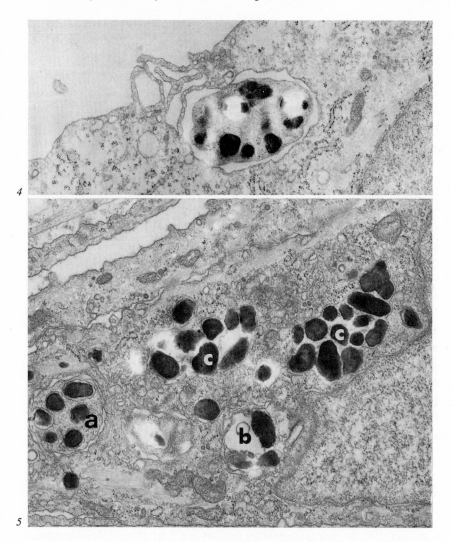

Fig. 4. A transmission electron microscopic picture showing a part of cultured epidermal cell. A cross section of a melanocyte dendrite which was enfolded with keratinocyte cytoplasm and several microvillus-like projections. ×16,000.

Fig. 5. A vertical section of epidermal cell culture. Several keratinocytes were piled up in layers, and one of these cells contained various types of packages of melanosomes. ×16,000. a = A package surrounded with two layers of membranes; b = a package surrounded with one outer membrane and one diminishing membrane, and c = packages surrounded with an apparently single membrane.

several villus-like cytoplasmic projections of this keratinocyte. Figure 5 shows a typical electron microscopic picture of the cultured cells obtained from adult guinea pig ear. The horizontal line indicates the surface of the Falcon plastic dish on which cells have grown. It seems to represent various stages of the melanosome transfer in cell culture system. One group of melanosomes, seen left, most 'a' was assumed to represent the phagocytized stage of the tip of the dendrite. There were two concentric layers of membranes. In this package, cytoplasmic constituents of melanocyte, like free ribosomes, outer membranes of melanosomes and fibrils were seen apparently intact. In the other type of group of melanosomes, 'b', seen in the lower middle, the outer membrane seemed to be intact, but the inner membrane and the outer membranes of individual melanosomes were vague, and the other cytoplasmic constituents of melanocyte seemed to be in digestion. Another type of the group of melanosomes is shown at the right, 'c'. Aggregate of melanosomes, in which no cytoplasmic constituents could be seen except melanosomes which do not possess their outer membranes, was surrounded by a single membrane. The changes in these membranes and cytoplasmic elements seemed to occur at the same time. There seems to be present a general tendency in distribution of these groups of melanosome aggregates. They were in sequence from periphery to nucleus; the enfolded tip of dendrite, the phagocytized dendrite in which the digestion of cytoplasmic constituents of melanocyte is in progress, and the aggregate of melanosomes which do not possess their outer membranes surrounded by a single membrane.

Hair Follicle Tissue Culture

Light microscopic observations: The newborn mouse hair isolated usually could survive and grow as long as for 8 h in the culture medium. Figure 6 shows a typical view of the hair follicular cells in tissue culture. As shown in figure 6, melanocytes were located in the upper part of the picture and extended their long dendritic processes among the cortical cells which were not visible under the transmission light microscope used. Several dendritic processes were seen to contain many melanosomes. The transfer of melanosomes was assumed to be in progress. Small package of melanosomes indicated with arrow, appeared to be transferred to the cytoplasm of the cortical cells.

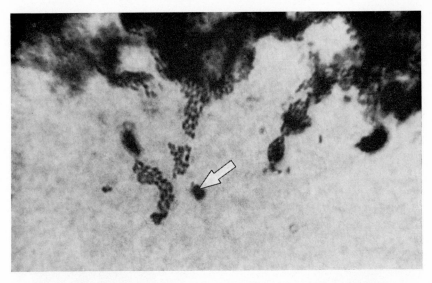

Fig. 6. Transmission light microscopic picture of cultured newborn mouse hair follicle. Melanocytes were located in upper part and extended their long dendritic processes among cortical cells which were not visible. The individual melanosomes were seen to be filled in these dendrites and a small package of melanosomes indicated by the arrow appeared to be transferred to the cytoplasm of the cortical cells. × 1,000.

Hair Follicle

Transmission electron microscopic observations: The cross section of hair bulb of C3H mouse was made and observed under the electron microscope in order to study the melanosome transfer processes from the melanocyte to the cortical cells in the hair. Figure 7 shows characteristic views of the melanocyte-keratinocyte interaction in the hair follicle. The slender dendritic process of melanocyte, which contained three round melanosomes, was located between two cortical cells. The upper cortical cell contained two packages of melanosomes, one of which was surrounded by two concentric layers of membranes and the cytoplasmic cell constituents were seemingly intact; the other of which showed that the inner membrane and the cytoplasmic constituents were assumed to be disintegrating. This cell also contained two single melanosomes with outer membranes. Figure 8 shows a part of cortical cell in which

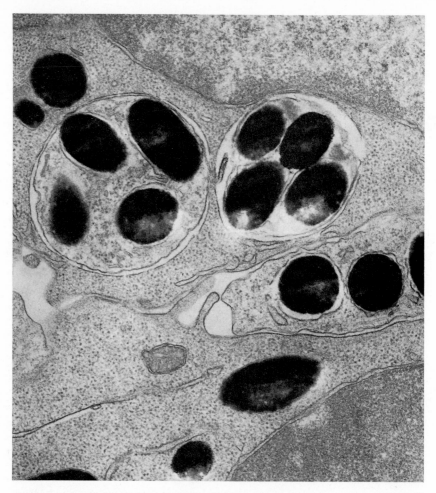

Fig. 7. A part of cross section of cortical cells in the C3H mouse hair bulb. The upper cortical cell contained two packages of melanosomes, one of which was surrounded by two concentric layers of membranes, and the other of which by a single membrane and the cytoplasmic constituents appeared to be in disintegration. ×33,000.

the dispersion process of melanosomes from the melanosome package was shown. On the upper right, there was a package of melanosomes which was surrounded by a single membrane, and cytoplasmic constituents were not seen between individual melanosomes and the outer membranes of these melanosomes were also not seen. Several single me-

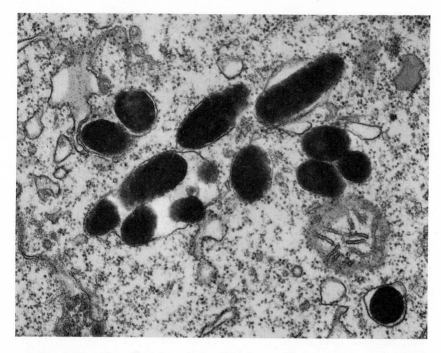

Fig. 8. The other part of cortical cell is shown. There are seen several single melanosomes and few melanosome complexes. They are assumed to be in the dispersion process. $\times$ 33,000.

lanosomes with outer membranes were scattered, and a melanosome complex was seen. In the case of hair follicle where keratinocytes are constructed in a highly organized fashion and melanocytes are well matured, the tip of dendrite of the melanocyte would be phagocytized by the cortical cell as a continuous minor event.

Discussion

The usual transmission light microscopic observation was extensively used in this series of time-lapse cinematography, so that behavior of the individual melanosome, as shown in figures 1, 2, and 6, could be observed clearly during the transfer process occurring between melanocyte and keratinocyte. It was revealed that individual melanosomes were

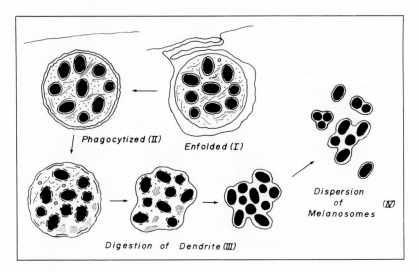

Fig. 9. Schematic illustration of melanosome transfer and dispersion.

never released from the dendritic processes but appeared to separate individually or as a group from the pouch in which melanosomes were
filled after it reached near the nucleus of the keratinocyte. The results
obtained at the light microscopic level showed definitely that the melanosome transfer process *in vitro* is, as has been inferred, a cytophagocyto-
lytic one. The cultured cells were fixed and embedded frequently during
light microscopic observations for transmission electron microscopic
studies. The serial thin sections were made in order to get the right sections where various steps of melanosome transfer and the dispersion
step of melanosomes are shown. The results, shown in figures 4, 5, 7,
and 8, will indicate the crucial evidence to support the hypothesis that
the melanosome transfer *in vivo* and *in vitro* is carried out with the cy-
tophagocytic mechanism. The tip of dendrite of melanocyte is assumed
to be enfolded, and a cluster of melanosomes is embedded in a cytoplasmic matrix surrounded by two membranes: one derived from the
melanocyte, and the other belonging to the epidermal cell. The dispersion
process is assumed to take place at the final stage, since melanosomes
were found to be distributed – small ones to be complexed, and large
ones to be dispersed singly in the cytoplasm of the recipient keratinocyte
[7, 14, 15, 17–20].

From these light and electron microscopic observations, the transfer mechanisms of melanosomes from melanocyte to keratinocyte *in vitro* and *in vivo* are assumed to take place as follows (fig. 9): The tip of the dendrite of melanocyte is penetrated into the keratinocyte, then it is enfolded for a while with the cell membrane of keratinocyte (enfolded, I). Then the dendrite appears to be squeezed and cut off by the keratinocyte to form a pouch filled with many melanosomes. The size of the pouch formed appears to depend on both the nature of melanocyte, mature or immature, and the situation of the keratinocyte (in cell culture or tissue) in which they are highly organized (phagocytized, II). There are two membranes; the inner membrane is derived from the melanocyte, and the outer one from the keratinocyte, surrounding a mass of melanosomes. Among melanosomes, there are present cytoplasmic constituents of the dendrite of melanocyte which are apparently intact. The resulting pouch gradually moves toward the nucleus of the keratinocyte, during which the digestive process is assumed to take place in this pouch (digestion of dendrite, III), i.e. the inner membrane derived from melanocyte and cytoplasmic constituents of melanocyte disintegrate, probably by lysosomes. At the end of this stage, the pouch can be found to consist of a single envelope membrane and aggregated melanosomes without their outer membranes. Then, aggregated melanosomes seem to release into the cytoplasm; melanosomes are scattered from the pouch individually and/or as a few groups depending on their sizes; larger melanosomes to be single and smaller ones to be complexed (dispersion of melanosomes, IV). Individual melanosomes appear to acquire their outer membranes again at the final stage.

Summary

Guinea pig ear epidermal cells and newborn mouse hair were grown in cell culture systems and observed with time-lapse cinematography and electron microscopy. In the monolayer cell culture, the tip of melanocyte dendrite contained numerous melanosomes, penetrated into the keratinocyte, and formed large balloon-like structures which were then pinched off by the keratinocyte. Under the electron microscope, large groups of melanosomes were found in the keratinocytes to be either enfolded dendrites or melanosome aggregates, which were then dispersed into cytoplasm singly or in complexes of several melanosomes. Keratinocytes and melanocytes in the hair are arranged in an organized fashion, thus melanosome transfer appeared to be carried out as a continuous regular minor event.

References

1   Cohen, J. and Szabo, G.: Study of pigment donation *in vitro*. Expl Cell Res. *50:* 418–434 (1968).

2   Cruckshank, C. N. D. and Harcourt, S. A.: Pigment donation *in vitro*. J. invest. Derm. *42:* 183–184 (1964).

3   Fitzpatrick, T. B. und Breathnach, A. S.: Das epidermale Melanin Einheit-System. Derm. Wschr. *147:* 481–488 (1963).

4   Hori, T.; Toda, K.; Pathak, M. A.; Clark, W. H., jr., and Fitzpatrick, T. B.: A fine structure study of the human epidermal melanosome complex and its acid phosphatase activity. J. Ultrastruct. Res. *25:* 109–120 (1968).

5   Klaus, S. N.: Post-transfer digestion of melanosome complexes and saltatory movement of melanin granules within mammalian epidermal cells. J. invest. Derm. *53:* 440–444 (1969).

6   Klaus, S. N.: Pigment transfer in mammalian epidermis. Archs Derm. *100:* 756–762 (1969).

7   Konrad, K. and Wolff, K.: Hyperpigmentation, melanosome size, and distribution patterns of melanosomes. Archs Derm. *107:* 853–860 (1973).

8   Moellmann, G.; MacGuire, J., and Lerner, A. B.: Intracellular dynamics and the fine structure of melanocytes with special reference to the effects of MSH and cyclic AMP of microtubules and 10-nm filaments. Yale J. Biol. Med. *46:* 337–360 (1973).

9   Mottaz, J. H. and Zelickson, A. S.: Melanin transfer: A possible phagocytic process. J. invest. Derm. *49:* 605–610 (1967).

10 Prunieras, M.: Interactions between keratinocytes and dendritic cells. J. invest. Derm. *52:* 1–17 (1969).

11 Ruprecht, K. W.: Pigmentierung der Dunenfeder von *Gallus domesticus* L. Licht- und elektronenmikroskopische Untersuchungen zur Melanosomen-übertragung. Z. Zellforsch. *112:* 396–413 (1971).

12 Szabo, G.: Photobiology of melanogenesis: cytological aspects with special sequence of differences in racial coloration; in Montagna and Hu The pigment system. Adv. Biol. Skin, vol. 8, pp. 379–396 (Pergamon Press, Oxford 1967).

13 Szabo, G.; Gerald, A. B.; Pathak, M. A., and Fitzpatrick, T. B.: Racial differences in the fate of melanosomes in human epidermis. Nature, Lond. *222:* 1081–1082 (1969).

14 Toda, K.; Pathak, M. A.; Parrish, J. A., and Fitzpatrick, T. B.: Nongenetic factors affecting melanosome complexes. J. invest. Derm. *56:* 255 (1971).

15 Toda, K.; Pathak, M. A.; Parrish, J. A., and Fitzpatrick, T. B.: Alteration of racial differences in melanosome distribution in human epidermis after exposure to ultraviolet light. Nature new Biol. *236:* 143–145 (1972).

16 Wikswo, M. A. and Szabo, G.: Effects of cytochalasin B on mammalian melanocytes and keratinocytes. J. invest. Derm. *59:* 163–169 (1972).

17 Wolff, K. and Konrad, K.: Melanin pigmentation: an *in vivo* model for studies of melanosome kinetics within keratinocytes. Science *174:* 1034–1035 (1971).

18 Wolff, K. and Konrad, K.: Phagocytosis of latex beads by epidermal keratinocytes *in vivo*. J. Ultrastruct. Res. *39:* 262–280 (1972).

19 WOLFF, K.: Melanocyte-keratinocyte interactions *in vivo:* the fate of melanosomes. Yale J. Biol. Med. *46:* 384–396 (1973).
20 WOLFF, K.; JIMBOW, K., and FITZPATRICK, T. B.: Experimental pigment donation *in vitro*. J. Ultrastruct. Res. *47:* 400–419 (1974).

M. SEIJI, MD, PhD, Department of Dermatology, Tohoku University School of Medicine, 1–1 Seiryo-machi, *Sendai* (Japan)

Glossary

ACTH. See Adrenocorticotrophic hormone.

Adenosine triphosphate (ATP). A nucleotide synthesized mainly in mitochondria, through the Embden-Meyerhof pathway; principal means of cellular energy transfer; present in cytoplasm and nucleus of the cell. Cyclic AMP is formed from ATP by adenyl cyclase. See Adenyl cyclase, Cyclic AMP, Embden-Meyerhof pathway, and Mitochondria.

Adenyl cyclases. A group of enzymes which catalyze the formation of cyclic AMP from ATP in response to specific hormones such as MSH, ACTH, epinephrine, glucagon, luteinizing hormone, antidiuretic hormone, and others. Normal melanocytes, and at least some melanoma cells, have adenyl cyclase systems which respond specifically to MSH. Non-MSH-responsive adenyl cyclases are found in other tissues. See Adenosine triphosphate, Cyclic AMP, ACTH, Ephinephrine, and MSH.

Adrenaline. See Epinephrine.

Adrenergic nerves. Postganglionic sympathetic nerves, activated by, or liberating norepinephrine (noradrenaline). The melanophores of teleost fishes are adrenergically innervated; their α-adrenergic receptors mediate melanosome aggregation, while their β-adrenergic receptors are involved in pigment dispersion. See Norepinephrine.

Adrenochrome. A red oxidation product of adrenaline.

Adrenocorticotrophic hormone (ACTH). Polypeptide hormone produced by the anterior lobe of the pituitary, in response to stressful stimuli, resulting in the production of corticosteroids by the adrenal cortex. The action of ACTH in stimulating the nutrition, growth, and function of the adrenal cortex is mediated by cyclic AMP. The first 13 amino acids in the ACTH polypeptide chain are identical with those of the α-melanocyte-stimulating hormone (MSH). See Corticosterone, MSH, and Cyclic AMP.

Albinism. Congenital absence or reduction of pigment. An inborn error of metabolism, inherited as an autosomal recessive trait, characterized by the partial or total absence of melanin in the skin, hair, and eyes. The melanocytes are structurally normal; however, there is probably a block of deficiency in the pathway between tyrosine and melanin. Albinos are rarely afflicted with melanoma, but have a high incidence of squamous cell carcinoma.

Allogeneic. Pertaining to genetically dissimilar individuals of the same species.

Allogeneic inhibition. The growth inhibitory effects on cells, due to an antigenic dissimilarity, which allogeneic cells exert on each other when in contact, both *in vitro* and *in vivo.*

Allograft. A graft derived from an allogeneic donor.

Amelanotic melanoma. Malignant neoplasm, derived from melanocytes, but not forming melanin. See Melanoma.

Aminophylline. One of the family of methylxanthines which inhibit phosphodiesterase; it is used in the measurements of adenyl cyclase activity to prevent hydrolysis of accumulating cyclic AMP. See Adenyl cyclases, Cyclic AMP.

Antibody-mediated immunity. Humoral immunity depending directly or indirectly on the capacity of circulating protective antibodies to intercept antigens, which are then neutralized or opsonized.

ATP. See Adenosine triphosphate.

Autochthonous. Found in the part of the body in which it originates, as in the case of an autochthonous tumor; a spontaneous tumor borne by the host of origin.

Autologous. Derived from the subject itself.

B-16 mouse melanoma. A spontaneous, metastasizing pigmented melanoma, which arose in the skin, at the base of the ear, in a C57BL/6J strain mouse in 1954. It is transplantable in the strain of origin. Most lines carry the LDH-elevating virus. See Melanoma, LDH-virus.

Basal cells. Cells forming the basal layer of the stratum germinativum of the epidermis. Basal cells are the principle dividing cell population, and are especially subject to actinic neoplastic transformation. Since melanocytes frequently accompany basal cell tumors, the pigment they produce may lead to an erroneous clinical diagnosis of melanoma. This is of prognostic importance since basal cell carcinomas are relatively benign compared with melano-carcinoma.

Birthmark. A circumscribed benign growth in the skin which is evident at birth and frequently pigmented. A congenital nevus of any type. See Nevus.

Bloch reaction. Development of melanin *in vitro*; observed in melanocytes following the addition of dopa, described by the Swiss dermatologist, B. BLOCH, 1878–1933.

Blue nevus. A nevus, covered by smooth skin, which appears to be blue, or blue-black. The lesion is composed of pigmented spindle cells in the lower dermis; the unusual color is due to the quantity of melanin and its location in the dermis. Clinically, there are several varieties; the Jadassohn-Tieche and the cellular blue nevus are the most common. The latter is sometimes misdiagnosed as melanosarcoma. Malignant blue nevi are extremely rare. See Nevus.

Carotenoids. Lipid soluble, yellow to orange-red pigments universally present in photosynthetic tissues of plants; also found in marine invertebrates, fish, amphibians and in feathers.

Catecholamine. Generic term for compounds containing a catechol group and an amine group, generally considered to be derivatives of β-phenylethylamine. The catecholamines, dopamine, epinephrine, and norepinephrine, are of importance in the sympathetic nervous system, and are melanin-aggregating agents when applied to adrenergically innervated fish melanophores.

Cell line M40. Derived from a human melanoma; has separate and distinct sites for fetal-associated and tumor-specific antigens.

Cell-mediated immunity. See Thymus-derived lymphocytes.

Chediak-Higashi syndrome. Pleiotrophic syndrome in man, characterized by autosomal recessive inheritance, dilution of pigmentation in eye, skin, and hair, giant granules in the melanocytes and leukocytes, photophobia, susceptibility to infection and early death.

Chloasma (mask of pregnancy). Abnormal collections of pigment covering a relatively large and diffuse skin area. Hyperpigmentation may occur as a result of the action of hormones, friction, heat, light, application of various irritant substances to the skin. Melasma is specifically associated with pregnancy, or systemic diseases such as tuberculosis, cancer, and endocrine diseases.

Cholinergic nerves. Postganglionic, parasympathetic nerves which secrete acetylcholine at their axon terminals. Adrenergic, rather than cholinergic nerves, are apparently involved in the innervated melanophores of fish. See Adrenergic nerves.

Chromatophores. Pigment-bearing cells of invertebrates and lower vertebrates, which are derived from the embryonic neural crest and are capable of effecting color changes by concentrating or dispersing their pigment granules. Specific examples are: erythrophores, iridophores, xanthophores, and melanophores.

Chromatotrophic hormone (CTH). Synonymous with MSH or intermedin; refers to actions on iridophores, as well as melanophores. See MSH.

Cloudman S-91 mouse melanoma. A classical, transplantable, metastasizing mouse melanoma discovered by A. M. CLOUDMAN in 1937. The original tumor arose in the skin at the base of the tail of a DBA strain female mouse. Melanotic and amelanotic variants are available. Most lines carry the LDH-elevating virus. See Melanoma.

Corticosterone. Steroid hormone produced by the adrenal cortex in response to ACTH production by the pituitary. Corticosterone is the major steroid produced in mice, rats, and other rodents; whereas cortisol is the major glucocorticoid in human beings. When elevated, these hormones have adverse effects upon the immunological system, including involution of lymph nodes, spleen, thymus, and a lymphocytopenia, with a resultant impairment of cell-mediated immunity. See Adrenocorticotropic hormone, Thymus-derived lymphocytes, and LDH-virus.

Cross syndrome. Oculocerebral syndrome encompassing hypopigmentation of hair and skin, gingival fibromatosis, microphthalmia, oligophrenia, spasticity, and athetoid movements.

Cyclic AMP (3',5'-cyclic adenosine monophosphate). Nucleotide formed from ATP by adenyl cyclases. Cyclic AMP mediates the effects of MSH upon melanocytes and melanophores, and is also the biochemical mediator of various other hormone-induced cellular responses. See Adenyl cyclase, Adenosine trophosphate, Adrenocorticotropic hormone, Cyclic nucleotide phosphodiesterase and MSH.

Cyclic nucleotide phosphodiesterase. Enzyme found in tissues containing adenyl cyclase, which catalyzes the conversion of cyclic 3',5'-AMP to

5'-AMP. This enzyme is inhibited by methylxanthines, such as caffeine, aminophylline and theophylline. See Adenyl cyclase, Cyclic AMP.

Dendrites. Elongated, branched protoplasmic processes characteristic of cells derived from the neural crest, including melanocytes, chromatophores and nerve cells. In the latter they conduct nerve impulses toward the cell body.

Deoxyribonucleic acid (DNA). Helical molecule constructed of a sequence of paired nucleotides on a deoxyribose backbone. DNA bears the genetic code, which is transcribed to messenger RNA, and carried to the ribosomes where it is translated into proteins. Substitution of synthetic nucleotides for naturally occurring ones has resulted in a lessening of tumorigenicity in some tumor cell lines. In melanoma cell lines, melanogenesis has also been suppressed by such substitution.

Dermal chromatophore unit. A compound functional unit which brings about color changes in fish and amphibians, consisting of the integrated response of melanophores, xanthophores, and iridophores, that provides the mechanism for integumental color change in response to hormonal stimulation either in the intact animal or *in vitro.*

Dermis (corium). The subepithelial connective tissue component of the skin, which is derived from the embryonic mesoderm. See Epidermis.

DNA. See Deoxyribonucleic acid.

Dopa (3,4-dihydroxyphenylalanine). Amino acid, intermediate product in the oxidation of tyrosine by oxidases (tyrosinase, dopa oxidase, peroxidase) to melanin. The naturally occurring amino acid is in the L-form. L-Dopa is also involved in the synthesis of catecholamines.

Dopa oxidase. The mammalian enzyme which converts dopa to dopaquinone in the process of melanin synthesis. Although the terms dopa oxidase and tyrosinase are used interchangeably, it has not been unequivocally established that mammalian dopa oxidase can use tyrosine as a substrate. See Raper theory, Tyrosinase, and Peroxidase.

Dopamine. A catecholamine intermediate in the formation of norepinephrine and epinephrine (adrenaline) from dopa. See Dopa, Epinephrine, and Norepinephrine.

DTIC (dimethyltriazeno imidazole carboxamide). Inhibits L-dopa oxidation *in vitro,* and has been used as a chemotherapeutic agent against melanoma.

Ectoderm. Outermost of the three primary embryonic germ layers, and source of neural tissue, the neural crest, sense organs, epidermis, melanocytes, and chromatophores. See Neural crest.

Embden-Meyerhof pathway. Metabolic, glycolytic pathway by which glucose is converted to alcohol or to lactic acid, yielding ATP, in the cell. See Adenosine triphosphate.

Endoplasmic reticulum (ER). A system of subcellular structures consisting of interconnected tubules and vesicles (cisternae) that occupy the cytoplasm of metabolically active cells. The microsome fraction obtained from disrupted cells is derived from the endoplasmic reticulum and has a high RNA content. The ER is postulated to be involved in the transfer of enzymes, including tyrosinase and dopa oxidase, from ribosomes to Golgi vesicles, in the formation of premelanosomes.

Ephelid. See Freckle.

Epidermal melanin unit. Melanocyte

plus an associated pool of keratinocytes (Malpighian cells) the number
of which may vary. The melanocyte
and the Malpighian cells appear to
operate closely together, with the melanocyte synthesizing the pigment and
donating it to the Malpighian cells.
They can be considered to comprise a
structural, as well as a functional unit
that is analogous in some respects to
other compound cellular functional
units such as the nephron. See Melanocyte, Keratinocyte.

Epidermis. Outer stratified squamous
keratinizing epithelium of the skin,
which is derived from the embryonic
ectoderm. In addition to being a protective covering for the entire body,
the epidermis gives rise to hair, feathers, scales, nails, hoofs, and several
types of glands. It is composed of
five layers. See Dermis.

Epinephrine (adrenaline). A catecholamine having hormone action, produced
by the adrenal medulla; it inhibits the
release of MSH and ACTH from the
pituitary, and causes melanin aggregation in teleost and amphibian melanophores. See Catecholamines.

Erythrophore. Chromatophore containing a red (pteridine or carotenoid)
pigment that occurs in some fishes
and crustaceans. See Carotenoid and
Pteridine pigment.

Eumelanin. The dark brown variety of
melanins, widely distributed in the tissues of animals and birds. The pigment is usually formed from tyrosine
or dopa under the catalytic influence
of tyrosinase (dopa oxidase). See
Phaeomelanin.

Eyestalk. Site of chromatophorotrophin
production in crustaceans.

Familial melanoma. Melanoma which
occurs in more than one member of
the same human family. Initial data
suggests that an autosomal dominant

gene with incomplete penetrance may
be involved.

Fortner hamster melanomas. A series of
'spontaneous' pigmented tumors
which arose over a period of time in
a colony of hamsters maintained in
the laboratory of J. G. FORTNER. Various melanotic and amelanotic lines
are maintained by transplantation in
Syrian golden hamsters.

Freckle (ephelid). A tan to brown macule found on areas of skin exposed
to sunlight. Freckles are not present
at birth, and do not appear until after
infancy, despite exposure to sunlight.
However, the role of sunlight in the
development of freckles is indisputa-
ble. There is an heritable tendency. See
Lentigo.

Gallophaeomelanins. Group of phaeomelanic pigments of high molecular
weight (2,000–50,000) which occur in
hair, fur, and feathers. They are insoluble in dilute acids, but dissolve in
alkalies giving yellow-brown solutions
which display no defined absorption
maxima in the ultraviolet and visible
region. See Phaeomelanins and Trichosiderins.

Genes for melanogenesis. Genes which
control the various synthetic steps, including enzymes, involved in melanogenesis. Abnormalities in any of these
genes can result in various pigmentation disorders. See Familial melanoma, Albinism, Cross, and Chediak-Higashi syndromes.

Gloger's rule. 'Darkest-colored animals
are generally found in the warm, hu-
mid tropics; grading to the lightest-co-
lored animals in the cold, dry arctic
regions.'

Golgi apparatus. Intracellular complex
of vesicles and fine tubules, adjacent
to the nucleus. Its function may include coating the products of exocrine
secretion with a protein envelope, and

the secretion of complex carbohydrates. The Golgi apparatus is postulated to be the site of origin of the enzymic components of the premelanosomes.

Guanophore. Chromatophore containing reflecting platelets which are partially composed of guanine. See Iridophore.

Halo nevus. A pigmented nevus surrounded by a halo of acquired leukoderma. Ultrastructural investigations indicate that the early inflammatory reaction consists of active stimulated lymphocytes and monocytes migrating from blood vessels to form close association with nevus cell nests. Nevus cell destruction is associated with macrophages involved in phagocytosis of cytoplasmic remnants and pigment granules. Antibodies against the cytoplasm of melanoma cells have been found in the sera of patients with regressing halo nevi.

Harding-Passey mouse melanoma. A classical, transplantable pigmented mouse tumor discovered in the laboratory of R. A. PASSEY in 1925. The original tumor arose spontaneously in the ear of a non-inbred mouse, and will grow in a variety of mouse strains. This tumor exhibits a high population of pigment-containing macrophages, and a low capacity for metastasizing. Most lines carry the LDH-elevating virus. See Melanoma.

Hermansky-Pudlak syndrome. Albinism associated with hemorrhagic diathesis, due to a platelet storage pool deficiency.

Hogben and Slome melanophore index. Measure of the degree of pigment dispersal in melanophores.

Humoral immunity. See Antibody-mediated immunity.

Hypothalamus. A region at the base of the brain, situated in close proximity to the pituitary. The hypothalamus produces a number of neuro-hormones which regulate the release of various pituitary hormones, including MSH. See MIF, MRF, and MSH.

Iglesias rat melanomas. Several spontaneous, transplantable pigmented tumors discovered by R. IGLESIAS, Santiago, Chile, in A×C strain rats. The first tumor was transplanted successfully in 1957. See Melanoma.

Intermedin. The same as MSH, a term used by some authors working with melanophores. The term was originally used to indicate that the hormone is produced by the pars intermedia of the hypophysis. See MSH.

Iridophore. Chromatophore containing iridescent guanine-containing granules, which occurs in the skin of cephalopods, fishes, and reptiles. See Guanophore.

Iridosomes (reflecting platelets). Granules containing guanine, found primarily in iridophores.

Keratinocyte (Malpighian cell). The epidermal cell which synthesizes keratin, stores melanin, and together with the melanocyte forms the binary cell system of the epidermis. The keratinocyte develops through successive stages of basal cell, prickle cell, and granular cell, eventually producing the noncellular, fibrillar material, keratin. See Epidermal melanin unit.

Langerhans' cell (suprabasal clear cell). Dendritic, star-shaped, nonpigmented cell situated in the epidermis. The Langerhans' cell contains nonmelanized disc-shaped organelles bearing some resemblance to melanosomes; however, it is tyrosinase and dopa-negative. It is considered by some to be a phagocytic cell which engulfs degenerate melanocytes in piebald and vitiligenous skin.

LDH-virus (lactate dehydrogenase-elevating virus). Benign RNA-virus ubiquitously distributed in materials routinely transplanted in mice, including transplantable melanomas. The virus infection causes an elevation in several plasma enzymes, including lactate dehydrogenase, from which its name is derived. Of greater experimental concern, this virus causes modifications of the immunological system which may compromise experimental results.

Lentigo. A well circumscribed, round, pigmented macular lesion ranging in color from light tan to dark brown or even black. Lentigos, in contrast to senile lentigo, are not dependent upon sunlight; they may appear on any part of the body and are often found at birth, which distinguishes them from freckles. They differ from junctional nevi in that they are not potentially malignant. See Freckle, Nevus.

Lipofuscin. Golden brown pigment, considered to be a derivative of lysosomes, and found in certain tissues of older animals, especially in neurones and the cells of the myocardium. Lipofuscin is considered to be a component of neuromelanin, but is also postulated to be a degenerate 'wear and tear' pigment. See Lysosome, Neuromelanin.

Lipophore. Older collective term for erythrophores and xanthophores, used because of the solubility of their pigments in lipid solvents.

Lymphotoxin. Factor obtained from tissues of tumor-bearing mice; has the ability to kill tumor cells *in vitro,* similar to the action of living spleen cells.

Malignant melanoma. The term 'malignant melanoma' is a redundancy, and should not be used since melanomas are assumed to be malignant, unless specifically designated as juvenile melanomas, or 'benign', as in some ocular varieties. See Melanoma.

Malpighian cells. Keratinocytes which are closely associated with melanocytes in the epidermal melanin unit. Melanosomes produced by melanocytes are transferred to the Malpighian cells, which were named after the Italian anatomist, histologist, and embryologist, M. MALPIGHI, 1628–1694. See Epidermal melanin unit, and Keratinocytes.

Melanin. A generic term for a wide variety of natural pigments responsible for shades of black and brown found in plants and animals. Melanin is an insoluble, high molecular weight polymer derived from the enzymic oxidation of phenols, starting with tyrosine. In the case of vertebrates, melanin is synthesized in melanosomes, a cellular organelle within melanocytes or melanophores. See Eumelanin and Phaeomelanin.

Melanin as semiconductor. Melanins have been demonstrated to be amorphous semiconductors; some melanin-binding drugs alter this conductivity, as well as the threshold switching properties of melanins.

Melanoblast. An immature pigment cell; a precursor of the melanocyte and melanophore. See Melanocyte, Melanophore.

Melanocyte. A pigment synthesizing cell. A secretory cell, derived from the neural crest, that produces a specialized organelle, the melanosome, containing enzymes (dopa oxidase, tyrosinase, peroxidase) which catalyze the oxidation of the natural precursor tyrosine to an insoluble, dense polymer, melanin.

Melanocyte-stimulating hormone. See MSH.

Melanogenesis. Formation of melanin is probably initiated in the premelanosome and continued in the melanosome of the melanocyte or melanophore. In the presence of tyrosinase, dopa oxidase, or peroxidase, tyrosine is first oxidized to dopa; the dopa is then oxidized to dopa-quinone, which in turn is converted through several intermediates into a pigmented polymer, melanin.

Melanoma. Malignant neoplasm, derived from melanocytes. Malignant amelanotic varieties occur, also originating from melanocytes but not forming melanin.

Melanoma-associated antigens. Isolated from melanoma cells grown *in vitro*; appear to be glycoproteins. The melanoma antigens are distinct from known murine transplantation antigens.

Melanophage. Macrophage which has ingested or phagocytized melanin. A confusing term which should be abandoned.

Melanophore. A dermal melanocyte of cold-blooded vertebrates, constituting the pigmentary effector system (aggregation and dispersion of melanosomes within these melanophores).

Melanosome. An organelle that is surrounded by a membrane and contains a highly organized internal structure of longitudinally oriented strands or concentric lamellae that have a regular pattern of dense particles with a characteristic periodicity. The organelle may be spherical or elipsoid and may be from 0.5 to 1.0 μm in length, and from 0.2 to 0.3 μm in diameter. Melanosomes contain the melanin-synthesizing enzyme dopa oxidase (tyrosinase). See Melanocyte.

Melanotrophin. Synonymous with MSH, intermedin, and chromatophorotrophin.

Melatonin (5-methoxy-N-acetyltryptamine). Hormone produced by the pineal gland which lightens MSH-darkened skin; effects are specific for melanophores, having no effect on iridophores. Melatonin is responsible for dark-adaptation in larval amphibians. See MSH.

Messenger RNA. A ribonucleic acid that carries the code for a particular protein from nuclear deoxyribonucleic acid (DNA), and acts as a template for the formation of that protein. See Nuclear acidic proteins.

Methylxanthines. A family of compounds which competitively inhibit the hydrolysis of cyclic AMP by phosphodiesterase. See Aminophylline, Cyclic AMP, Phosphodiesterases.

Microtubules. Cellular organelles which, in melanocytes, appear to be involved in melanin aggregation in *Fundulus* melanophores, and possibly also in frog and other melanophores.

MIF. See MSH-release-inhibiting factor.

Mitochondria. Subcellular organelles of various size and shape, limited by an outer smooth membrane and an inner membrane showing infoldings (cristae mitochondriales). Mitochondria are the major sites of energy transduction and ATP synthesis in the cell. They possess cytochrome oxidase and other Krebs' cycle enzymes. See Adenosine triphosphate, and Embden-Meyerhof pathway.

Mole (lay term for intradermal nevus). A pigmented lesion in the skin, usually benign, resulting from the proliferation of melanocytes. See Nevus.

MRF. See MSH-releasing factor.

MSH (melanocyte-stimulating hormone, also known as intermedin). A polypeptide hormone of 13–22 amino acid residues, produced by the pars intermedia of the pituitary. MSH stimulates melanocytes and melanophores to produce pigment. In lower vertebrates, MSH effects melanin dispersion in melanophores, and is the only hormone of major importance in regulating iridophore responses. These effects are mediated by cyclic AMP. There are two types of MSH, α and β. MSH is related chemically to ACTH. See ACTH, Cyclic AMP.

MSH-releasing factor (MRF). Postulated hypothalamic hormone which may release MSH from the pars intermedia of the pituitary. See MSH.

MSH-release-inhibiting factor (MIF). Hypothalamic hormone which inhibits the release of MSH from the pituitary. See MSH.

Neural crest. Ectodermal embryonic site, lateral to the neural tube, from which cells of the adrenal medulla, nerve cells, and other dendritic cell arise.

Neural pigments. See Neuromelanin, and Lipofuscin.

Neuromelanin. Intraneuronal pigment; considered to be melanized lipofuscin. See Lipofuscin.

Nevus. A general term applied to discolored patches in the skin. Pigmented nevi may be either congenital or acquired lesions, and are due to benign melanocyte proliferation; pigmented nevi may become wholly or partially amelanotic. Certain pigmented nevi have malignant potential. Epithelial nevi are congenital hyperplastic lesions of epidermal cells which may appear to be pigmented as a consequence of the activity of associated melanocytes. Connective tissue nevi are congenital lesions in which there is a localized thickening of the dermis. Vascular nevi are those due to malformations of cutaneous blood vessels. Junctional, intradermal, and compound nevi are important clinical classifications.

Norepinephrine (noradrenaline). A catecholamine; precursor of epinephrine produced by the adrenal medulla; also principal transmitter substance in sympathetic adrenergic neuro-effector junctions; a vasoconstrictor; reverses the effects of MSH upon teleost melanophores.

Nuclear acidic proteins (NAP). Proteins associated with chromatin which are believed to be associated with genetic expression. MSH treatment of Cloudman mouse melanoma cells *in vitro* results in differences in the NAP as well as increased melanin content.

Oncorna viruses. Oncogenic RNA viruses with 70S RNA, RNA-directed DNA polymerase, and a particle density of 1.16–1.19 g/ml. These viruses have been found in various animal melanomas, and similar particles have been detected in human melanomas. Their etiological relationship to human tumors is uncertain. See RNA, RNA viruses.

Parkinson's disease. Paralysis agitans, a disease of the central nervous system which is associated with loss of pigment by the cells of the substantia nigra of the brain. This disease responds in some cases to the therapeutic administration of L-dopa.

Peroxidase. Enzyme catalyzing the oxidation of various substances, such as diphenols, aromatic amines, and peroxides. Peroxidase may be involved in the oxidation of tyrosine to dopa during melanin and/or catecholamine synthesis in mammals. Peroxidase has been detected in some melanoma preparations.

Phaeomelanins. The term includes all red, yellow, orange and brown pigments which are formed by a deviation of the eumelanin pathway involving interreaction of cysteine with dopa quinones produced by the enzymatic oxidation of tyrosine. See Gallophaeomelanins and Trichosiderins.

Phenylalanine ammonia-lyase. Enzyme which degrades the amino acid phenylalanine, and inhibits the growth of B-16 melanoma *in vivo*.

Phosphodiesterases. Enzymes found in tissues containing adenyl cyclase; these enzymes are involved in the biochemical mechanisms for converting cyclic AMP to 5′-AMP. They are also found in snake venom. See Cyclic AMP, Cyclic nucleotide phosphodiesterase, MSH.

Piebaldism. Localized hypomelanosis of skin and hair, which may be inherited either as an autosomal dominant or recessive trait, and histologically characterized by the complete absence of melanocytes, or by the presence of abnormal melanocytes, in contrast to the morphologically normal melanocytes found in albinism.

Pineal gland (epiphysis). Endocrine gland rising from the roof of the third ventricle of the brain, which produces serotonin and melatonin. See Melatonin.

Pituitary (hypophysis). An endocrine gland attached to the infundibulum of the brain, which is under the general control of the hypothalamus. The anterior portion of the pituitary secretes ACTH and other hormones, while the closely related MSH is produced by the pars intermedia. See MSH, ACTH.

Pleiotrophic syndrome. See Chediak-Higashi syndrome.

Premelanosome. An immature melanosome. A cytoplasmic granule in melanocytes which is the site of melanin formation. See Melanosome.

Primordial organelle. Postulated chromatophore organelle of lower vertebrates which may develop into a melanosome, pterinosome, or iridosome, depending upon specific developmental cues.

Prosencephalon. The anterior division of the embryonic brain, which forms the cerebral hemispheres.

Pteridine pigments. Yellow crystalline bicyclic bases found in pterinosomes; for example, xanthopterin (2 amino, 4′,6′-dihydro pteridine). Pteridine pigments were first discovered in the wings of butterflies (Greek *pteron*, wing). See Pterinosomes, Erythrophores, and Xanthophores.

Pterinosomes. Granules containing pteridine pigments, found in lower vertebrate erythrophores.

Purine pigments. Principal pigments of iridophores (guanine, hypoxanthine and adenine). See Iridophores, Iridosomes.

Quinones. Intermediates in the formation of melanin from tyrosine.

Raper theory. The biochemical scheme proposed by H. S. RAPER in 1927, to account for the metabolic pathway leading from tyrosine to melanin.

Reflecting platelet. See Iridosome.

Retinal pigment epithelium. Innermost layer of the eye, which synthesizes melanosomes in embryonic life. The cells of the retinal pigment epithelium are interdigitated with the rods and cones of the neural retina.

Retinal pigment hormones. Crustacean hormones that regulate pigment movements in the retina.

Ribonucleic acid (RNA). Single or double stranded chains of ribonucleotides. The three major types of ribonucleic acid in cells are messenger RNA, ribosomal RNA, and transfer RNA. RNA is concerned with the transfer of the genetic code, carried in DNA, to the cellular site of protein synthesis. Certain viruses possess the only known double stranded RNA. See Deoxyribonucleic acid.

Ribosomes. RNA-rich, cytoplasmic granules that function in protein and enzyme synthesis; site of tyrosinase/dopa oxidase synthesis.

RNA. See Ribonucleic acid.

RNA C-type viruses. RNA viruses which have been detected in many animal tumor cell lines, including Greene hamster melanoma cells.

RNA viruses. See RNA C-type viruses, Oncorna viruses, LDH-virus.

Serotonin (5-hydroxytryptamine). Pineal indole, which acts to disperse melanin in *Xenopus* melanophores. See Melatonin.

Substantia nigra. See Parkinson's disease.

Syngeneic (isogenic, isologous). Implies a degree of genetic identity between mammals of the same species, enabling acceptance of homografts. Occurs naturally in identical twins and may be achieved experimentally in mice by about 20 successive generations of brother-sister mating.

Tanning. Uniform darkening of the skin following exposure to sunlight or other effective radiation. Following irradiation, there appear to be two effects: (1) an immediate oxidation of existing melanin in the skin, making it darker; (2) after a few days an increase in tyrosinase/dopa oxidase activity, resulting in the formation of more melanin. Increased proliferation of latent epidermal melanocytes or stem cells may also occur.

Thymus-derived lymphocytes (T cells). Effector lymphocytes of cell-mediated immunity. T cells act against malignant cells, including melanoma cells. T cells can be separated from other leukocytes on the basis of their receptors for sheep RBCs. These small lymphocytes are usually long-lived, and recirculate through the blood stream and the cortical areas of the lymphoid tissues, returning to the blood via lymphatic vessels.

Trichosiderins. Group of phaeomelanic pigments, originally considered to contain iron (hence the name), which occur in hair, fur and feathers. Most trichosiderins have characteristic pH-dependent colors and display well-defined absorption maxima in the visible and ultraviolet region. In contrast to gallophaeomelanins, they are soluble in both dilute acids and alkalies. See Phaeomelanins and Gallophaeomelanins.

Tyrosinase (dopa oxidase). Aerobic oxidase; copper-protein complex found in plants and insects which catalyzes the oxidation of both tyrosine and dopa. Although the term 'tyrosinase' has been used interchangeably with dopa oxidase in reference to mammalian melanogenesis, the role and characterization of mammalian 'tyrosinase' is also called catechol oxidase, polyphenol oxidase, and phenolase. The systematic name and number is 1.10.3.1 *o*-diphenol:oxygen oxidoreductase. The recommended trivial name is *o*-diphenol oxidase. See Dopa oxidase, Peroxidase.

Tyrosine phenol-lyase. An enzyme which degrades the amino acid tyrosine, and has inhibitory effects on the growth of B-16 melanoma *in vivo.*

Vitiligo (leukoderma). Condition in which there are patches of depigmentation of the skin. Postulated to be due to replacement of melanocytes in the basal layer of the epidermis by Langerhans' cells. Vitiligo is non-congenital. See Langerhans' cells.

Xanthophore. Chromatophore occurring in fishes, amphibians, and certain reptiles, containing yellow pigment, composed of pteridines, flavines and carotenoids.

Author Index

Subject Index

Acid phosphatase
  in Golgi complex 142, 144, 149
  in lysosomes of keratinocytes during pigment transfer 138–149
ACTH, acceleration of development of amphibian melanophores 285, 290
Actinomycin D, induction of yellow pigment in hair bulbs 179, 180, 182
Adenosine-3′,5′monophosphate, see Cyclic AMP
Adenyl cyclase
  activation, effects on embryonic development of amphibian melanophores 285
  stimulation, by catecholamines 341
Adenylate cyclase
  activation by MSH, ACTH, Ca⁺⁺ requirement for 272, 277–281
  activation by MSH in *Xenopus* melanophores 275–281
    related to Na⁺ influx 281
    resulting in increased cyclic AMP 275, 281
  activation by PGE 237, 251, 278–281
Adrenaline, in human
  biosynthesis 99, 103
  metabolic products 99–101
  not precursor of melanin 103, 104
Adrenergic receptors of chromatophores
  stimulation, by catecholamines 266, 267, 269–273, 276–279, 323–334, 337–341, 343

in teleost melanophores
  alpha 256, 262, 322, 323, 329–334, 336, 337
  beta 256, 322–343
in teleosts
  alpha, in xanthophores 256, 262
  in light-reflecting cells 262
in *Xenopus*, beta, involved in MSH action 276, 277
Adrenoreceptors, see Adrenergic receptors
Albinism in man
  associated with abnormal vision resulting from retinal hypopigmentation 202–205, 209, 217
    with sensitivity to ethanol 206, 209
  Hermansky-Pudlak, lipid storage defect 207
    serious bleeding, following aspirin blocking of release of storage pool-deficient platelet arachidonic endoperoxide 206–209
  recessive oculocutaneous and dominant tyrosinase-positive oculocutaneous, associated with alteration in melanization of melanosomes 372, 373, 376
  tyrosinase-negative, Hermansky-Pudlak, and yellow mutant oculocutaneous, effects of prostaglandins upon 250–252
  tyrosinase-positive, induction of pigmentation by prostaglandins, precursor and intermediates 247–252